RESEARCH AND PERSPECTIVES IN ALZHEIMER'S DISEASE
Fondation Ipsen

W0051406

Editor

Yves Christen, Fondation Ipsen, Paris (France)

Pierre-Marie Sinet, Hôpital Necker, Paris (France)
Peter St George-Hyslop, University of Toronto, Toronto (Canada)
Robert Terry, University of California, La Jolla (USA)
Henry Wisniewski, Institute for Basic Research in Development Disabilities, Staten Island (USA)
Edouard Zarifian, Centre Hospitalier Universitaire, Caen (France)

C.L. Masters K. Beyreuther M. Trillet
Y. Christen (Eds.)

Amyloid Protein Precursor in Development, Aging and Alzheimer's Disease

With 55 Figures and 13 Tables

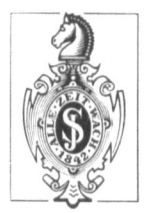 Springer-Verlag Berlin Heidelberg GmbH

Masters, C.L., M.D.
Department of Pathology
The University of Melbourne and
The Mental Health Research Institute of Victoria
Parkville, Victoria 3052, Australia

Beyreuther, K., Ph.D.
Center for Molecular Biology
University of Heidelberg
Im Neuenheimer Feld 282
69120 Heidelberg, Germany

Trillet, M., Prof.
Hôpital Neurologique
59, Bld Pinel
69003 Lyon, France

Christen, Y., Ph.D.
Fondation IPSEN
24, rue Erlanger
75781 Paris, France

ISBN 978-3-662-01137-9   ISBN 978-3-662-01135-5 (eBook)
DOI 10.1007/978-3-662-01135-5

Library of Congress Cataloging-in-Publication Data. Amyloid protein precursor in development, aging, and Alzheimer's disease/C.L. Masters . . . [et al.] (eds.). p. cm. — (Research and perspectives in Alzheimer's disease) "Fondation IPSEN pour la recherche therapeutique." "Proceedings of the Ninth "Colloque médecine et recherche" . . . held in Lyon on June 21, 1993"—Pref. Includes bibliographical references and index. ISBN 3-540-57788-2 — ISBN 0-387-57788-2 1. Alzheimer's disease—Pathophysiology—Congresses. 2. Amyloid beta-protein precursor—Congresses. I. Masters, Colin L. II. Fondation IPSEN pour la recherche thérapeutique. III. Colloque médecine et recherche (9th : 1993 : Lyon, France) IV. Series. [DNLM: 1. Alzheimer's Disease—congresses. 2. Amyloid beta—Protein Precursor—congresses. WM 220 A531 1994] RC523.A49 1994 616.8'3107—dc20 DNLM/DLC for Library of Congress 94-4461

Originally published by Springer-Verlag Berlin Heidelberg New York in 1994

Softcover reprint of the hardcover 1st edition 1994

Typesetting: Macmillan India Ltd., Bangalore-25
SPIN: 10465846   27/3130/SPS – 5 4 3 2 1 0 – Printed on acid-free paper

Preface

This volume contains the proceedings of the ninth "Colloque médecine et recherche" of the Fondation IPSEN devoted to research on Alzheimer's disease. This symposium was held in Lyon on June 21, 1993, on the topic, "Amyloid Protein Precursors in Development, Aging and Alzheimer's Disease". The choice of this venue and of this particular subject was not a matter of chance. As far as the history of medicine and neurology is concerned, Lyon is doubtless one of the most famous cities in France and the Fondation IPSEN had to organize one of its meetings in this city which has been regarded for centuries as a major crossroads. Regarding the topic, the amyloid story is at the center of the debate in the field of Alzheimer's studies.

For nearly 10 years, "alzheimerology" has more or less been intertwined with "amyloidology". The purification and the sequencing of the beta/A4 peptide in amyloid congophilic angiopathy (Glenner and Wong 1984) and in Alzheimer's disease (Masters et al. 1985) were the first steps toward the numerous successes realised in the last few years. The discovery of the amyloid precursor protein (APP), the localisation of its gene on chromosome 21 and the sequencing of its cDNA in 1987 (Kang et al. 1987; Goldgaber et al. 1987; Robakis et al. 1987) were the next major breakthroughs. Let us recall that the Fondation IPSEN started its series on Alzheimer's disease at this same time, and it organized its first meeting focused on the amyloid story (Pouplard-Barthelaix et al. 1988). Since this date, many important discoveries have been made concerning the splicing of APP, the existence of a whole class of APP-related homologue genes, the biological role of the APP protein and its cleaving and processing, the mechanism of amyloid deposition in Alzheimer's disease, the regulation of APP gene activity, the mutations in the APP genes which cause hereditary early onset Alzheimer's disease (Goate et al. 1991), transgenic animals and experimental models, etc. All of these discoveries open new perspectives, not only for the understanding of the disease and some fundamental processing which takes place in the nervous system, but also for future therapeutic intervention. Since it is very clear that the most important advances in the field of Alzheimer's disease research are related to basic science, the next meeting of this series of Colloque médecine et recherche will also be devoted to a fundamental topic. It will be entitled "Alzheimer's Disease: the Lessons of Cell Biology". This meeting will be organized by Ken Kosik and

Dennis Selkoe from Harvard Medical School, along with Yves Christen, and will be held in Paris on April 25, 1994.

Yves Christen
Marc Trillet

Acknowledgements. The editors wish to express their gratitude to Mary Lynn Gage for her editorial assistance and Jacqueline Mervaillie for the organization of the meeting.

References

Glenner GG, Wong CW (1984) Alzheimer's disease: initial report of the purification and characterization of a novel cerebrovascular amyloid protein. Biochem Biophys Res Comm 120: 885–890

Goate A, Chartier-Harlin MC, Mullan MJ, Brown J, Crawford F, Fidiani L, Gioffra L, Haynes A, Irving N, James L, Mant R, Newton P, Rooke K, Roques P, Talbot C, Pericak-Vance M, Roses A, Williamson R, Rossor M, Owen M, Hardy JA (1991) Segregation of a missence mutation in the amyloid precursor protein gene with familial Alzheimer's disease. Nature 349: 704–706

Goldgaber D, Lerman MI, McBride OW, Saffiotti U, Gajdusek DC (1987) Characterization and chromosomal localization of a cDNA encoding brain amyloid of Alzheimer's disease. Science 235: 877–880

Kang J, Lemaire HG, Unterbeck A, Salbaum JM, Masters CL, Grzeschik KH, Multhaup G, Beyreuther K, Müller-Hill B (1987) The precursor of Alzheimer's disease amyloid A4 protein resembles a cell-surface receptor. Nature 325: 733–736

Masters CL, Simms G, Weinman NA, Multhaup G, McDonald BL, Beyreuther K (1985) Amyloid plaque core protein in Alzheimer disease and Down syndrome. Proc Nat Acad Sci USA 82: 4245–4249

Pouplard-Barthelaix A, Emile J, Christen Y (eds) (1988) Immunology and Alzheimer's Disease. Springer Verlag, Heidelberg

Robakis NK, Wisniewski HM, Jenkins EC, Devin-Gage EA, Houch GE, Yao XL, Ramakrishna N, Wolfe G, Silverman WP, Brown WT (1987) Chromosome 21q21 sublocalisation of gene encoding beta-amyloid peptide in cerebral vessels and neuritic (senile) plaques of people with Alzheimer disease and Down syndrome. Lancet 1: 384–385

Contents

Contributors

Aigaki, T.
Department of Biology, Tokyo Metropolitan University, Minamiohsawa Hachiohji-shi, Tokyo 192–03, Japan

Allinquant, B.
CNRS, URA 1414, ENS, 46 rue d'Ulm, Paris, France

Allsop, D.
SmithKline Beecham Pharmaceuticals, Department of Molecular Neuropathology, Coldharbour Road, The Pinnacles, Harlow, Essex CM19 5AD, UK, and Division of Biochemistry, The Queen's University of Belfast, Medical Biology Centre, 97 Lisburn Road, Belfast BT9 7BL, Northern Ireland, UK

Beal, M. F.
Neurology Service, Neurochemistry Laboratory, Massachusetts General Hospital, Boston, MA 02114, USA

Bennett, C.
Suncoast Alzheimer's Disease Research Group, Department of Psychiatry, University of South Florida, Tampa, FL 33613 USA

Beyreuther, K.
Center for Molecular Biology, University of Heidelberg, Im Neuenheimer Feld 282, 69120 Heidelberg, Germany

Bogdanovic, N.
Alzheimer's Disease Research Centre, Department of Geriatric Medicine, Huddinge University Hospital, The Karolinska Institute, 14186 Huddinge, Sweden

Borchelt, D. R.
Department of Pathology, The Johns Hopkins University School of Medicine, Baltimore, MD 21205–2196, USA

Bouillot, C.
CNRS, URA 1414, ENS, 46 rue d'Ulm, Paris, France

Bowling, A. C.
Neurology Service, Neurochemistry Laboratory, Massachusetts General Hospital, Boston, MA 02114, USA

Bush, A. I.
Laboratory of Genetics and Aging, Neuroscience Center, Department of Neurology, Harvard Medical School, Massachusetts General Hospital East, Building 149, 13th Street, Charlestown, MA 02129, USA

Cai, X.-D.
Division of Neuropathology, Institute of Pathology, Case Western Reserve University, Cleveland, OH 44106, USA

Chartier-Harlin, M.-C.
Cerebral Ageing and Neurodegeneration Laboratory, U156 INSERM, Place de Verdun, 59045 Lille Cedex, France

Cheung, T. T.
Division of Neuropathology, Institute of Pathology, Case Western Reserve University, Cleveland, OH 44106, USA

Clarris, H.
Department of Pathology, The University of Melbourne, and The Mental Health Research Institute, Parkville, Victoria 3052, Australia

Clements, A.
Division of Biochemistry, The Queen's University of Belfast, Medical Biology Centre, 97 Lisburn Road, Belfast BT9 7BL, Northern Ireland, UK

Cordell, B.
Scios Nova Inc., 2450 Bayshore Parkway, Mountain View, CA 94043, USA

Cowburn, R.
Alzheimer's Disease Research Centre, Department of Geriatric Medicine, Huddinge University Hospital, The Karolinska Institute, 14186 Huddinge, Sweden

Crawford, F.
Suncoast Alzheimer's Disease Research Group, Department of Psychiatry, University of South Florida, Tampa, FL 33613 USA

Crook, R.
Suncoast Alzheimer's Disease Research Group, Department of Psychiatry, University of South Florida, Tampa, FL 33613, USA and Alzheimer's Disease Research Group, Departments of Biochemistry and Neurology, St. Mary's Hospital Medical School, London W2 1PG, UK

Crowley, A.
Laboratory of Genetics and Aging, Neuroscience Center, Department of Neurology, Harvard Medical School, Massachusetts General Hospital East, Building 149, 13th Street, Charlestown, MA 02129, USA

Diaz, P.
Suncoast Alzheimer's Disease Research Group, Department of Psychiatry, University of South Florida, Tampa, FL 33613 USA

Duff, K.
Suncoast Alzheimer's Disease Research Group, Department of Psychiatry, University of South Florida, Tampa, FL 33613 USA

Dutar, P.
Laboratoire de Physiopharmacologie du Système Nerveux, INSERM U 161, 2 rue d'Alésia, 75014 Paris, France

Fidani, L.
Department of Neurology, A.H.E.P.A. Aristotelian University of Thessaloniki, Thessaloniki, Greece

Gandy, S.
Department of Neurology and Neuroscience, Cornell University Medical College, 1300 York Avenue, and The Rockefeller University, 1230 York Avenue, New York, NY 10021, USA

Gaston, S.
Laboratory of Genetics and Aging, Neuroscience Center, Department of Neurology, Harvard Medical School, Massachusetts General Hospital East, Building 149, 13th Street, Charlestown, MA 02129, USA

Gearhart, J. D.
Department of Obstetrics and Gynecology, The Johns Hopkins University School of Medicine, Baltimore, MD 21205–2196, USA

Gittner, A.
Developmental Neurobiology Group, Department of Medicine, University of Cambridge, Addenbrooke's Hospital, Hills Road, Cambridge CB2 QQ, UK

Goate, A.
Alzheimer's Disease Research Group, Department of Psychiatry, Washington University, St. Louis, MO 63110, USA

Golde, T. E.
Division of Neuropathology, Institute of Pathology, Case Western Reserve University, Cleveland, OH 44106, USA

Greengard, P.
Laboratory of Molecular and Cellular Neuroscience, The Rockefeller University, 1230 York Avenue, New York, NY 10021, USA

Gurubhagavatula, S.
Laboratory of Genetics and Aging, Neuroscience Center, Department of Neurology, Harvard Medical School, Massachusetts General Hospital East, Building 149, 13th Street, Charlestown, MA 02129, USA

Haines, J.
Laboratory of Genetics and Aging, Neuroscience Center, Department of Neurology, Harvard Medical School, Massachusetts General Hospital East, Building 149, 13th Street, Charlestown, MA 02129, USA

Hardy, J.
Suncoast Alzheimer's Disease Research Group, Department of Psychiatry, University of South Florida, Tampa, FL 33613, USA

Hendriks, L.
Laboratory of Neurogenetics, Born Bunge Foundation, University of Antwerp (UIA), Department of Biochemistry, 2610 Antwerp, Belgium

Higgins, L.
Scios Nova Inc., 2450 Bayshore Parkway, Mountain View, CA 94043, USA

Hilbich, C.
Center of Molecular Biology, University of Heidelberg, Im Neuenheimer Feld 282, 69120 Heidelberg, Germany

Houlden, H.
Suncoast Alzheimer's Disease Research Group, Department of Psychiatry, University of South Florida, Tampa, FL 33613 USA and
Alzheimer's Disease Research Group, Departments of Biochemistry and Neurology, St. Mary's Hospital Medical School, London W2 1PG, UK

Jin, L.-W.
Department of Neurosciences, 0624, School of Medicine and Center for Molecular Genetics, University of California, San Diego, La Jolla, CA 92093, USA

Johnston, J.
Alzheimer's Disease Research Centre, Department of Geriatric Medicine, Huddinge University Hospital, The Karolinska Institute, 14186 Huddinge, Sweden

Kennedy, H.
Division of Biochemistry, The Queen's University of Belfast, Medical Biology Centre, 97 Lisburn Road, Belfast BT9 7BL, Northern Ireland, UK

Kisters-Woike, B.
Center for Molecular Biology, University of Heidelberg, Im Neuenheimer Feld 228, 69120 Heidelberg, Germany. Present address: Institute of Genetics, University of Cologne, Weyertal 121, 50931 Cologne, Germany

Koo, E. H.
Center for Neurologic Disease, Brigham and Women's Hospital, Boston, MA 02115, USA

Kovacs, D.
Laboratory of Genetics and Aging, Neuroscience Center, Department of Neurology, Harvard Medical School, Massachusetts General Hospital East, Building 149, 13th Street, Charlestown, MA 02129, USA

Lamb, B. T.
Department of Obstetrics and Gynecology, The Johns Hopkins University School of Medicine, Baltimore, MD 21205-2196, USA

Lamour, Y.
Laboratoire de Physiopharmacologie du Système Nerveux, INSERM U 161, 2 rue d'Alésia, 75014 Paris and Service d'Explorations Fonctionnelles du Système Nerveux, Hôpital Lariboisière, 2 rue Ambroise Paré, 75010 Paris, France

Lannfelt, L.
Alzheimer's Disease Research Centre, Department of Geriatric Medicine, Huddinge University Hospital, The Karolinska Institute, 14186 Huddinge, Sweden

Lo, A. C. Y.
Department of Neuroscience and the Neuropathology Laboratory,
The Johns Hopkins University School of Medicine, Baltimore,
MD 21205-2196, USA

Luo, L.
Department of Physiology and Biochemistry, Howard Hughes Medical
Institute, University of California, San Francisco, CA 94143, USA

Martin, L. J.
Department of Pathology, The Johns Hopkins University School of
Medicine, Baltimore, MD 21205–2196, USA

Masliah, E.
Department of Neurosciences, 0624, School of Medicine and Center for
Molecular Genetics, University of California, San Diego, La Jolla,
CA 92093, USA

Masters, C. L.
Department of Pathology, The University of Melbourne, and The Mental
Health Research Institute of Victoria, Parkville, Victoria 3052, Australia

Mills, W.
Developmental Neurobiology Group, Department of Medicine,
University of Cambridge, Addenbrooke's Hospital, Hills Road,
Cambridge CB2 QQ, UK

Monastirioti, M.
Biology Department and Center for Complex Systems, Brandeis University,
Waltham, MA 02254, USA

Moya, K. L.
CNRS URA 1285 and INSERM U 334, SHFJ-CEA, 4 Place du Géneral
Leclerc, Orsay, France

Mullan, M.
Suncoast Alzheimer's Disease Research Group, Department of Psychiatry,
University of South Florida, Tampa, FL 33613 USA

Multhaup, G.
Center for Molecular Biology, University of Heidelberg, Im Neuenheimer
Feld 228, 69120 Heidelberg, Germany

Ninomiya, H.
Department of Neurosciences, 0624, School of Medicine and Center for
Molecular Genetics, University of California, San Diego, La Jolla,
CA 92093, USA

Nurcombe, V.
Department of Anatomy and Cell Biology, The University of Melbourne, Parkville, Victoria 3052, Australia

Otero, D. A. C.
Department of Neurosciences, 0624, School of Medicine and Center for Molecular Genetics, University of California, San Diego, La Jolla, CA 92093, USA

Paradis, M.
Laboratory of Genetics and Aging, Neuroscience Center, Department of Neurology, Harvard Medical School, Massachusetts General Hospital East, Building 149, 13th Street, Charlestown, MA 02129, USA

Parfitt, M.
Cerebral Ageing and Neurodegeneration Laboratory, U156 INSERM, Place de Verdun, 59045 Lille Cedex, France

Peppercorn, J.
Laboratory of Genetics and Aging, Neuroscience Center, Department of Neurology, Harvard Medical School, Massachusetts General Hospital East, Building 149, 13th Street, Charlestown, MA 02129, USA

Pettingell, W.
Laboratory of Genetics and Aging, Neuroscience Center, Department of Neurology, Harvard Medical School, Massachusetts General Hospital East, Building 149, 13th Street, Charlestown, MA 02129, USA

Potier, B.
Laboratoire de Physiopharmacologie du Système Nerveux, INSERM U 161, 2 rue d'Alésia, 75014 Paris, France

Price, D. L.
Neuropathology Laboratory, The Johns Hopkins University School of Medicine, 558 Ross Research Building, 720 Rutland Avenue, Baltimore, MD 21205–2196, USA

Prochiantz, A.
CNRS, URA 1414, ENS, 46 rue d'Ulm, Paris, France

Prusiner, S. B.
Departments of Neurology and of Biochemistry and Biophysics, University of California, San Francisco, CA 94143, USA

Reed, G.
Department of Pathology, The University of Melbourne, and The Mental
Health Research Institute, Parkville, Victoria 3052, Australia

Richards, S.-J.
Developmental Neurobiology Group, Department of Medicine,
University of Cambridge, Addenbrooke's Hospital, Hills Road,
Cambridge CB2 QQ, UK

Roch, J.-M.
Department of Neurosciences, 0624, School of Medicine and Center for
Molecular Genetics, University of California, San Diego, La Jolla,
CA 92093, USA

Romano, D.
Laboratory of Genetics and Aging, Neuroscience Center, Department of
Neurology, Harvard Medical School, Massachusetts General Hospital East,
Building 149, 13th Street, Charlestown, MA 02129, USA

Roques, P.
Alzheimer's Disease Research Group, Departments of Biochemistry and
Neurology, St. Mary's Hospital Medical School, London W2 1PG, UK

Rossor, M.
Alzheimer's Disease Research Group, Departments of Biochemistry and
Neurology, St. Mary's Hospital Medical School, London W2 1PG, UK

Saitoh, T.
Department of Neurosciences, 0624, School of Medicine and Center for
Molecular Genetics, University of California, San Diego, La Jolla,
CA 92093, USA

Samtani, V.
Developmental Neurobiology Group, Department of Medicine,
University of Cambridge, Addenbrooke's Hospital, Hills Road,
Cambridge CB2 QQ, UK

Shoji, M.
Division of Neuropathology, Institute of Pathology, Case Western Reserve
University, Cleveland, OH 44106, USA

Sisodia, S. S.
Neuropathology Laboratory, The Johns Hopkins University School of
Medicine, 558 Ross Research Building, 720 Rutland Avenue, Baltimore,
MD 21205-2196, USA

Slunt, H. H.
Neuropathology Laboratory, The Johns Hopkins University School of Medicine, Baltimore, MD 21205-2196, USA

Small, D. H.
Department of Pathology, The University of Melbourne, and The Mental Health Research Institute, Parkville, Victoria 3052, Australia

St George-Hyslop, P.
Department of Medicine, Centre for Research in Neurodegenerative Disease, Tanz Neuroscience Building, 6 Queen's Park Crescent, Toronto, Ontario, M5S 1A8 Canada

Tanzi, R. E.
Laboratory of Genetics and Aging, Neuroscience Center, Department of Neurology, Harvard Medical School, Massachusetts General Hospital East, Building 149, 13th Street, Charlestown, MA 02129, USA

Thinakaran, G.
Neuropathology Laboratory, The Johns Hopkins University School of Medicine, 558 Ross Research Building, 720 Rutland Avenue, Baltimore, MD 21205-2196, USA

Thorpe, A.
Developmental Neurobiology Group, Department of Medicine, University of Cambridge, Addenbrooke's Hospital, Hills Road, Cambridge CB2 QQ, UK

Van Broeckhoven, C.
Laboratory of Neurogenetics, Born Bunge Foundation, University of Antwerp (UIA), Department of Biochemistry, 2610 Antwerp, Belgium

Van Koch, C.
Department of Neuroscience and the Neuropathology Laboratory, The Johns Hopkins University School of Medicine, Baltimore, MD 21205-2196, USA

Walker, L. C.
Department of Pathology, The Johns Hopkins University School of Medicine, Baltimore, MD 21205-2196, USA

Walsh, D.
Division of Biochemistry, The Queen's University of Belfast, Medical Biology Centre, 97 Lisburn Road, Belfast BT9 7BL, Northern Ireland, UK

Wasco, W.
Laboratory of Genetics and Aging, Neuroscience Center, Department of Neurology, Harvard Medical School, Massachusetts General Hospital East, Building 149, 13th Street, Charlestown, MA 02129, USA

White, K.
Biology Department and Center for Complex Systems, Brandeis University, Waltham, MA 02254, USA

Williams, C.
Division of Biochemistry, The Queen's University of Belfast, Medical Biology Centre, 97 Lisburn Road, Belfast BT9 7BL, Northern Ireland, UK

Yamamoto, K.
Department of Neurosciences, 0624, School of Medicine and Center for Molecular Genetics, University of California, San Diego, La Jolla, CA 92093, USA

Younkin, S. G.
Division of Neuropathology, Institute of Pathology, Case Western Reserve University, Cleveland, OH 44106, USA

Strategic Thoughts on the Alzheimer's Disease Amyloid Protein Precursor: The Way Forward

*C. L. Masters** and *K. Beyreuther*

A survey of the contributions in this volume provides an unparalleled vision of the state of knowledge of the Alzheimer's disease amyloid protein precursor (APP) as of 1993. This represents the culmination of a decade of research on this topic, starting with the first serious attempts to characterise the AD-associated amyloid (Allsop et al. 1983). Within this volume we can see a strategic plan emerging, one which has the potential of leading to a rational therapeutic intervention for Alzheimer's disease.

The Biophysical Basis for βA4 Amyloidosis

Even without knowledge of the precise proteolytic events which generate the βA4 molecule, its innate tendency to polymerize into amyloid filaments has been sufficiently well-characterised (Hilbich et al., this volume; Hilbich et al. 1991a,b, 1992; Jarrett and Lansbury 1993) to enable the synthetic analogs of βA4 to be used successfully to model amyloidogenesis *in vitro*. There is every prospect of designing peptides or compounds which can inhibit the polymerization of βA4, either through nucleation-dependent processes (lag time, critical concentration, seeding efficiency; Jarrett and Lansbury 1993) or through altering the kinetics of fibril growth by affecting hydrophobic interactions (Hilbich et al., this volume).

The toxicity of aggregated βA4 remains enigmatic (Potier et al., this volume), or by altering conditions relating to metal catalyzed oxidation (Dyrks et al. 1992) or to direct metal–βA4 interactions (Bush et al. this volume). Despite much effort, a consensus has not emerged since Yankner et al. (1989) first proposed that specific regions of βA4 were neurotoxic, and hence were capable of explaining, at least in part, the dramatic loss of neuronal function associated with Alzheimer's disease. The mechanism of synaptic loss (Masliah et al. 1989) and neuronal dysfunction, central to our understanding of Alzheimer's disease, might well involve the generation of βA4 or the impairment of the normal function of APP, but the simplistic notion that βA4, either as a monomer or as a polymerized fibril, is a direct neurotoxin seems unlikely.

---

* Department of Pathology, The University of Melbourne, and The Mental Health Research Institute of Victoria, Parkville, Victoria 3052, Australia

C.L. Masters et al. (Eds.)
Amyloid Protein Precursor in Development,
Aging and Alzheimer's Disease
© Springer-Verlag Berlin Heidelberg 1994

The Structure and Function of the APP Superfamily

In addition to the APP products generated by the splicing of exons, 7, 8 and 15 (Kitaguchi et al. 1988; König et al. 1992), the discovery of two separate classes of APP-related homologue genes (APLP1 and APPH/APLP2; Sisodia et al., this volume; Wasco et al. 1992, 1993; Sprecher et al. 1993) adds a completely novel layer of complexity (Figs. 1 and 2). This is particularly apparent in all attempts to quantitate the various gene products by use of immunoassays. Antibodies which reliably distinguish between the amyloidogenic and non-amyloidogenic members of the APP superfamily are now urgently required. It is also likely that these APP homologues will interfere with our ability to produce a phenotype in mice where the APP gene is ablated. Nevertheless, the existence of the superfamily should facilitate the elucidation of function based on the preservation of motifs in common between the members of this family (Fig. 2).

If, as predicted (Kang et al. 1987), APP is a receptor, then the definition of its ligand(s) will surely reveal its function. To date, the identification of heparin domains (Small et al., this volume; Multhaup, this volume), the inhibitory serine protease domain (Kitaguchi et al. 1990) and zinc binding domains (Bush et al. 1993) has provided useful leads in conceptualising the function of APP. Yet one suspects that the principal ligand is yet to be discovered. Functional mappings of APP (Saitoh et al., this volume) and APP-related products in phylogenetically lower species (Okado and Okamoto 1992; White et al., this volume) are but preliminary steps in this process. Other approaches include the clearer definition

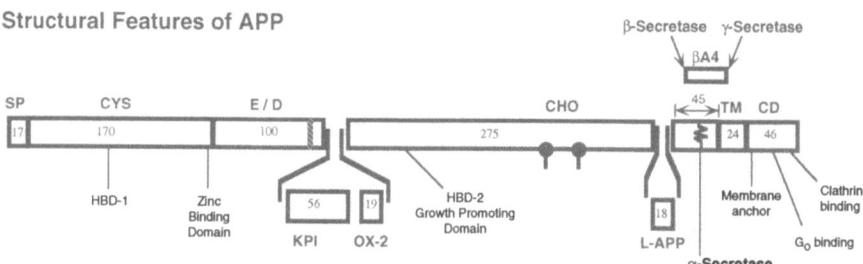

Fig. 1. Diagrammatic representation of the major structural domains of APP. The 17 residue signal peptide (SP) is followed by 170 residues with 12 cysteines (Cys); within this region is a heparin binding domain (HBD-1) and a zinc binding domain. The next 100 residues are largely acidic (E/D; glu/asp) with an unusual poly-threonine area (shaded bar). Exon 7 (the 56 residue KPI domain) and exon 8 (the 19 residue OX.2 domain) are subject to alternative splicing events. The next region of APP contains the second heparin binding domain (HBD-2), which is coincident with a growth promoting domain, and two N-linked carbohydrate attachment sites. The 18 residues of exon 15 are spliced out for the L-APP isoforms. The α-secretase site occurs within the βA4 domain, which itself is generated by the loosely defined β- and γ- secretase regions. The γ-secretase releases the C-terminus of βA4, which is within the transmembrane domain (TM). The TM is anchored in the lipid bilayer and is followed by a short cytoplasmic domain (CD) which contains both G_o and clathrin binding motifs. (Truncated, non-amyloidogenic forms of APP_{365} and APP_{563} are not shown in this diagram.)

APP Superfamily

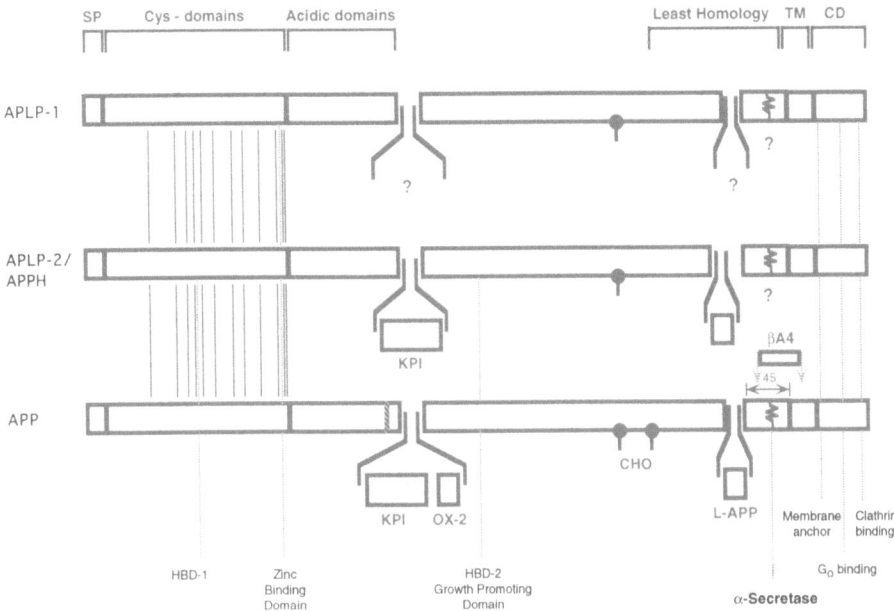

Fig. 2. Diagrammatic representation of the mammalian APP superfamily. There is an extraordinary conservation of the cysteine residues. An OX-2 related domain has not yet been defined in APPH/APLP-2, and the existence of both KPI and OX-2 related domains in APLP-1 is unknown. The HBD-2 and growth promoting domains are preserved in APPH/APLP-2, and at least one of the N-linked glycosylation sites is present in all members. Between this region and the transmembrane domain (TM) is the area with least homology. A small exon is known to be subject to alternate splicing in APPH/APLP-2, perhaps analogous to the events which relate to exon 15 of APP. Whether secreted/released forms of APPH/APLP-2, and APLP-2 occur is not yet known. The βA4 domain is present only in APP. The cytoplasmic domain (CD) is highly conserved, suggesting that previous studies which have employed immunoassays based on C-terminal epitopes need to be re-evaluated

of the metabolic pools of APP and their membrane traffic and cycling pathways (Gandy and Greengard; this volume; Allinquant et al., this volume; Cole et al. 1989; Buxbaum et al. 1990; Bush et al. 1990; Oltersdorf et al., 1990; Haass et al. 1992a,b; Hung et al. 1992). The observation that soluble forms of βA4 may be released from cells during normal processing events (Golde et al., this volume; Haass et al. 1992, 1993a,b; Seubert et al. 1992; Shoji et al. 1992; Busciglio et al. 1993; Dovey et al. 1993) has wide implications.

The cleavage events which surround this process (the relative balance between the α-secretase and the β- and γ-secretases) are now amenable to an in-depth analysis. For the first time, it will now be possible to examine a wide range of variables which can influence the production and aggregation of the βA4 molecule (Bush et al., this volume; Bowling and Beal, this volume; Siman et al. 1993; Fukushima et al. 1993).

Regulation of the APP Gene Activity

The importance of a gene regulation strategy is emphasised by the gene dosage effect of Alzheimer's disease that occurs in all cases of Down's syndrome. Despite the cloning of the promoter of APP (Salbaum et al. 1988; Yoshikai et al. 1990), there has been only modest progress in determining the major events which govern the transcriptional and translational control of the APP gene and mRNA. While some of the APP gene regulatory elements have been defined (Lahiri and Robakis 1991; Pollwein 1993; Pollwein et al. 1992; Quitschke and Goldgaber 1992), no specific transcriptional factors have yet been identified. Only a handful of defined growth factors and cytokines have been found to affect mRNA levels (Donnelly et al. 1990; Goldgaber et al. 1989; König et al. 1990; Mobley et al. 1988; Smith et al. 1991; Ohyagi and Tabira 1993), whereas more generalised phenomena such as heat shock, ischemia (Abe et al. 1991a,b) and neurotoxicity (Solá et al. 1993) clearly affect APP gene transcription. Even less is known about the factors which relate to the alternate splicing events, particularly those pertaining to the KPI and L-APP domains, which may play a role in the restriction of βA4 amyloid deposition to the central nervous system. This may yet prove to be a critical area for Alzheimer's disease research.

Identification of Environmental Risk Factors

The remarkable age-related incidence of Alzheimer's disease points strongly to a widespread environmental factor operating decades before the onset of clinical disease. Our analyses indicate that a preclinical phase of approximately 30 years is likely, based on the rate of evolution of the disease in Down's Syndrome (Rumble et al. 1989) and on the rate of racemization of amyloid (Shapira et al. 1988). In many respects, Alzheimer's disease has features in common with the process of atherosclerosis, in which a few well-defined genetic factors operate in combination with the effects of widespread dietary and occupational insults to the body's vascular system. The preclinical phase of atherosclerosis begins in early adult-hood, decades before the clinical onset of the typical forms of disease which occur in later life.

In Alzheimer's disease, no convincing environmental risk factors have yet emerged. Our strategy has been to examine the structure and metabolism of APP in the hope of finding a clue which professional epidemiologists might use. First, we have identified an effect of zinc and other metals on APP (Bush et al. 1993) and on βA4 amyloid itself (Bush et al., this volume; Mantyh et al. 1993; Exley et al. 1993); second, we are currently investigating the effect of carbohydrate metabolism on how the body processes APP (Whyte, Gilbert, Beyreuther and Masters, unpublished data). There are intriguing preliminary studies suggesting that the risk for Alzheimer's disease is increased 3-fold in meat consumers (Giem et al. 1993) and that the incidence of brain amyloid deposition is decreased in at least one developing country, Nigeria

(Osuntokun et al. 1994). Together, these studies suggest future areas of research which might identify the major environmental risk factors.

Genetic Factors in the Causation of Alzheimer's Disease

Our current state of knowledge of the causative link between APP mutations and Alzheimer's disease is summarised admirably in this volume (see chapters by Tanzi et al., Hendriks et al., Lannfelt et al., Hardy et al.). The incontrovertible linkage of critical mutations within or close to the βA4 domain of APP identifies for the first time the pre-eminence of APP/βA4 in the pathogenesis of Alzheimer's disease. But there are clearly multiple genetic pathways which can lead to Alzheimer's disease. Currently, much interest surrounds the association of the apolipoprotein E type 4 allele with both sporadic and familial late-onset Alzheimer's disease (Corder et al. 1993; Rebeck et al. 1993). An 8- to 9-fold relative risk associated with this allele suggests that this gene has a profound effect. Whether it operates through the βA4/APP pathway remains to be determined (Wisniewski et al. 1993). There remains yet another genetic locus for early-onset familial Alzheimer's disease on chromosome 14 (Schellenberg et al. 1992), but the precise genetic defect at this locus has not yet been determined.

Experimental Animal Models of Alzheimer's Disease

Still elusive, the full-blown lesions of Alzheimer's disease have not yet been re-created in a genetically engineered mouse (see Cordell and Higgins, this volume; Price et al., this volume). Nevertheless, the success of this strategy in closely related disease processes (Prusiner, this volume) gives encouragement for continued efforts. While in vitro and cell-culture models of βA4 amyloidogenesis have now been developed, only the faithful reproduction of the disease in experimental animals will allow the full testing of potential therapeutic agents.

Future Therapeutic Strategies for Alzheimer's Disease

Based on this decade of research effort, what does the future hold for a rational therapeutic intervention for Alzheimer's disease? Obviously, if an environmental risk factor is identified, then avoidance of this factor will override other direct therapeutic interventions. If genetic factors prove to be intractable to environmental modulation, then novel therapeutic strategies based on our knowledge of APP/βA4 amyloidogenesis will remain as prime targets. At present, these strategies fall into 4 major categories:

1) inhibition of βA4 amyloid aggregation
2) mobilisation of βA4 amyloid from the brain
3) modulation of the APP-βA4 amyloidogenic pathway, based on the characterisation of APP ligands, APP secretases, and APP processing steps in general

4) genetic manipulation of APP synthesis or associated metabolic pathways ("gene therapy").

We hope that the information contained in this volume will provide the impetus for future research directed at an eventual therapeutic intervention. If progress in this field is maintained at the rate that we have witnessed over the last decade, we are confident that an effective treatment or prevention strategy will emerge during the next decade.

References

Abe K, St George-Hyslop PH, Tanzi RE, Kogure K (1991a) Induction of amyloid precursor protein mRNA after heat shock in cultured human lymphoblastoid cells. Neurosci Lett 125:169–171

Abe K, Tanzi RE, Kogure K (1991b) Selective induction of Kunitz-type protease inhibitor domain-containing amyloid precursor protein mRNA after persistent focal ischemia in rat cerebral cortex. Neurosci Lett 125:172–174

Allsop D, Landon M, Kidd M (1983) The isolation and amino acid composition of senile plaque core protein. Brain Res 259:348–352

Busciglio J, Gabuzda DH, Matsudaira P, Yankner BA (1993) Generation of β-amyloid in the secretory pathway in neuronal and nonneuronal cells. Proc Natl Acad Sci USA 90:2092–2096

Bush AI, Martins RN, Rumble B, Moir R, Fuller S, Milward E, Currie J, Ames D, Weidemann A, Fischer P, Multhaup G, Beyreuther K, Masters CL (1990) The amyloid precursor protein of Alzheimer's disease is released by human platelets. J Biol chem 265:15977–15983

Bush AI, Multhaup G, Moir RD, Williamson TG, Small DH, Rumble B, Pollwein P, Beyreuther K, Masters CL (1993) A novel zinc (II) binding site modulates the function of the βA4 amyloid protein precursor of Alzheimer's disease. J Biol Chem 268:16109–16112

Buxbaum JD, Gandy SE, Cicchetti P, Ehrlich ME, Czernik AJ, Fracasso RP, Ramabhadran TV, Unterbeck AJ, Greengard P (1990) Processing of Alzheimer β/A4 amyloid precursor protein: modulation by agents that regulate protein phosphorylation. Proc Natl Acad Sci USA 87:6003–6006

Cole GM, Huynh TV, Saitoh T (1989) Evidence for lysosomal processing of amyloid β-protein precursor in cultured cells. Neurochem Res 14:933–939

Corder EH, Saunders AM, Strittmatter WJ, Schmechel DE, Gaskell PC, Small GW, Roses AD, Haines JL, Pericak-Vance MA (1993) Gene dose of apolipoprotein E type allele and the risk of Alzheimer's disease in late onset families. Science 261:921–923

Donnelly RJ, Friedhoff AJ, Beer B, Blume AJ, Vited MP (1990) Interleukin-1 stimulates the beta-amyloid precursor protein promoter. Cell Mol Neurobiol 10:485–495

Dovey HF, Suomensaari-Chrysler S, Lieberburg I, Sinha S, Keim PS (1993) Cells with a familial Alzheimer's disease mutation produce authentic β-peptide. Neuro Report 4:1039–1042

Dyrks T, Dyrks E, Hartman T, Masters CL, Beyreuther K (1992) Amyloidogenecity of βA4 and βA4-bearing APP fragments by metal catalysed oxidation. J Biol Chem 267:18210–18217

Exley C, Price NC, Kelly SM, Birchall JD (1993) An interaction of β-amyloid with aluminium in vitro. FEBS Letts 324:293–295

Fukushima D, Konishi M, Maruyama K, Miyamoto T, Ishiura S, Suzuki K (1993) Activation of the secretory pathway leads to a decrease in the intracellular amyloidogenic fragments generated from the amyloid protein precursor. Biochem Biophys Res Commun 194:202–207

Giem P, Beeson WL, Fraser GE (1993) The incidence of dementia and intake of animal products: preliminary findings from the Adventist Health Study. Neuroepidemiology 12:28–36

Goldgaber D, Harris HW, Hla T, Maciag T, Donnelly RJ, Jacobsen JS, Vitek MP, Gajdusek DC (1989) Interleukin 1 regulates synthesis of amyloid β-protein precursor mRNA in human endothelial cells. Proc Natl Acad Sci USA 86:7606–7610

Haass C, Koo EH, Mellon A, Hung AY, Selkoe DJ (1992a) Targeting of cell-surface β-amyloid precursor protein to lysosomes: alternative processing into amyloid-bearing fragments. Nature 357: 500–503

Haass C, Schlossmacher MG, Hung AY, Vigo-Pelfrey C, Mellon A, Ostaszewski BL, Lieberburg I, Koo EH, Schenk D, Teplow DB, Selkoe DL (1992b) Amyloid β-peptide is produced by cultured cells during normal metabolism. Nature 359: 322–325

Haass C, Hung AY, Schlossmacher MG, Oltersdorf T, Teplow DB, Selkoe DJ (1993a) Normal cellular processing of the β-amyloid precursor protein results in the secretion of the amyloid β-peptide and related molecules. Ann NY Acad Sci 695: 109–116

Haass C, Hung AY, Schlossmacher MG, Teplow DB, Selkoe DJ (1993b) β-amyloid peptide and a 3-kDa fragment are derived by distinct cellular mechanisms, J Biol Chem 268: 3021–3024

Hilbich C, Kisters-Woike B, Reed J, Masters CL, Beyreuther K (1991a) Aggregation and secondary structure of synthetic amyloid βA4 peptides of Alzheimer's disease. J Mol Biol 218: 149–163

Hilbich C, Kisters-Woike B, Reed J, Masters CL, Beyreuther K (1991b) Human and rodent sequence analogs of Alzheimer's amyloid βA4 share similar properties and can be solubilized in buffers of pH 7.4. Eur J Biochem 201: 61–69

Hilbich C, Kisters-Woike B, Reed J, Masters CL, Beyreuther K (1992) Substitutions of hydrophobic amino acids reduce the amyloidogenicity of Alzheimer's disease βA4 peptides. J Mol Biol 228: 460–473

Hung AY, Koo EH, Haass C, Selkoe DJ (1992) Increased expression of β-amyloid precursor protein during neuronal differentiation is not accompanied by secretory cleavage. Proc Natl Acad Sci USA 89: 9439–9443

Jarrett JT, Lansbury PT Jr (1993) Seeding "one-dimensional crystallization" of amyloid: a pathogenic mechanism in Alzheimer's disease and scrapie? Cell 73: 1055–1058

Kang J, Lemaire H, Unterbeck A, Salbaum JM, Masters CL, Grzeschik K, Multhaup G, Beyreuther K, Müller-Hill B (1987) The precursor of Alzheimer's disease amyloid A4 protein resembles a cell-surface receptor. Nature 325: 733–736

Kitaguchi N, Takahashi Y, Tokushima Y, Shiojiri S, Ito H (1988) Novel precursor of Alzheimer's disease amyloid protein shows protease inhibitory activity. Nature 331: 530–532

Kitaguchi N, Takahashi Y, Oishi K, Shiojiri S, Tokushima Y, Utsunomiya T, Ito H (1990) Enzyme specificity of proteinase inhibitor region in amyloid precursor protein of Alzheimer's disease: different properties compared with protease nexin I. Biochim Biophys Acta 1038: 105–113

König G, Masters CL, Beyreuther K (1990) Retinoic acid induced differentiated neuroblastoma cells show increased expression of the βA4 amyloid gene of Alzheimer's disease and an altered splicing pattern. FEBS Lett 269: 305–310

König G, Mönning U, Czech C, Prior R, Banati R, Schreiter-Gasser U, Bauer J, Masters CL, Beyreuther K (1992) Identification and differential expression of a novel alternative splice isoform of the βA4 amloid precursor protein (APP) mRNA in leukocytes and brain microglial cells. J Biol Chem 267: 10804–10809

Lahiri D, Robakis NK (1991) The promoter activity of the gene encoding Alzheimer β-amyloid precursor protein (APP) is regulated by two blocks of upstream sequences. Mol Brain Res 9: 253–257

Mantyh PW, Ghilardi JR, Rogers S, DeMaster E, Allen CJ, Stimson ER, Maggio JE (1993) Aluminum, iron, and zinc ions promote aggregation of physiological concentrations of β-amyloid peptide. J Neurochem 61: 1171–1174

Masliah E, Terry RD, DeTeresa RM, Hansen LA (1989) Immunohistochemical quantification of the synapse-related protein synaptophysin in Alzheimer disease. Neurosci Lett 103: 234–239

Mobley WC, Neve RL, Prusiner SB, McKinley MP (1988) Nerve growth factor increases mRNA levels for the prion protein and the β-amyloid protein precursor in developing hamster brain. Proc Natl Acad Sci USA 85: 9811–9815

Ohyagi Y, Tabira T (1993) Effect of growth factors and cytokines on expression of amyloid β protein precursor mRNAs in cultured neural cells. Mol Brain Res 18: 127–132

Okado H, Okamoto H (1992) A *Xenopus* homologue of the human β-amyloid precursor protein: developmental regulation of its gene expression. Biochem Biophys Res Commun 189:1561–1568

Oltersdorf T, Ward PJ, Henriksson T, Beattie EC, Neve R, Lieberburg I, Fritz LC (1990) The Alzheimer amyloid precursor protein: identification of a stable intermediate in the biosynthetic/degradative pathway. J Biol Chem 265:4492–4497

Osuntokun BO, Ogunniyl A, Akang EEV, Aghadiuno PU, Ilori A, Bamgboye EA, Beyreuther K, Masters C (1994) βA4-amyloid in the brains of non-demented Nigerian Africans. Lancet 343:56

Pollwein P (1993) Overlapping binding sites of two different transcription factors in the promoter of the human gene for the Alzheimer amyloid precursor protein. Biochem Biophys Res Commun 190:637–647

Pollwein P, Masters CL, Beyreuther K (1992) The expression of the amyloid precursor protein (APP) is regulated by two GC-elements in the promoter. Nucleic Acids Res 20:63–68

Quitschke WW, Goldgaber D (1992) The amyloid β-protein precursor promoter: a region essential for transcriptional activity contains a nuclear factor binding domain. J Biol Chem 267:17362–17368

Rebeck GW, Reiter J, Strickland DK, Hyman BT (1993) Apolipoprotein E in sporadic Alzheimer's disease: allelic variation and receptor interactions. Neuron 11:575–580

Rumble B, Retallack R, Hilbich C, Simms G, Multhaup G, Martins R, Hockey A, Montgomery P, Beyreuther K, Masters CL (1989) Amyloid A4 protein and its precursor in Down's Syndrome and Alzheimer's disease. N Engl J Med 320:1446–1452

Salbaum JM, Weidemann A, Lemaire H, Masters CL, Beyreuther K (1988) The promoter of Alzheimer's disease amyloid A4 precursor gene. EMBO J 7:2807–2813

Schellenberg GD, Bird TD, Wijsman EM, Orr HT, Anderson L, Nemens E, White JA, Bonnycastle L, Weber JL, Alonso ME, Potter H, Heston LL, Martin GM (1992) Genetic linkage evidence for a familial Alzheimer's disease locus on chromosome 14. Science 258:668–671

Seubert P, Vigo-Pelfrey C, Esch F, Lee M, Dovey H, Davis D, Sinha S, Schlossmacher M, Whaley J, Swindlehurst C, McCormack R, Wolfert R, Selkoe D, Lieberburg I, Schenk D (1992) Isolation and quantification of soluble Alzheimer's β-peptide from biological fluids. Nature 359:325–327

Shapira R, Austin GE, Mirra SS (1988) Neuritic plaque amyloid in Alzheimer's disease is highly racemized. J Neurochem 50:69–74

Shoji M, Golde TE, Ghiso J, Cheung TT, Estus S, Shaffer LM, Cai X, McKay DM, Tintner R, Frangione B, Younkin SG (1992) Production of the Alzheimer amyloid β protein by normal proteolytic processing. Science 258:126–129

Siman R, Mistretta S, Durkin JT, Savage MJ, Loh T, Trusko S, Scott RW (1993) Processing of the β-amyloid precursor. Multiple proteases generate and degrade amyloidogenic fragments. J Biol Chem 268:16602–16609

Smith CJ, Wion D, Brachet P (1991) Nerve growth factor induces differential splicing of β-amyloid precursor mRNAs in the PC12 cell line. In: Hefti F, Brachet PH, Will B, Christen Y, eds. Growth factors and Alzheimer's disease, Berlin: Springer-Verlag, pp 216–221

Solá C, García-Landon FJ, Mengod G, Probst A, Frey P, Palacios JM (1993) Increased levels of the Kunitz protease inhibitor-containing βAPP mRNAs in rat brain following neurotoxic damage. Mol Brain Res 17:41–52

Wasco W, Bupp K, Magendantz M, Gusella JF, Tanzi RE, Solomon F (1992) Identification of a mouse brain cDNA that encodes a protein related to the Alzheimer disease-associated amyloid β protein precursor. Proc Natl Acad Sci USA 89:10758–10762

Wasco W, Gurubhagavatula S, d Paradis M, Romano DM, Sisodia SS, Hyman BT, Neve RL, Tanzi RE (1993) Isolation and characterization of the human APLP2 encoding a homologue of the Alzheimer's associated amyloid β protein precursor. Nature Genet 5:95–100

Wisniewski T, Golabek A, Matsubara E, Ghiso J, Frangione B (1993) Apolipoprotein E: binding to soluble Alzheimer's β-amyloid. Biochem Biophys Res Commun 192:359–365

Yankner BA, Dawes LR, Fisher S, Villa-Komaroff L, Oster-Granite ML, Neve RL (1989) Neurotoxicity of a fragment of the amyloid precursor associated with Alzheimer's disease. Science 245:417–420

Yoshikai S, Sasaki H, Doh-ura K, Furuya H, Sakaki Y (1990) Genomic organization of the human amyloid beta-protein precursor gene. Gene 87:257–263

Drosophila Appl Gene and APPL Protein: A Model System to Study the Function of the APP Protein Family

K. White*, L. Luo, T. Aigaki, and *M. Monastirioti*

Summary

Drosophila Amyloid precursor protein-like (*Appl*) gene encodes a protein product, APPL, similar to the β-amyloid precursor protein (APP) associated with Alzheimer's disease. The *Drosophila* APPL protein is neural-specific and is first detected in developing neurons concomitant with axonogenesis. APPL immunoreactivity is observed in neuronal cell bodies and in axons of both immature and mature neurons. Similar to APP, APPL is synthesized as a membrane-associated glycosylated precursor protein that is rapidly converted into a secreted form that lacks the cytoplasmic domain.

To understand the *in vivo* function of the APPL protein, we have taken a neurogenetic approach. Flies deleted for the *Appl* gene have been generated. These flies are viable, fertile and morphologically normal, yet they exhibit subtle behavioral deficits. The fast phototaxis defect in mutant *Appl* flies that lack APPL protein can be partially rescued by transgenes expressing the wild-type APPL protein. Furthermore, transgenes expressing the human APP protein show a level of rescue similar to the transgenes expressing APPL. Our analyses suggest a conserved ancestral function for the APP class of proteins in the nervous system. We discuss the implications of current functional studies on the APP proteins and how the *Drosophila* system could facilitate the *in vivo* analysis of the function of this class of proteins.

Introduction

The discovery of the amyloid β protein precursor (APP) gene provided the first direct tangible molecular handle to the pathology of Alzheimer's disease. Since then, the scientific community has vigorously pursued the study of this gene and its protein products and has accumulated a vast body of information relating to its biosynthesis, processing and subsequent degradation (reviewed in Selkoe

* Biology Department and Center for Complex Systems, Brandeis University, Waltham, MA 02254, USA

C.L. Masters et al. (Eds.)
Amyloid Protein Precursor in Development,
Aging and Alzheimer's Disease
© Springer-Verlag Berlin Heidelberg 1994

1991). The main stimulus for these studies derives from the questions related to the pathogenesis of Alzheimer's disease: What are the differences in the processing of APP molecules in normal and disease conditions? How do the AβP cores form? Are the senile plaques causal to the neuronal cell death observed in Alzheimer's condition? What is the normal function of APP and is this function affected in the disease condition?

When it was first discovered, APP$_{695}$ was a novel protein (Kang et al. 1987). The amino acid sequence predicted an integral membrane protein with a single membrane-spanning segment, a large extracellular domain and a small cytoplasmic domain; AβP spanned the extracellular-membrane border. Subsequently, several additional APP isoforms that are products of alternatively spliced RNAs and contain exons that code a Kunitz-type protease inhibitor domain were identified (Ponte et al. 1988; Tanzi et al. 1988; Kitaguchi et al. 1988). Recently, it has become evident that APP is a member of a protein family that is evolutionarily conserved in domain structure and function, as two other mammalian genes, APLP1 and APLP2, have been identified that show a high degree of conservation to the APP gene (Wasco et al. 1992, 1993). Moreover, these three remarkably conserved members of the APP family are likely to be co-expressed within at least some and perhaps many neurons (Wasco et al. 1993). These findings further complicate the functional analysis of any individual member of the APP protein family, as not only are there a multiplicity of isoforms encoded by each gene, but there are also proteins encoded by closely related genes.

We serendipitously identified a *Drosophila* transcript that encoded a protein that demonstrated striking sequence homology with the APP$_{695}$ protein in two large extracellular domains, in the cytoplasmic domain and in the overall structure (Fig. 1, E1, E2 and C; Rosen et al. 1989). We christened the new gene

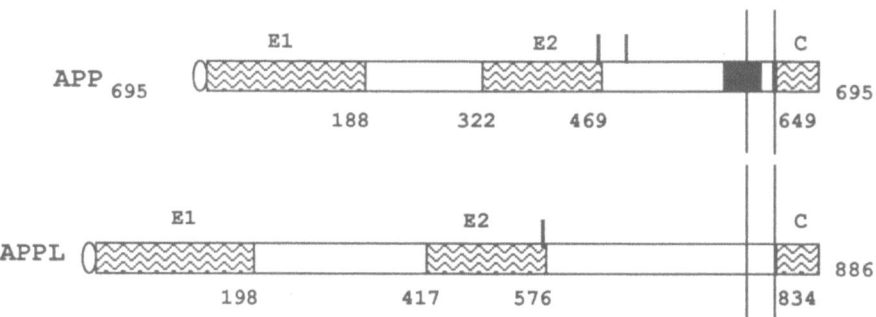

Fig. 1. Diagrammatic representation of *Drosophila* APPL and human APP. The model of APP is adapted from Kang et al (1987) and the analogous APPL polypeptide is presented. The N terminus is at the left; the circles at the N terminus represent the presumed signal sequences. The regions of homology E1, E2 and C between APPL and APP are drawn as open rectangles; the loops in APPL represent the regions of non-homology. Asterisks note putative N-glycosylation sites

defined by this transcript *Amyloid β protein precursor-like* (*Appl*) and its protein product, APPL (Martin-Morris and White 1990). Unlike APP, which shows a broad tissue distribution, *Drosophila Appl* gene is expressed in a neural-specific fashion. We undertook to characterize the *Drosophila* APPL protein and analyze its function, with the expectation that the *Appl* gene, with its single transcript and neural-specific expression, might help elucidate the basic function provided by the APP class of molecules in the nervous system. We felt that the *Drosophila* system brought special advantages to this analysis through the scalpel it provides by its mutational genetic analysis, and the opportunity it provides to study in vivo function provided by transgenes in the absence of the wild type gene (Rubin 1988; Miklos 1993). Thus, one can study a gene's function by genetically removing the gene product and also genetically add back wild-type and in vitro-mutated genes to the mutant fly and observe the consequences. Moreover, other molecular players involved in the same biological process can be discovered by identifying other genes that genetically interact with the gene of interest. In our studies, reviewed below, we have attempted to answer the following basic questions: How is the APPL protein processed? Where is the APPL protein localized? What are the consequences of complete absence of APPL protein to the fly? Is there functional homology between APPL and APP proteins?

Drosophila Appl Gene and APPL Protein

Drosophila Appl gene spans ∼ 38 kb of genomic DNA; the single mature transcript of ∼ 6.5 kb predicts an 886 amino acid protein. In situ RNA localization data show that the *Appl* transcripts are found exclusively in post-mitotic neurons in all stages of development. They are not observed in neuronal precursor cells or in at least some and perhaps all glia. *Appl* transcripts are first observed in differentiating neurons, concomitant with axonal outgrowth, and continue to be expressed in mature neurons (Martin-Morris and While 1990). This finding is similar to mammalian APP transcripts that are abundant in fetal tissues and in adult stages (Kitaguchi et al. 1988; Tanzi et al. 1988). These observations have been substantiated by immunolocalization of the APPL protein using α-APPL serum. APPL protein is observed in neuronal cell bodies and in neuronal processes (Luo et al. 1990). Figure 2 shows APPL immunoreactivity in the photoreceptors in developing eye primordia; the developing eye primordia is connected to the optic lobes in the central nervous system by the optic nerve. During *Drosophila* eye development, a morphogenetic furrow separates the differentiated and undifferentiated epithelium; the undifferentiated cells ahead of the furrow are devoid of APPL immunoreactivity. But behind the furrow, the newly differentiating photoreceptors show high levels of APPL immunoreactivity. APPL immunoreactivity is also observed in the developing photoreceptor axons in the optic stalk.

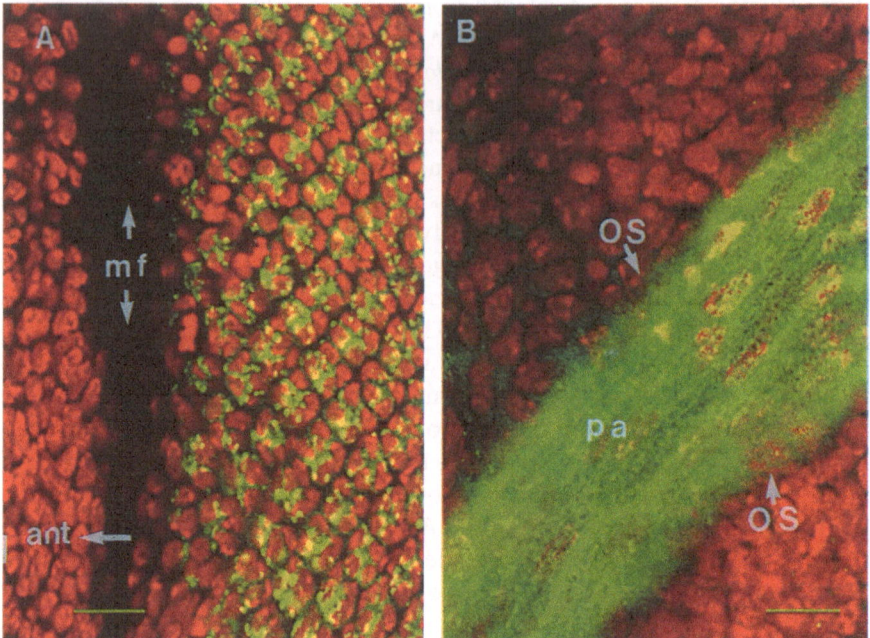

Fig. 2. APPL immunoreactivity in the developing eye primordia. Optic sections through the developing *Drosophila* eye imaginal disc (A) and the optic stalk carrying the photoreceptor axons (B). Green color represents APPL-immunoreactivity and red color represents propidium iodide staining used to visualize all nuclei. Note that only the differentiated photoreceptors posterior to the morphogenetic furrow (mf) show APPL immunoreactivity and that the undifferentiated cells anterior to the furrow are devoid of APPL immunoreactivity. Also note that the axons of the differentiating photoreceptors (pa) traversing the optic stalk (OS) are highly APPL immunoreactive. Scale bar, 10 microns

We have identified two forms of APPL protein in *Drosophila*: a 145-kDa membrane-associated form and a 130-kDa soluble form that lacks the cytoplasmic domain (Fig. 3, lane 2; Luo et al. 1990). Pulse-chase experiments in *Drosophila* tissue culture cells transfected with APPL cDNA show that: 1) the 145-kDa membrane-bound protein is a precursor to the 130-kDa secreted protein, 2) this conversion is very rapid, and 3) both forms are N-glycosylated. In tissue extracts from either embryos or adult heads, the 145-kDa precursor and the 130-kDa soluble form are present in roughly equal abundance, suggesting that if the half life of the precursor *in vivo* is similar to that in the tissue culture, the soluble form does not accumulate but is instead rapidly turned over. APPL cDNA has been expressed in the baculovirus system where APPL protein undergoes cleavage as in *Drosophila* tissue culture cells (Aigaki and White, unpublished observations).

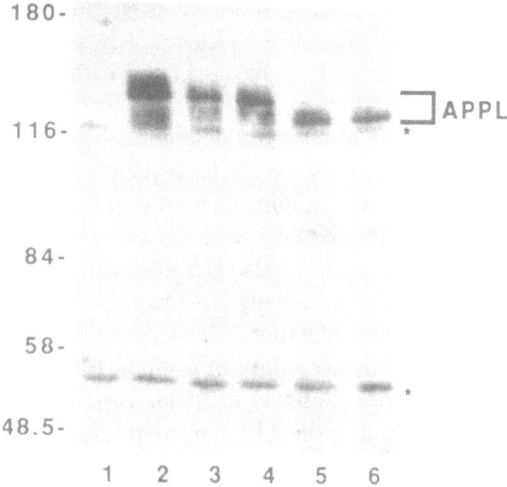

Fig. 3. Immunoblot of APPL proteins in different *Appl* related genotypes (figure taken from Luo et al 1992). Lane 1, APPL deficient genotype *Appl^d/Y*; lane 2, an APPL$^+$ genotype *Appl^d/m^{52}Y*; lanes 3 and 4, APPL$^+$ genotype where APPL protein is supplied by the *hsp-Appl$^+$* transgenes (*Appl^d/Y; 3a2/ +* and *Appl^d/Y; 3a3/ +* , *3a2* and *3a3* represent transgenes bearing *hsp-Appl$^+$*); lanes 5 and 6, genotypes where APPL protein is supplied by a mutated *Appl* gene, *hsp-Appl^{sd}* which carries a 30 amino acid deletion that disrupts secretion (*Appl^d/Y; 2c1/ +* ; *Appl^d/Y; 3c2/ +* , *2c1 and 3c2* represent transgenes bearing *hsp-Appl^{sd}* transgene). Note the absence of the two APPL bands from lane 1, and a single major band in lanes 5 and 6. The single major band and its size are consistent with secretion defective phenotype from a deletion mutant. Asterisks mark background bands

Similarities and Differences Between APPL and APP

Similar to APP, APPL has a membrane-spanning domain close to its C terminus (APP, 24 amino acid membrane spanning domain, 47 amino acid cytoplasmic domain; APPL, 23 amino acid membrane-spanning domain, 53 amino acid cytoplasmic domain). Strong sequence homology was observed between APP_{695} and APPL in three regions. An N-terminus domain E1 (APP_{695}, 1–198; APPL, 1–188), that shows 38% identity, has 12 conserved cysteine residues and harbors a highly conserved stretch of 19 amino acids with 15 identities. A second extracellular domain E2 (APP_{695}, 322–469; APPL, 417–576), that shows 37% identity, contains one conserved N-glycosylation site and has a highly conserved stretch of 71 amino acid residues. Finally, the cytoplasmic domain is 47% identical and contains a conserved nonapeptide that includes a tetrameric motif NPXY required for coated pit-mediated internalization.

APP is known to be processed in at least two major pathways: a secretory pathway (Weidemann et al. 1989) and an endosomal-lysosomal pathway (Estus et al. 1992; Golde et al. 1992; Haass et al. 1992). The processing of APPL through the secretory pathway is similar to that of APP. Both are synthesized as integral membrane glycoproteins that are then cleaved to yield secreted forms. The preservation of the cleavage suggests that it is physiologically significant event that is likely to be associated with the function of the protein. We do not yet know if APPL is also processed through the endosomal-lysosomal pathway.

There are also several differences between APPL and APP, the most notable of these being that there is no sequence similarity in the region of AβP, although the membrane-spanning character in that region is maintained. It is worthwhile to note in this context that the two other mammalian genes related to APP, APLP1 and APLP2, also lack the AβP domain (Wasco et al. 1992, 1993). Thus APP is unique in having AβP peptide in the APP family of proteins that have thus far been identified. A second difference is that *Appl* does not encode a Kunitz protease inhibitor domain that has been identified in both APP and APLP2 genes (Ponte et al. 1988; Tanzi et al. 1988; Wasco et al. 1993). A third difference is that the APPL protein is larger than APP, APLP1 and APLP2; the functional significance of regions of non-homology is currently unknown. Finally, unlike its mammalian relatives that show a broad tissue distribution, APPL is specifically expressed in the nervous system. Absence of the protease inhibitor domain and the expression pattern make APPL most similar to the APP_{695}, an APP isoform that is enriched in the nervous system (Ponte et al. 1988; Tanzi et al. 1988).

Functional Analyses of *Appl* Gene

We have investigated APPL's function using a neurogenetic approach (Luo et al. 1992). As a first step, we generated mutant APPL-deficient flies ($Appl^d$) that carried a synthetic interstitial deletion within the *Appl* gene, and thus were devoid of any APPL protein (Fig. 3, lane 1). These $Appl^d$ flies, congenitally deprived of APPL protein, develop into morphologically normal adults that appear to enjoy a normal life span and are fertile under laboratory conditions. Thus the function of APPL protein does not seem to be essential for the development of the adult fly. This could imply that either APPL does not play any role in processes vital for fly development, or that the process that it is engaged in is not uniquely essential.

We argued that APPL protein must be important to nervous system function because it is expressed in most and perhaps all neurons in the developing and mature fly nervous system, and because of the evolutionary retention of the sequence and domain structure during arthropod and chordate lineages. We therefore initiated a behavioral analysis of the $Appl^d$ flies (Luo et al. 1992). Among the behaviors we tested, $Appl^d$ flies have reduced performance index in a learning paradigm-shock associated odor avoidance classical conditioning assay (Tully and Quinn 1985). The fact that they also exhibit reduced shock reactivity (running away after an electric shock), though, prevents us from concluding that the reduced learning index was specifically due to the classical conditioning per se. $Appl^d$ flies were poor performers in fast phototaxis; both shock reactivity and fast phototaxis involve locomoter reactivity (Benzer 1967; Meehan and Wilson 1987). In fast phototaxis, flies are repeatedly asked to respond to light after they have been physically banged down and allowed to recover for a few seconds. Independent tests showed that although the *Appl^d* flies were deficient in fast phototaxis, their defect was not in vision. Since *Appl^d* flies were also poor performers in shock reactivity tests that involve escape response induced by a noxious stimulus, we believe that the behavioral deficit is in locomoter reactivity.

To demonstrate that the fast phototaxis behavioral deficit is indeed caused by the absence of APPL protein, an *Appl* minigene constructed using *Appl* cDNA expressed under the control of a *Drosophila* heat shock promoter (*hsp-Appl^+*) was used (Fig. 3, lanes 3 and 4). *Appl^d* flies and *Appl^d* flies that also carried one copy of *hsp-Appl^+* transgene were tested in fast phototaxis assays. The deficit observed in the behavior of *Appl^d* flies was partially rescued by the transgene expressing wild type APPL protein, as the transgene-bearing flies showed about 50% rescue of the mutant phenotype. As a negative control another transgene, *hsp-appl^sd*, that encodes a mutant APPL protein with a 30-amino acid deletion in the extracellular region near the membrane-spanning domain and abolishes the secretion of the APPL protein was used (lanes 5 and 6). *Appl^d* flies that carried one copy of *hsp-Appl^sd* transgene showed no rescue of the mutant phenotype.

A limitation of our analysis is that the functional rescue we obtain is partial (Luo et al. 1992). At least part of the reason for this observed inadequacy of the wild-type APPL expressing transgene is likely to be due to the fact that, instead of a genomic transgene, we used a minigene in which *Appl* cDNA was expressed under the heat shock promoter. This was necessitated by the large size of the *Appl* gene (at least 38 kb) and because the promoter region of the *Appl* gene was not defined. To allow construction of transgenes that mimic the expression pattern of the endogenous gene, we are currently using *Appl* promoter-*lacZ* fusion constructs to define the *Appl* promoter. Presumably, a transgene that expresses *Appl* cDNA under its own promoter will provide an improvement over the *hsp-Appl* transgene used in our functional studies.

Human APP$_{695}$ is a Functional Homologue of APPL

The fast phototaxis assay described above was used to test the ability of APP$_{695}$ to provide the biological function of APPL. A transgene that expresses APP$_{695}$ cDNA under the hsp promoter (*hsp*-APP$_{695}$), as was used to express APPL, was introduced into the fly genome, and expression and processing of APP$_{695}$ were ascertained using immunoblots (Luo et al. 1992). Then *Appl^d* flies that carried one copy of *hsp*-APP$_{695}$ transgene were tested in fast phototaxis assays along with *Appl^d* flies and *Appl^d* flies that also carried one copy of *hsp-Appl^+* transgene. The results of these tests showed that the APP$_{695}$ expressing transgenes are able to rescue the fast phototaxis deficit of *Appl^d* flies to the same extent as the APPL expressing transgenes (Luo et al. 1992).

Cellular Functions of APP and APPL

Our ultimate goal is to contribute to the understanding of the cellular functions of the APP family of proteins. Initially, the structure of APP protein suggested that it may serve as a cell surface receptor (Kang et al. 1987). One concrete role assignable to some APP isoforms is that of a protease inhibitor, by virtue of their identity to the protease Nexin II (Oltersdorf et al. 1989; Van Nostrand et al. 1989). Over the years, however, heterogeneous functional roles have been proposed for APP and its domains. Several studies have suggested that APP may be involved in cell-cell or cell-matrix interactions (e.g., Schubert et al. 1988, 1989; Klier et al. 1990) and in general promote cell adhesion. It has been proposed that these interactions may be mediated through an integrin-like cell surface receptor molecule (Ghiso et al. 1992). Secreted forms of APP have been demonstrated to have a growth-promoting effect on fibroblasts (Saitoh et al. 1989). Data suggesting that the secreted form of APP with the protease inhibitor domain is a core protein of a chondroitin sulfate proteoglycan have been presented (Shioi et al. 1992). Certain regions of the APP molecule have been shown to have neurotoxic properties (Yankner et al. 1990). Secreted APP has been suggested to play excitoprotective and intraneuronal calcium regulating roles (Mattson et al. 1993). A metalloproteinase inhibitor domain has been recently identified in the C terminal glycosylated region of the secreted APP (Miyazaki et al. 1993). While the multidomain organization of APP is conducive to it being a multifunctional protein, it is unlikely that in vivo APP isoforms perform all the varied functions that have been implied by these studies.

A recent report shows that the cytoplasmic domain of APP may associate with G_0 and be involved in G_0 activation (Nishimoto et al. 1993). This finding goes back to the original cell surface receptor proposal. The notion of APP being a G_0 coupled receptor is attractive, as it offers a functional involvement for both the extracellular and cytoplasmic domains of APP, and thus explains evolutionary pressures to preserve large domains of homology on both sides of the membrane. This postulate will gather strength if other aspects of the signaling process become evident. These findings make it reasonable to suggest that the primordial APP protein served as a receptor, with the cleavage being an obligatory step in the process. It is easy to envision that the secreted protein could have acquired additional functions as organisms evolved and that perhaps, in some instances, this was followed by evolution of ligands to procure regulated secretion. This latter notion will accommodate some of the functions postulated for the secreted form of APP molecules.

We are asking focused questions of the *Drosophila Appl* gene that all revolve around the physiological function of the 145-kDa membrane-associated form and the 130-kDa secreted form in the nervous system. An important finding is that flies can develop without any APPL protein and these flies appear relatively normal. Such a finding is not necessarily surprising as current estimates suggest that two-thirds of the fly's genome is likely to encode functions that fall into this category, i.e., absence of the gene function does not lead to any readily observable phenotype (Miklos 1993). Many instances of genes for which null-mutations do not result in obvious phenotypes are known in *Drosophila*. Among genes expressed in the nervous system some examples are *Amalgam* (Seeger et al. 1988), *Fasciclin I* and *Fasciclin III* (Elkins et al. 1990). Neither is this situation unique to *Drosophila*; in yeast as much as 70% of genes are not essential for cell division or growth (Goebl and Petes 1986), and there are examples where mice lacking a particular protein develop normally (e.g., Prp knock out, Büeler et al. 1992; MyoD knock out, Rudnicki et al. 1992). This portion of the genome is likely to be made up of at least two sets of genes: those genes that when changed lead to only subtle changes in the organism's development or behavior and those that are redundant. Absence of APPL leads to subtle deficits in behavior, implying that APPL is essential for optimal function of the nervous system. This is consistent with the temporal and spatial expression of APPL.

We recognize that the behavioral defect in itself does not yield any direct clues regarding the cellular processes in which APPL engages. Nevertheless, the functional assay developed with transgenes expressing wild-type APPL protein can now be used for assessing *in vivo* function of mutant APPL proteins. For example, one can ask if mutant *Appl* transgenes that express just the membrane-associated form or just the secreted form can also be functional. In fact, the negative control used in our studies consisted of an APPL mutant transgene (*hsp-APPL^{sd}*) that synthesized a secretion-defective protein because of a 30-amino acid deletion that presumably deleted the cleavage site. *hsp-APPL^{sd}* was unable to provide any APPL function in the fast phototaxis behavioral paradigm (Luo et al. 1992). Therefore, secretion appears to be physiologically significant, with the caveat that the deleted amino acids could be per se structurally required for the biological activity.

A great strength of *Drosophila* is that one can use mutants to assess *in vivo* consequences of alterations in a single molecule. Additionally, current molecular and genetic methodologies allow identification of other molecules that interact with a given molecule. An important generalization that has emerged from the explosion in our understanding of cellular mechanisms is that molecules engaged in similar processes in different organisms are often structurally related and possibly share common ancestry. Moreover, interacting classes of molecules unearthed in one system are likely to participate in the same process in other systems. Recent studies in the signal transduction process mediated by receptor tyrosine kinases provide a striking example of how knowledge from different organismal systems can be synergistic and lead to better understanding of a key biological process – in this case – the activation of Ras by receptor tyrosine kinases (reviewed in McCormick 1993). In these studies one sees the convergence of research from *Drosophila* photoreceptor R7 development, *Caenorhabditis elegans* vulval development, and the mammalian signal transduction/oncogene field. When it was discovered that the *Drosophila sevenless* gene encoded a receptor tyrosine kinase similar to many proto-oncogenes (Hafen et al. 1987), it became possible to identify other molecules involved in this signaling process. Over the years, the genetic analysis of this process has not only identified the ligand for the sevenless receptor (Kramer et al. 1991), but also downstream elements such as Ras, guanine nucleotide exchange factor Sos, and SH2/SH3 domain containing factor drk (Simon et al. 1991, 1993; Oliver et al. 1993). Biochemical experiments both in *Drosophila* and in mammalian tissue culture cells demonstrate a universal pathway in activation of Ras by receptor tyrosine kinases (e.g., see Egan et al. 1993; Rozakis-Adcock et al. 1993; Li et al. 1993; Simon et al. 1993; Olivier et al. 1993). Examples like this make it reasonable for us to suggest that in future it should be possible to unearth molecules that interact with APPL in *Drosophila*, and also to use the *Drosophila* system to test physiological roles of interacting molecules implicated in APP function.

Acknowledgments. This work is supported by NIH grant NS29826 to K.W. We thank Patricia Parmenter for help in manuscript preparation.

References

Benzer S (1967) Behavioral mutants of *Drosophila* isolated by countercurrent distribution. Proc Natl Acad Sci USA 58:1112–1119

Büeler H, Fischer M, Lang Y, Bluethmann H, Lipp H-P, DeArmond SJ, Prusiner SB, Aguet M, Weissmann C (1992) Normal development and behaviour of mice lacking the neuronal cell surface PrP protein. Nature 356:577–582

Elkins T, Zinn K, McAllister L, Hoffman FM, Goodman CS (1990) Genetic analysis of a *Drosophila* neural cell adhesion molecule: interaction of fasciclin I and Abelson tyrosine kinase mutations. Cell 60:565–575

Estus S, Golde TE, Kunishita T, Blades D, Lowery D, Eisen M, Usiak M, Qu X, Tabira T, Greenberg BD, Younkin SG (1992) Potentially amyloidogenic, carboxy-terminal derivatives of the amyloid protein precursor. Science 255:726–728

Egan SE, Giddings BW, Brooks MW, Buday L, Sizeland AM, Weinberg RA (1993) Association of Sos Ras exchange protein with Grb2 is implicated in tyrosine kinase signal transduction and transformation. Nature 363:45–51

Ghiso J, Rostagno A, Gardella JE, Liem L, Gorevic PD, Frangione B (1992) A 109-amino-acid C-terminal fragment of Alzheimer's-disease amyloid precursor protein contains a sequence, –RHDS–, that promotes cell adhesion. Biochem J 288:1053–1059

Goebl MG, Petes TD (1986) Most of the yeast genomic sequences are not essential for cell growth and division. Cell 46:983–992

Golde TE, Estus S, Younkin LH, Selkoe DJ, Younkin SG (1992) Processing of the amyloid protein precursor to potentially amyloidogenic derivatives. Science 255:728–730

Haass C, Koo EH, Mellon S, Huang AY, Selkoe DJ (1992) Targeting of cell-surface β-amyloid precursor protein to lysosomes: alternative processing into amyloid-bearing fragments. Nature 357:500–503

Hafen EM, Basler K, Edstroem JE, Rubin GM (1987) *Sevenless*, a cell-specific homeotic gene of *Drosophila*, encodes a putative transmembrane receptor with a tyrosine kinase domain. Science 236:55–63

Kang J, Lemaire HG, Unterbeck A, Salbaum JM, Masters CL, Grzeschik KH, Multhaup G, Beyreuther K, Müller-Hill B (1987) The precursor of Alzheimer's disease amyloid A4 protein resembles a cell-surface receptor. Nature 325:733–736

Kitaguchi N, Takahashi Y, Tokushima Y, Shiojiri S, Ito H (1988) Novel precursor of Alzheimer's disease amyloid protein shows protease inhibitory activity. Nature 331:530–532

Klier FG, Cole G, Stallcup W, Schubert D (1990) Amyloid β-protein precursor is associated with extracellular matrix. Brain Res 515:336–342

Kramer H, Cagan RL, Zipursky SL (1991) Interaction of *bride of sevenless* membrane bound ligand and the *sevenless* tyrosine kinase receptor. Nature 352:207–212

Li N, Batzer A, Daly R, Yajnik V, Skolnik E, Chardin P, Bar-Sagi D, Margolis B, Schlessinger J (1993) Guanine-nucleotide-releasing factor hSos 1 binds to Grb2 and links receptor tyrosine kinases to Ras signalling. Nature 363:85–87

Luo L, Martin-Morris LE, White K (1990) Identification, secretion, and neural expression of APPL, a *Drosophila* protein similar to human amyloid protein precursor. J Neurosci 10:3849–3861

Luo L, Tully T, White K (1992) Human amyloid precursor protein ameliorates behavioral deficit of flies deleted for *Appl* gene. Neuron 9:595–605

Martin-Morris LE, White K (1990) The *Drosophila* transcript encoded by the β-amyloid protein precursor-like gene is restricted to the nervous system. Development 110:185–195

Mattson MP, Cheng B, Culwell AR, Esch FS, Lieberburg I, Rydel RE (1993) Evidence for excitoprotective and intraneuronal calcium-regulating roles for secreted forms of the β-amyloid precursor protein. Neuron 10:243–254

McCormick R (1993) How receptors turn Ras on. Nature 363:15–16

Meehan MJ, Wilson R (1987) Locomotor activity in the *Tyr-1* mutant of *Drosophila melanogaster*. Behav Genet 17:503–512

Miklos GLG (1993) Molecules and cognition: The latterday lessons of levels, language, and *lac*. Evolutionary overview of brain structure and function in some vertebrates and invertebrates. J Neurobiol 24:842–890

Miyazaki K, Hasegawa M, Funahashi K, Umeda M (1993) A metalloproteinase inhibitor domain in Alzheimer amyloid protein precursor. Nature 362:839–841

Nishimoto I, Okamoto T, Matsuura Y, Takahashi S, Okamoto T, Murayama Y, Ogata E (1993) Alzheimer amyloid protein precursor complexes with brain GTP-binding protein G_0. Nature 362:75–79

Oltersdorf T, Fritz LC, Schenk DB, Lieberburg I, Johnson-Wood KL, Beattie EC, Ward PJ, Blacher RW, Dovey HF, Sinha S (1989) The secreted form of Alzheimer's amyloid precursor protein with the Kunitz domain is protease nexin-II. Nature 341:144–147

Olivier JP, Raabe T, Henkemeyer M, Dickson B, Mbamalu G, Margolis B, Schlessinger J, Hafen E, Pawson T (1993) A *Drosophila* SH2-SH3 adaptor protein implicated in coupling the sevenless tyrosine kinase to an activator of Ras guanine nucleotide exchange, Sos. Cell 73:179 191

Ponte P, Gonzalez-DeWhitt P, Schilling J, Miller J, Hsu D, Greenberg B, Davis K, Wallace W, Lieberburg I, Fuller F, Cordell B (1988) A new A4 amyloid mRNA contains a domain homologous to serine proteinase inhibitors. Nature 331:525–527

Rosen DR, Martin-Morris L, Luo L, White K (1989) A *Drosophila* gene encoding a protein resembling the human β-amyloid protein precursor. Proc Natl Acad Sci USA 86:2478–2482

Rozakis-Adcock M, Fernley R, Wade J, Pawson T, Bowtell D (1993) The SH2 and SH3 domains of mammalian Grb2 couple the EGF receptor to the Ras activator mSos1. Nature 363:83–85

Rubin GM (1988) *Drosophila melanogaster* as an experimental organism. Science 240:1453–1459

Rudnicki MA, Braun T, Hinuma S, Jaenisch R (1992) Inactivation of *MyoD* in mice leads to up-regulation of the myogenic HLH gene *Myf-5* and results in apparently normal muscle development. Cell 71:383–390

Saitoh T, Sundsmo M, Roch J-M, Kimura N, Cole G, Schubert D, Oltersdorf T, Schenk DB (1989) Secreted form of amyloid β protein precursor is involved in the growth regulation of fibroblasts. Cell 58:615–622

Schubert D, Schroeder R, LaCorbiere M, Saitoh S, Cole G (1988) Amyloid β protein precursor is possibly a helparan sulfate proteoglycan core protein. Science 241:223–226

Schubert D, LaCorbiere M, Saitoh T, Cole G (1989) Characterization of an amyloid β precursor protein that binds heparin and contains tyrosine sulfate. Proc Natl Acad Sci USA 86:2066–2069

Seeger MA, Hattley L, Kaufman TC (1988) Characterization of *Amalgam*, member of the immunoglobulin superfamily from *Drosophila*. Cell 55:589–600

Selkoe DJ (1991) The molecular pathology of Alzheimer's disease. Neuron 6:487–498

Shioi J, Anderson JP, Ripellino JA, Robakis NK (1992) Chondroitin sulfate proteoglycan form of the Alzheimer's β-amyloid precursor. J Biol Chem 267:13819–13822

Simon MA, Bowtell DDL, Dodson GS, Laverty TR, Rubin GM (1991) Ras1 and a putative guanine nucleotide exchange factor perform crucial steps in signaling by the sevenless protein tyrosine kinase. Cell 67:701–716

Simon MA, Dodson GS, Rubin GM (1993) An SH3-SH2-SH3 protein is required for p21$^{Ras 1}$ activation and binds to sevenless and Sos proteins in vitro. Cell 73:169–177

Tanzi RE, McClatchey AI, Lamperti ED, Villa-Komaroff L, Gusella JF, Neve RL (1988) Protease inhibitor domain encoded by an amyloid protein precursor mRNA associated with Alzheimer's disease. Natue 331:528–530

Tully T, Quinn WG (1985) Classical conditioning and retention in normal and mutant *Drosophila melanogaster*. J Comp Physiol 157:263–277

Van Nostrand WE, Wagner SL, Suzuki M, Choi BH, Farrow JS, Geddes JW, Cotman CW, Cummingham DD (1989) Protease nexin-II, a potent anti-chymotrypsin, shows identity to amyloid β-protein precursor. Nature 341:546–549

Wasco W, Bupp K, Magendantz M, Gusella JF, Tanzi RE, Solomon F (1992) Identification of a mouse brain cDNA that encodes a protein related to the Alzheimer disease-associated amyloid β protein precursor. Proc Natl Acad Sci USA 89:10758–10762

Wasco W, Gurubhagavatula S, d. Paradis M, Romano DM, Sisodia SS, Hyman BT, Neve RL, Tanzi RE (1993) Isolation and characterization of the human APLP2 gene encoding a homologue of the Alzheimer's associated amyloid β protein precursor. Nature Genet 5:95–100

Weidemann A, Konig G, Bunke D, Fischer P, Salbaum JM, Masters CL, Beyreuther K (1989) Identification, biogenesis, and localization of precursors of Alzheimer's disease A4 amyloid protein. Cell 57:115–126

Yankner BA, Duffy LK, Kirschner DA (1990) Neurotrophic and neurotoxic effects of amyloid β protein: reversal by tachykinin neuropeptides. Science 250:279–282

Amyloid βA4 of Alzheimer's Disease: Structural Requirements for Folding and Aggregation

C. Hilbich*, B. Kisters-Woike, C. L. Masters, and *K. Beyreuther*

Summary

Alzheimer's disease is known to be the most common cause for a dementia in elderly people. Its specific pathological markers are extracellular protein depositions (i.e., amyloid) in the brain. The main component of this amyloid is "βA4," a peptide comprising 43 amino acids. It is highly insoluble under physiological conditions and aggregates into dense clusters of filaments. We have used βA4 isolated from amyloid plaque cores as well as synthetic peptides corresponding to the natural βA4 sequence and analogue peptides to determine requirements for aggregation and the secondary structure of βA4. Infrared and circular dichroism spectroscopy of βA4 peptides showed that their secondary structure consists of a β-turn flanked by two strands of β-sheet. Purified βA4 peptides are soluble in water and are precipitated by the addition of salts, suggesting that aggregation depends upon a hydrophobic effect. Accordingly, the substitution of hydrophobic residues led to βA4 variants with reduced amyloidogenicity. Analogues showed lower β-sheet contents after solubilization in water and in the solid state. Although still forming filaments, some variants did not aggregate into the highly condensed depositions that are typical for amyloid; they could also be solubilized in 200 mM NaCl and KCl. When mixed with βA4 peptides bearing the natural sequence, two analogues could inhibit the formation of filaments *in vitro*. They may open the opportunity for a rational therapy of Alzheimer's disease.

Introduction

Alzheimer's disease is the most prominent cause of dementia in elderly people. It is triggered by degenerative processes in the brain. Its histopathology is characterized by a degeneration of neurons, gliosis and the deposition of highly insoluble proteins in the brain, the latter classifying Alzheimer's disease as an

* Center of Molecular Biology, University of Heidelberg, Im Neuenheimer Feld 282, 69120 Heidelberg, Germany

C.L. Masters et al. (Eds.)
Amyloid Protein Precursor in Development,
Aging and Alzheimer's Disease
© Springer-Verlag Berlin Heidelberg 1994

amyloidosis. Proteinacious deposits appear as neurofibrillary tangles (NFT), amyloid plaque cores (APC) and amyloid of the congophilic angiopathy (ACA; for reviews see Reisberg 1983; Selkoe 1989; Müller-Hill and Beyreuther 1989).

In contrast to NFT and ACA, amyloid plaques are found in the brains of all Alzheimer's disease victims and are therefore regarded as the main criterion in the pathological diagnosis of this disease. The major constituent of both APC and ACA has been shown to be a 4.5 kD peptide denoted as βA4. βA4 consists, in its longest form, of 43 amino acids (Glenner and Wong 1984a,b; Wong et al. 1985; Masters et al. 1985a,b; Kang et al. 1987; Mori et al. 1992; Roher et al. 1993). All kinds of amyloid βA4 deposits contain considerable amounts of amino(N)-terminally truncated peptides. APC comprises the carboxy(C)-terminal amino acid 42 and, in 5 to 25% of the material, also residue 43. C-terminally truncated sequences ending at amino acid 40 or 39 were reported for ACA in Alzheimer's disease and for the amyloid of cerebral hemorrhage with amyloidosis of Dutch type, both of which are found within blood vessel walls of the brain (Prelli et al. 1988a,b; Joachim et al. 1988). This "raggedness" of βA4 peptides from natural sources is summarized in Figure 1. Electron microscopy has revealed similar ultrastructural features of APC and ACA. Besides minor amounts of other proteins, they contain βA4 in the form of straight filaments having a diameter of 5 to 10 nm (Terry et al. 1964; Schlote 1965).

Amyloid βA4 is proteolytically derived from a transmembrane protein whose function still remains unclear. Different splice-forms of this amyloid precursor protein (APP) are encoded by a widely expressed gene (for reviews see, Selkoe 1991; Hardy and Allsop 1991). βA4 comprises the last 28 residues of the

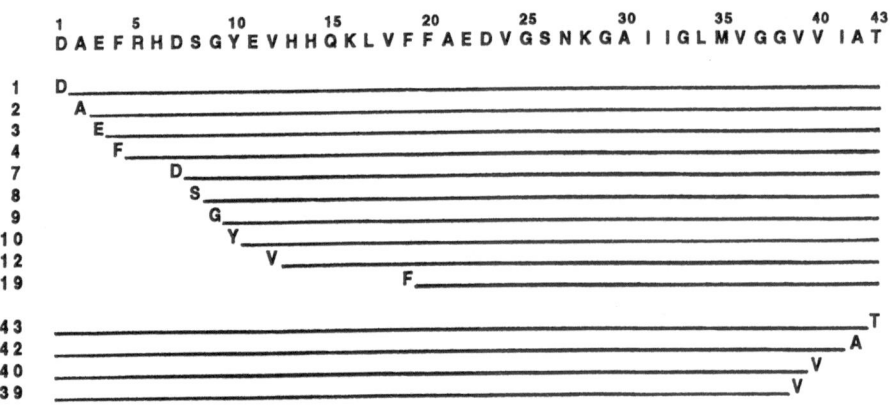

Fig. 1. βA4 and its naturally occurring variants. The numbers of N- or C-terminal residues, respectively, are indicated. N- and C-terminally truncated peptides are shown for otherwise intact sequences; *in vivo*, further variants appear due to simultaneous degradation at both termini

extramembraneous part of APP and the first 14 residues of its transmembrane domain. During normal secretion (Weidemann et al. 1989), APP is cleaved within the βA4 region, thus preventing the formation of amyloid (Sisodia et al. 1990; Esch et al. 1990). Intact βA4 peptides are released by a minor, alternative processing pathway (Haass et al. 1992; Seubert et al. 1992, 1993).

Cell biological experiments have presented clues to the neurotoxicity of βA4 peptides (Yankner et al. 1990; Mattson et al. 1992). Moreover, mutants of the APP gene have been isolated from patients suffering from familial Alzheimer's disease. Several amino acid substitutions have been identified in different families. Common to them all is their location close to or even within the βA4 region (Hardy 1992 (review); Citron et al. 1992; Carter et al. 1992). Together these results strongly support the hypothesis that Alzheimer's disease is due to a metabolic defect of APP which results in the formation of βA4 aggregates which, in turn, cause damage to growing neurons.

This line of evidence leads to the question of why βA4 peptides aggregate at all, that is: are there structural features causing this peptide to form highly insoluble filaments under physiological conditions, where most "normal" proteins or peptides are soluble?

An initial report addressing this question employed X-ray diffraction of oriented filaments obtained from a natural APC preparation. It indicated that the peptides adopt a cross-β conformation, i.e., an extended β-pleated sheet structure, whose hydrogen bonds are located parallel to the long axis of the filament (Kirschner et al. 1986).

A classical method for the detection of all kinds of amyloid in histological sections employs the dye Congo red. After staining, amyloid shows a green birefringence when inspected under polarized light (Bennhold 1922; Divry and Florkin 1927; Puchtler et al. 1962; Cooper 1974). This property is correlated to the existence of extended β-pleated sheet structure within insoluble peptide aggregates: it is also detected in poly-L-lysine when it adopts a β-sheet structure after heating (Glenner et al. 1972). These results further corroborate the assumption that a β-pleated sheet conformation (leading to the formation of filamentous aggregates) is the ultrastructural commonality behind all types of amyloid (for reviews see Glenner 1980; Castaño and Frangione 1988).

Further experiments have used chemically synthesized peptides comprising partial sequences of βA4 to identify structural as well as environmental requirements for βA4 aggregation (Castaño et al. 1986; Gorevic et al. 1987; Kirschner et al. 1987; Hollosi et al. 1989; Halverson et al. 1990; Spencer et al. 1991). On the following pages, we will describe our results presenting a comprehensive model of βA4 structure and aggregation.

Results

The Secondary Structure of Naturally Occurring Amyloid βA4

In our first attempt to characterize the structure of amyloid βA4 we used a sample of amyloid plaque cores isolated from a patient who had suffered from Alzheimer's disease. The plaque cores were purified according to previously published procedures (Masters et al. 1985a). We chose infrared (IR) spectroscopy as a fast approach giving accurate information about secondary structures (Krimm and Bandekar 1986) without requiring the high purity and high amounts of samples necessary even for low resolution X-ray analysis or NMR spectroscopy.

Figure 2 shows an IR spectrum obtained from 0.2 mg of an APC isolate dispersed in a micropellet (0.2 mg) of dry KBr. It was recorded at a resolution of 4 cm^{-1} on a 20 SDX FTIR spectrometer (Nicolet).

The absorption spectrum shows an unequivocal maximum at 1630 cm^{-1} in the amide I region as well as peaks at 1550 cm^{-1} (amide II) and 1235 cm^{-1} (amide III). All three signals prove the existence of an antiparallel β-pleated sheet as the major structural feature of APC constituents. The weak shoulder centered around 1665 cm^{-1}, like the amide III signals at 1280, 1350, 1385 and 1400 cm^{-1}, indicate the existence of β-turns. No α-helical structures could be detected.

In summary, the spectrum confirms the (preliminary) data of Kirschner et al. (1986) who were the first to report a cross-β structure for an APC isolate. Our results demonstrate that the β-sheets are arranged in an antiparallel manner. In the following paragraphs, we will show that this is also in agreement with results obtained using synthetic βA4 peptides.

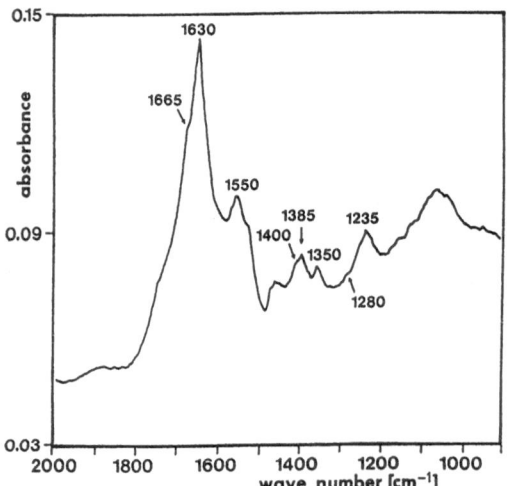

Fig. 2. Fourier transform infrared spectrum of an APC isolate dispersed in dry KBr

Peptides Bearing the Natural βA4 Sequence

The next steps in our study dealt with the characterization of peptides corresponding to naturally occurring βA4 variants (Hilbich et al. 1991a). Peptides have been synthesized bearing amino acid 1, 2, 4, 8, 9, 10 and 12 of the entire βA4 sequence as their N-terminal residue. They contain threonine 43 as C-terminal residue, thus corresponding to the longest variants of βA4 (Kang et al. 1987; Mori et al. 1992). Collectively these peptides will be denoted as "X-43."

Solid phase peptide synthesis was performed using N^{α}-t-Boc-protected amino acid derivatives transformed into symmetrical anhydrides by reaction with dicyclohexylcarbodiimid. After cleavage from the resin and deprotection of side chain functional groups (by reaction with neat hydrogen fluoride) the peptides were solubilized in 70% formic acid and purified by size exclusion chromatography in the same solvent. A second size exclusion chromatography was performed in 1 nM acetic acid. Identity and purity of the peptides were monitored by amino acid analysis and automated Edman degradation.

As expected, the X-43 peptides show all properties characteristic of natural amyloid βA4 and of amyloid in general. 1) After staining with the dye Congo red, the peptides show a green or (at very high peptide concentrations) yellow birefringence. 2) They aggregate in the form of filaments with a length of at least 100 nm and a diameter of about 5 nm. 3) At physiological ionic strength and pH values (e.g., phosphate buffered saline (PBS), pH 7.4), more than 90% of the material form an insoluble aggregate, whereas only a small fraction (5 to 10%) can be solubilized.

In contrast, the peptides could be solubilized to more than 90% in distilled water. Upon addition of salts (e.g., 50 mM NaCl) or organic solvents, βA4 peptides can be quantitatively precipitated.

The solubilities of βA4 peptides were expressed only in relative values determined at peptide concentrations of 0.5 to 2 mg/ml. When a suspension of this concentration is centrifuged and the supernatant is removed from the pellet and incubated alone, a new equilibrium between precipitated and solubilized peptides will form. Thus, the solubilized peptide fractions cannot be regarded as stable solutions. Based on these results, we concluded that solubilized forms of βA4 should also appear *in vivo*, if an aggregate, i.e., APC or ACA, is present (Hilbich et al. 1991). This conclusion was confirmed by the detection of βA4 in cell culture media, blood plasma and cerebrospinal fluid (Seubert et al. 1992).

A characterization of βA4 has thus to discriminate between its solubilized and precipitated (solid) states. Both the detection of birefringence after Congo red staining as well as electron microscopy of filaments characterize high molecular weight aggregates, i.e., βA4 in its precipitated form. Secondary structure in the solid state was examined by IR spectroscopy of peptides dispersed in dry KBr. The X-43 peptides adopt mainly an antiparallel β-sheet conformation. Additional signals are due to β-turns and sequences lacking a definite secondary structure. Together with the green birefringence of polarized light after Congo red staining, these results prove an antiparallel β-pleated sheet as the main structural feature of βA4 peptides in the solid state. This finding has also been confirmed by low resolution X-ray analysis of filaments prepared from a peptide 1–42 (Fraser et al. 1991).

The secondary structure of solubilized βA4 peptides was determined by circular dichroism (CD) spectroscopy. When solubilized in distilled water, peptide 10–43 contains an amount of 80% β-sheet, 10% turn (of type I) and 10% random coil conformations. An increase in ionic strength causes a decrease in the fraction of solubilized peptides. Their secondary structure changes as well: up to concentrations of 30 mM NaF (used because of its low UV absorbance), the β-sheet conformation remains preserved; between 40 and 50 mM the β-sheet content is reduced sharply and reaches a level of 24% in 60 mM NaF. The amount of random coil conformations increases to 51%. In 500 mM NaF, β-sheet content is as low as 6%. Size exclusion chromatography of solubilized peptides shows that only dimers exist in distilled water, whereas βA4 peptides are monomeric in 500 mM NaF. Similar results were also obtained using other types of ions.

These data can be summarized as follows (see Fig. 3). Peptides solubilized in distilled water adopt mainly a β-pleated sheet conformation containing a β-turn. The β-sheet is stabilized by dimerization of the peptides. Addition of salts or other substances that remove the peptides' hydrate shell and break up the regular structure of pure water causes the peptides to precipitate. In contrast to the precipitation of many proteins which are soluble under physiological

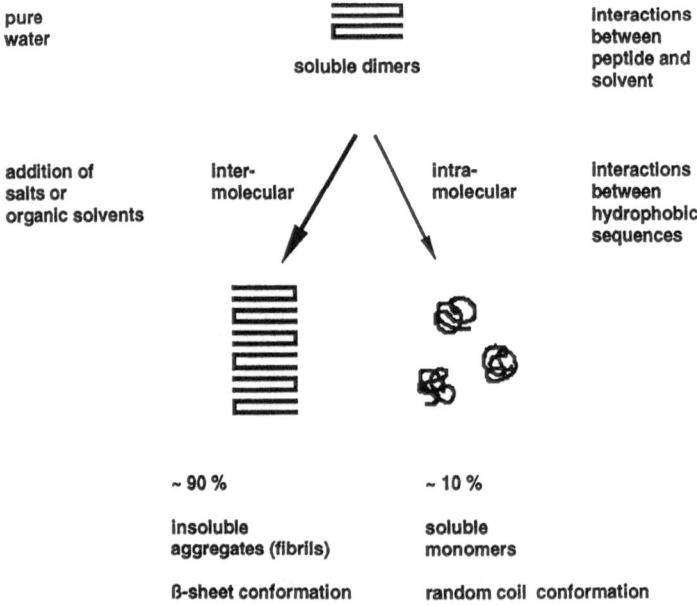

Fig. 3. Aggregation of βA4 peptides *in vitro* (see text for comments)

conditions, βA4 aggregates in the form of filaments, thus building up highly ordered structures. Within this aggregated fraction that contains at least 90% of the peptide material, the β-pleated sheet is conserved and stabilized by inter-molecular interactions. The remaining 10% of the peptides are solubilized; they adopt monomeric random coil conformations. Intramolecular interactions might possibly stabilize some kind of tertiary structure.

The fact that βA4 aggregation is due to an increase in ionic strength clearly demonstrates that interaction between βA4 peptides is based upon a hydropho-bic effect, i.e., the exclusion of hydrophobic parts of the molecule from an (aqueous) solvent. This can be easily understood regarding the large number of hydrophobic amino acid side chains, especially within the C-terminal part of βA4 that stems from the transmembrane domain of APP.

Characterization of Distinct Parts of the βA4 Sequence

Secondary structure determinations have demonstrated that the X-43 peptides, besides their antiparallel β-sheet, contain minor amounts of β-turns and unor-dered regions. To assign these structures to distinct parts of the sequence, we compared different members of the X-43 group and examined some analogue peptides.

The fact that all X-43 peptides form filaments *in vitro* already shows that the N-terminal residues are not necessary for βA4 aggregation. A comparison of filaments prepared from peptides 1–, 2– and 4–43 to preparations from peptides 8–, 9–, 10– and 12–43 demonstrates differences between these two groups. While the morphology of single filaments cannot be distinguished, filaments of peptides 1–, 2– and 4–43 seem to be tightly coiled around each other and form dense clusters. Filaments prepared from the shorter X-43 peptides show only loosely connected networks. This suggests that the N-terminal residues are located at the surface of filaments and mediate interactions between individual filaments.

Such a model is in accordance with the results of IR spectroscopy. NH-groups nonbonded within hydrogen bonds are detected by a signal at 3450 cm^{-1} and result from peptide regions lacking secondary structure. Among the X-43 peptides, the amount of these "free" NH-groups increases with increas-ing peptide length. Similarly, CD spectroscopy revealed an amount of 10% random coil conformations in peptide 10–43 after solubilization in distilled water. Peptide 2–43 shows an amount of 38% random coil and only 58% β-sheet under the same conditions.

The X-43 peptides also differ in their solubilities. In 5 mM NaCl, peptides 1–, 2– and 4–43 show soluble fractions of 50 to 58%; for peptides 8–, 9– and 10–43 this fraction is as low as 8 to 10%. Peptide 12–43 again shows an increased solubility of 20 to 25%, thus indicating that residues 11 and 12 influence the stability of βA4 aggregates. In contrast, amino acids 1 to 9 contrib-ute mainly to the solubility of βA4 peptides. This region is supposed to be localized at the filament surface and might mediate interactions between individual filaments. *In vivo*, they could also be involved in the binding of other proteins that are found in amyloid in minor amounts.

The sequence of residues 10 to 43 is sufficient to show all typical properties of βA4 peptides, while residues 1 to 9 have only modulating functions. Likewise, threonine 43 does not exert a substantial influence on the peptides' behaviour. Thus, a peptide 10–42 can be used as a prototype of βA4.

Both IR and CD spectroscopy demonstrate the existence of a β-turn within the structure of X-43 peptides. According to secondary structure predictions it should be found in the region of residues Ser 26/Lys 28 (Gorevic et al. 1987). To define the exact position of such a turn is certainly a task for X-ray crystallography; however, this would need the preparation of crystals–a kind of aggregate that βA4 has failed to form until today.

To develop a model that is based at least on biochemical data, analogues of the prototype peptide 10–43 have been synthesized in which several possible localizations of the β-turn were stabilized by the introduction of a disulfide bridge. Amino acids i − 1 and i + 4 (the postulated β-turn comprizes residues i to i + 3) were substituted by a cystine crosslink. The three resulting analogue peptides were suspended in phosphate buffer and subjected to digestion by leucine aminopeptidase: only one of the analogues is degraded to the same extent as peptide 10–43 bearing the natural sequence. In this analogue, a turn should be formed by residues 26 to 29.

This model is again corroborated by results of IR spectroscopy. It demonstrates that peptide 12–43 contains the lowest amount of unordered structure of all members of the X-43 group. We therefore postulated that a central β-turn would connect two strands of β-pleated sheet that have exactly the same length in this peptide. In the resulting model, the turn would as well be localized at residues Ser 26 – Asn 27 – Lys 28 – Gly 29.

The central β-turn is flanked by two regions that are supposed to adopt mainly β-sheet conformations. They were synthetically prepared by peptides 10–23 and 29–42 (both bearing amidated C-termini). In addition, peptides were examined comprising residues 1–27 and 4–27 (Hilbich et al. 1991a,b). Following Congo red staining, all four peptides show the typical green birefringence of polarized light. Peptides 1–27, 4–27 and 10–23 form filaments, whereas peptide 29–42, due to its extremely low solubility, aggregates in amorphous form. However, Halverson et al. (1990) demonstrated filament formation of a peptide 34–42; thus it can be stated that both regions situated N- and C-terminal of the postulated β-turn are capable of forming highly ordered aggregates.

IR spectroscopy demonstrates that all four peptides contain substantial amounts of antiparallel β-pleated sheet structure. In comparison to the X-43 peptides, they also contain higher amounts of β-turns and unordered structure. The different β-sheet regions of the entire βA4 molecule are obviously stabilized by mutual interactions. This also applies to the secondary structure of solubilized βA4. If peptides 1–27, 4–27 and 10–23 are solubilized in distilled water or 10 mM Na-phosphate (pH 7,4), they show random coil conformations, irrespective of their solubility. Hence, the C-terminal, hydrophobic stretch of the sequence is necessary to stabilize a β-sheet conformation in solubilized βA4 peptides.

It is thus not recommended that a βA4 peptide like "1–28" be used to determine physiological properties of amyloid βA4.

The analysis of βA4 partial sequences and analogues leads us to propose a structural model of a βA4 monomer within an aggregate (Fig. 4). A central β-turn formed by residues 26 to 29 is flanked by two β-pleated sheet regions of approximately equal length. Residues 1 to 9 protrude from this hairpin-like structure. In the direction of the long axis of filaments, aggregation is due to the formation of antiparallel β-sheets. The hydrogen bonds are arranged parallel to the filament axis, forming a cross-β conformation. The filament diameter results from the length of β-pleated sheet strands as well as from stacking of several layers of β-sheets onto each other. This stacking is stabilized by interactions between amino acid side chains. Interactions between hydrophobic side chains mediate the hydrophobic effect and lead to the formation of a hydrophobic core that might extend through the length of a filament. In summary, this model shows commonalities with a model proposed for the structure of paired helical filaments, whose main component is thought to be the microtubule-associated protein tau (Kirschner et al. 1986).

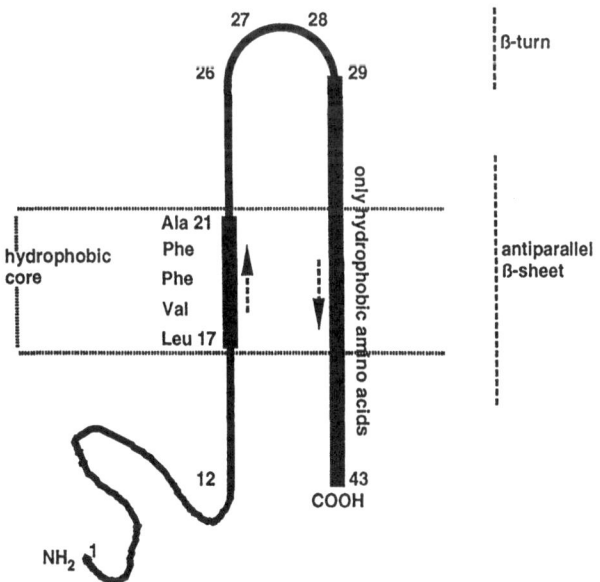

Fig. 4. Model of the conformation of a βA4 peptide within an aggregate (see text for comments)

Substitutions of Hydrophobic Amino Acids within βA4

A peptide covering residues 10–43 or 10–42 can serve well as a prototype for βA4, but a peptide 10–23 also forms filaments and shows essentially the same solubility profile as peptides comprising the whole βA4 sequence. The 10–23 peptide contains a region of hydrophobic amino acids which could serve as structural basis of a hydrophobic effect. First support for this assumption came from an analogue of peptide 10–23 in which the two phenylalanine residues had been substituted by an isoleucine in position 19 and a glycine residue in position 20 (residue numbers correspond to the entire βA4 sequence). This analogue showed a markedly increased solubility under physiological conditions and did not form filaments *in vitro* (Hilbich et al. 1991a).

However, the formation of a stable β-sheet structure requires the inclusion of the C-terminal, hydrophobic residues 29 to 42 of βA4 into model peptides (see above). As should have been expected, this sequence also leads to a further decrease in solubility compared to the 10–23 peptide (Hilbich et al. 1991b). To test whether the effects seen with analogues of the 10–23 sequence were also detectable in peptides comprising residues 10–42/43, we synthesized analogue peptides corresponding to this βA4 prototype sequence (Hilbich et al. 1992). Twelve different analogues were prepared, each bearing two amino acid substitutions within the region of residues Leu 17, Val 18, Phe 19 and Phe 20 (Fig. 5). Different types of amino acids were introduced: threonine (uncharged, polar), isoleucine (large, unpolar), and glycine or alanine (small, unpolar).

The solubility of each analogue was determined in a set of different solvents. All of the purified analogues are soluble to 90–99% in 1 M acetic acid and in distilled water and only to about 5–15% in PBS, pH 7.4. In these solvents, solubilities seem not to differ significantly between analogues and peptides bearing the naturally occurring sequence. To find out whether such differences exist, solubilities were determined in solvents of varying ionic strength and weakly acidic pH values. Here, increasing salt concentrations also lead to

```
               10      15  17    20        25        30        35      40  42 43
10-42 (43)     Y E V H H Q K L V F F A E D V G S N K G A I I G L M V G G V V I A (T)

10-43/FF->AG   _____ L V A G _____
10-43/FF->IG   _____ L V I G _____
10-43/FF->GI   _____ L V G I _____
10-43/FF->II   _____ L V I I _____
10-42/FF->TG   _____ L V T G _____
10-43/FF->GT   _____ L V G T _____
10-43/FF->TT   _____ L V T T _____
10-42/LTTF     _____ L T T F _____
10-42/TTFF     _____ T T F F _____
10-42/LTFT     _____ L T F T _____
10-42/TVTF     _____ T V T F _____
10-42/TVFT     _____ T V F T _____
```

Fig. 5. Sequences and designations of βA4 analogues bearing substitutions of hydrophobic residues

precipitation of peptides, but in comparison to peptide 10–43, elevated solubilities could be demonstrated. Analogues FF → TT and TVTF showed the highest relative solubilities of all analogues in 200 mM NaCl (74,8 and 91,4%) and 200 mM KCl (87,2 and 91,1%). In contrast, variants FF → AG and TVFT were almost as insoluble as βA4 peptides bearing the natural sequence.

βA4 peptides aggregate even under the usually denaturing conditions of SDS-polyacrylamide gel electrophoresis (PAGE): the X-43 peptides always show two bands of similar intensity, corresponding to a monomer and a tetramer. Among most of the analogues, the monomeric form strongly prevails: only at high peptide concentrations (40 μg/slot), the analogues give rise to very weak tetrameric bands, which are easily washed out from the gel.

To test the tendency of the peptides to aggregate in the absence of detergents, CD spectra of the analogues in distilled water were recorded. Here, peptide 10–43 bearing the natural sequence adopted conformations consisting of 80% β-sheet, 10% β-turn of type I, and 10% random coil (Hilbich et al. 1991a). None of the analogues showed the same high degree of β-sheet structure: β-sheet contents did not even reach 60% and were as low as 34% for LTTF and 28% for TVTF. For most of the analogues, the addition of salts caused a further decrease of β-sheet content. However, for LTTF and TVTF an increase of β-sheet structure at NaF concentrations of 20–60 mM was detected. This is reminiscent of "normal" soluble proteins that require a certain ionic strength to fold into their native conformation. In the solid state, a reduced β-sheet conformation of analogue peptides is demonstrated by IR spectroscopy of peptides dispersed in dry KBr.

Increased solubility and reduced β-sheet content result in a lack of aggregation under the conditions of SDS-PAGE; they can, however, be compensated under conditions closer to physiological ionic strength and pH. The analogues still form filaments in PBS (pH 7.4). Like filaments of peptides bearing the natural sequence, they have diameters of about 5 nm. Their length distribution differs; the shortest (< 50–100 nm) filaments are found in preparations of peptides LTTF and TVTF. These samples also lack the clustering of individual filaments that appears in most filament preparations of βA4 peptides. Unexpected results were obtained using mixtures of an analogue and an equimolar amount of peptide 10–43 or 10–42 bearing the natural sequence. Most of these mixtures also produce filaments, again showing diameters of about 5 nm and a length of more than 100 nm. But filamentous aggregates can scarcely be detected in mixtures of FF → GI and FF → TT with peptide 10–43. Besides some globular structures, again of about 5 nm in diameter, most of the peptide material precipitates in amorphous form. Obviously, these mixtures show an inhibition of filament formation.

This must be due to an interaction between an analogue and a peptide bearing the natural sequence. One could envisage that such interactions are mediated by the C-terminal, hydrophobic sequence that has not been altered in the analogues. Within resulting mixed oligomers, the most hydrophobic sequences might form a β-sheet core structure flanked by the more hydrophilic parts. In mixtures with variants FF → GI and FF → TT, oligomers have obviously lost their ability to interact with another βA4 peptide and prohibit an ongoing association. The globular structures appearing in these mixtures might correspond to such oligomers that are supposedly even unstable *per se*, since the bulk material forms amorphous precipitates.

The variants FF → GI and FF → TT are the ones possessing the highest amounts of β-sheet structure according to CD spectroscopy (59%). This correlation can be easily understood: an interaction between analogues and peptides of the natural sequence would be impossible without a certain degree of structural similarity.

All types of amyloid show a green birefringence under polarized light if they are stained with the dye Congo red. Synthetic βA4 peptides show the same property that is also shared by several analogues described here. In contrast, variants FF → GI, FF → TT, LTTF, and TVTF can be stained by Congo red, but do not exhibit any change of colour when inspected under polarized light. Thus they have lost an essential feature of amyloid peptides.

The peptides' birefringence can be correlated to their solubilities. The four analogues negative for birefringence show the highest solubilities in NaCl solutions and are the only ones that are solubilized significantly in KCl solutions. Since Congo red staining is done using suspensions of peptides in solutions of high salt concentration where all analogues are only poorly soluble (i.e., in PBS or 80% ethanol saturated with NaCl), birefringence cannot have been influenced directly by solubilization of a peptide. Instead, both solubility in NaCl and KCl solutions and the lack of birefringence obviously reflect alterations of three-dimensional structure which are effectively reducing amyloid properties of these βA4 analogues.

In all of the βA4 variants described here, hydrophobic amino acid residues have been substituted by more hydrophilic ones, often by threonine. Yet it is not simply the overall hydrophobicity that governs the behaviour of βA4 analogues, but their three-dimensional structure. This is illustrated by three pairs of analogues with identical amino acid composition and, hence, identical hydrophobicities. Peptides FF → GI, LTTF and TVTF exhibit reduced amyloidogenicity, whereas their counterparts FF → IG, LTFT and TVFT show low solubilities and the typical green/yellow birefringence after Congo red staining. In the case of peptides FF → GI and FF → IG, inversion of the substituting residues even decides whether the resulting analogue can inhibit filament formation.

In summary, the results clearly demonstrate that a well-preserved hydrophobic core around amino acids 17 to 20 of βA4 is crucial for the formation of both the β-sheet structure and the amyloid properties of βA4. In analogues FF → GI, FF → TT, LTTF and TVTF, substitutions of hydrophobic residues have lead to βA4 variants with markedly reduced amyloidogenicity. If APP contained two threonine residues instead of phenylalanine in position 19 and 20 of the βA4 region, Alzheimer's disease (being an amyloidosis) would presumably not be known. βA4-homologue peptides would only form diffuse plaques or preamyloid, and the disease would be halted at a stage where clinical symptoms are relatively rare and endurable.

However, as this hydrophobic region is of high importance for the structure of βA4, substitutions might also result in variants with increased amyloidogenicity. In a family suffering from Alzheimer's disease and cerebral hemorrhage, Hendrick et al. (1992) identified an APP mutation that leads to a substitution of alanine 21 by glycine. It might well be that this substitution results in a stabilization of the hydrophobic core and, consequently, of βA4 aggregates.

The synthesis of βA4 analogue peptides FF → GI and FF → TT which can inhibit filament formation *in vitro* opens a possibility for therapeutic approaches. They may serve as lead substances in the design of analogues that should retain the ability to inhibit filament formation, but should be more soluble and less vulnerable towards protease digestion. They could thus represent an opportunity for a rational therapy aimed at inhibiting amyloid formation in Alzheimer's disease.

Acknowledgements. We thank Fa. Nicolet (Offenbach, FRG) for giving us access to a FTIR spectrometer. The collaboration of J. Reed as well as the technical assistance of C. Grund and S. Pinto are gratefully acknowledged. This work was supported by the Federal Ministry of Science and Technology and the "Fonds der Chemischen Industrie".

References

Bennhold H (1992) Eine spezifische Amyloidfärbung mit Kongorot. Münch Med Wochenschr 69:1537

Carter DA, Desmarais E, Bellis M, Campion D, Clerget-Darpoux F, Brice A, Agid Y, Jaillard-Serradt A, Mallet J (1992) More missense in amyloid gene: Nature Genet. 2:255–256

Castaño EM, Frangione B (1988). Biology of disease: human amyloidosis, Alzheimer disease and related disorders. Lab Invest. 58:122–132

Castaño, EM, Ghiso J, Prelli F, Gorevic PD, Migheli A, Frangione B (1986) *In vitro* formation of amyloid fibrils from two synthetic peptides of different lengths homologous to Alzheimer's disease β-protein. Biochem Biophys Res Comm 141:782–789

Citron M, Oltersdorf T, Haass C, McConlogue L, Hung AY, Seubert P, Vigo-Pelfrey C, Lieberburg I, Selkoe DJ (1992) Mutation of the β-amyloid precursor protein in familial Alzheimer's disease increases β-protein production. Nature 360:672–674

Cooper JH (1974). Selective amyloid staining as a function of amyloid composition and structure. Lab Invest 3:232–238

Divry P, Florkin M (1927) Sur les propriétées optiques de l'amyloide. CR Soc Biol 97:1808

Esch F, Keim PS, Beattie EC, Blacher RW, Culwell AR, Oltersdorf T, McClure D, Ward P (1990) Cleavage of amyloid β peptide during constitutive processing of its precursor. Science 248:1122–1124

Fraser PE, Duffy LK, O'Malley MB, Nguyen J, Inouye H, Kirschner DA (1991) Morphology and antibody recognition of synthetic β-amyloid peptides. J Neurosci Res 28:474–485

Glenner GG (1980). Amyloid deposits and amyloidosis. New Engl J Med 302:1283–1292

Glenner GG, Wong CW (1984a) Alzheimer's disease: initial report of the purification and characterization of a novel cerebrovascular amyloid protein. Biochem Biophys Res Comm 120:885–890

Glenner GG, Wong CW (1984b) Alzheimer's disease and Down's syndrome: sharing of a unique cerebrovascular amyloid fibril protein. Biochem Biophys Res Comm 122:1131–1135

Glenner GG, Eanes ED, Page LD (1972) The relation of the properties of Congo red-stained amyloid fibrils to the β-conformation. J Histochem Cytochem 20:821–826

Gorevic PD, Castaño EM, Sarma R, Frangione B (1987) Ten to fourteen residue peptides of Alzheimer's disease protein are sufficient for amyloid formation and its characteristic X-ray diffraction pattern. Biochem Biophys Res Comm 147:854–862

Haass C, Schlossmacher MG, Hung AY, Vigo-Pelfrey C, Mellon A, Ostaszewski BL, Lieberburg I, Koo EH, Schenk D, Teplow DB, Selkoe DJ (1992) Amyloid β-peptide is produced by cultured cells during normal metabolism. Nature 359:322–325

Halverson K, Fraser PE, Kirschner DA, Lansbury PT (1990) Molecular determinants of amyloid deposition in Alzheimer's disease: conformational studies of synthetic β-protein fragments. Biochemistry 29:2639–2644

Hardy J (1992) Framing β-amyloid. Nature Genet 1:233–234

Hardy J, Allsop D (1991). Amyloid deposition as the central event in the aetiology of Alzheimer's disease. Trends Pharmacol Sci 12:383–388

Hendriks L, van Duijn CM, Cras P, Cruts M, van Hul W, van Harskamp F, Warren A, McInnis MG, Antonarakis SE, Martin J-J, Hofman A, van Broeckhoven C (1992) Presenile dementia and cerebral hemorrhage linked to a mutation at codon 692 of the β-amyloid precursor protein gene. Nature Genet. 1:218–221

Hilbich C, Kisters-Woike B, Reed J, Masters CL, Beyreuther K (1991a). Aggregation and secondary structure of amyloid βA4 protein of Alzheimer's disease. J Mol Biol 218:149–163

Hilbich C, Kisters-Woike B, Reed J, Masters CL, Beyreuther K (1991b). Human and rodent sequence analogs of Alzheimer's disease amyloid βA4 share similar properties and can be solubilized in buffers of pH 7.4. Eur J Biochem 201:61–69

Hilbich C, Kisters-Woike B, Reed J, Masters CL, Beyreuther K (1992) Substitutions of hydrophobic amino acids reduce the amyloidogenicity of Alzheimer's disease βA4 peptides. J Mol Biol 228:460–473

Hollosi M, Otvos L, Kajtar J, Percel A, Lee VM-Y (1989) Is amyloid deposition in Alzheimer's disease preceded by an environment-induced double conformational transition? Peptide Res 2:109–113

Joachim CL, Duffy LK, Morris JH, Selkoe DJ (1988) Protein chemical and immunocytochemical studies of meningovascular β-amyloid protein in Alzheimer's disease and normal aging. Brain Res 474:100–111

Kang J, Lemaire H-G, Unterbeck A, Salbaum J-M, Masters CL, Grzeschik K-H, Multhaup G, Beyreuther K, Müller-Hill B (1987) The precursor of Alzheimer's disease amyloid A4 protein resembles a cell-surface receptor. Nature 325:733–736

Kirschner DA, Abraham C, Selkoe DJ (1986) X-ray diffraction from intraneuronal paired helical filaments and extraneuronal amyloid fibers in Alzheimer disease indicates cross-β conformation. Proc Natl Acad Sci USA 83:503–507

Kirschner DA, Inouye H, Duffy LK, Sinclair A, Lind M, Selkoe DJ (1987) Synthetic peptide homologous to β-protein from Alzheimer disease forms amyloid-like fibrils in vitro. Proc Natl Acad Sci USA 84:6953–6957

Krimm S, Bandekar J (1986) Vibrational spectroscopy and conformation of peptides, polypeptides, and proteins. Adv Prot Chem 38:181–364

Masters CL, Simms G, Weinman NA, Multhaup G, McDonald BL, Beyreuther K (1985a) Amyloid plaque core protein in Alzheimer disease and Down syndrome. Proc Natl Acad Sci USA 82:4245–4249

Masters CL, Multhaup G, Simms G, Pottgiesser J, Martins RN, Beyreuther K (1985b) Neuronal origin of cerebral amyloid: neurofibrillary tangles of Alzheimer's disease contain the same protein as the amyloid of plaque cores and blood vessels. EMBO J 4:2757–2763

Mattson MP, Cheng BC, Davis D, Bryant K, Lieberburg I, Rydel RE (1992) β-amyloid peptides destabilize calcium homeostasis and render human cortical neurons vulnerable to excitoxicity. J Neurosci 12, 376–389

Mori H, Takio K, Ogawara M, Selkoe DJ (1992) Mass spectrometry of purified amyloid β protein in Alzheimer's disease. J Biol Chem 267:17082–17086

Müller-Hill B, Beyreuther K (1989) Molecular biology of Alzheimer's disease. Ann Rev Biochem 58:287–307

Prelli F, Castaño EM, van Duinen SG, Bots G, Luyendijk W, Frangione B (1988a) Different processing of Alzheimer's β-protein precursor in the vessels walls of patients with hereditary cerebral hemorrhage with amyloidosis – Dutch type. Biochem Biophys Res Comm 151:1150–1155

Prelli F, Castaño E, Glenner GG, Frangione B (1988b). Differences between vascular and plaque core amyloid in Alzheimer's disease. J Neurochem 51:648–651

Puchtler H, Sweat F, Levine M (1962) On the binding of Congo red by amyloid. J Histochem Cytochem 10:355–364

Reisberg B (ed) (1983) Alzheimer's disease, The Free Press, New York

Roher AE, Lowenson JD, Clarke S, Wolkow C, Wang R, Cotter RJ, Reardon IM, Zürcher-Neely HA, Heinrikson RL, Ball MJ, Greenberg BD (1993) Structural alterations in the peptide backbone of β-amyloid core protein may account for its deposition and stability in Alzheimer's disease. J Biol Chem 268:3072–3083

Schlote W (1965) Die Amyloidnatur der kongophilen, drusigen Entartung der Hirnarterien (Scholz) im Senium. Act Neuropathol 4:449–468

Selkoe DJ (1989) Biochemistry of altered brain proteins in Alzheimer's disease. Ann Rev Neurosci 12:463–490

Selkoe DJ (1991) The molecular pathology of Alzheimer's disease. Neuron 6:487–498

Seubert P, Vigo-Pelfrey C, Esch F, Lee M, Dovey H, Davis D, Sinha S, Schlossmacher MG, Whaley J, Swindlehurst C, McCormack R, Wolfert R, Selkoe D, Lieberburg I, Schenk D (1992) Isolation and quantification of soluble Alzheimer's β-peptide from biological fluids. Nature 359:325–327

Seubert P, Oltersdorf T, Lee MG, Barbour R, Blomquist C, Davis DL, Bryant K, Fritz LC, Galasko D, Thal LJ, Lieberburg I, Schenk DB (1993) Secretion of β-amyloid precursor protein cleaved at the amino terminus of the β-amyloid peptide. Nature 361:260–263

Sisodia S, Koo EH, Beyreuther K, Unterbeck A, Price DL (1990) Evidence that β-amyloid protein in Alzheimer's disease is not derived by normal processing. Science 248:492–495

Spencer RGS, Halverson KJ, Auger M, McDermott AE, Griffin RG, Lansbury PT (1991) An unusual peptide conformation may precipitate amyloid formation in Alzheimer's disease: application of solid-state NMR to the determination of protein secondary structure. Biochemistry 30:10382–10387

Terry RD, Gonatas NK, Weiss M (1964) Ultrastructural studies in Alzheimer' presenile dementia. Am J Pathol 44:269–297

Weidemann A, König G, Bunke D, Fischer P, Salbaum JM, Masters CL, Beyreuther K (1989) Identification, biogenesis, and localization of precursors of Alzheimer's disease A4 amyloid protein. Cell 57:115–126

Wong CW, Quaranta V, Glenner GG (1985) Neuritic plaques and cerebrovascular amyloid in Alzheimer's disease are antigenically related. Proc Natl Acad Sci USA 82:8729–8732

Yankner B, Duffy LK, Kirschner DA (1990) Neurotrophic and neurotoxic effects of amyloid β protein: reversal by tachykinin neuropeptides. Science 250:279–282

Production of Amyloid β Protein from Normal and Mutated Amyloid β Protein Precursors

T. E. Golde*, X.-D. Cai, T.-T. Cheung, M. Shoji, and S. G. Younkin

Introduction

In patients with Alzheimer's disease (AD), large numbers of senile plaques are found throughout the neuropil of the cerebral neocortex and hippocampus. These senile plaques, which are present in small numbers in the brains of aged mammals and normal elderly individuals, are observed in large numbers only in AD and thus represent a change that is quite specific for this disorder. "Classic" senile plaques consist of a spherical cluster of abnormal neurites surrounding an extracellular amyloid core composed of 5–10 nm fibrils that can be visualized on light microscopy by staining with Congo Red or Thioflavin S (Terry 1985). In most cases of AD, amyloid fibrils are also found in the walls of cerebral vessels (Glenner 1983).

The principal proteinaceous component of the amyloid deposited in AD is a ~ 4 kDa (39–43 residue) polypeptide (amyloid β protein, Aβ) that has been isolated both from plaque cores and meningeal blood vessels of AD brains (Glenner and Wong 1984; Prelli et al. 1988; Masters et al. 1985; Selkoe et al. 1986; Kang et al. 1987; Mori et al. 1991). Using oligonucleotides based on the Aβ sequence, several groups (Kang et al. 1987; Goldgaber et al. 1987; Tanzi et al. 1987; Robakis et al. 1987) isolated cDNA clones that encode the Aβ as part of a much larger amyloid β protein precursor (βAPP) and, with these clones, they mapped the βAPP gene to the long arm of chromosome 21.

Aβ is an Internal Peptide Located Close to the COOH Terminus of the βAPP

The βAPP gene produces at least six different mRNAs (Kitaguchi et al. 1988; Ponte et al. 1988; Tanzi et al. 1988; Jacobsen et al. 1991; De Sauvage and Octave 1989; Golde et al. 1990), all of which encode proteins that are identical in their amino terminal region. Two of these mRNAs encode proteins of 365 (Jacobsen et al. 1991) and 563 (De Sauvage and Octave 1989) amino acids that do not

* Division of Neuropathology, Institute of Pathology, Case Western Reserve University, Cleveland, OH 44106, USA

C.L. Masters et al. (Eds.)
Amyloid Protein Precursor in Development,
Aging and Alzheimer's Disease
© Springer-Verlag Berlin Heidelberg 1994

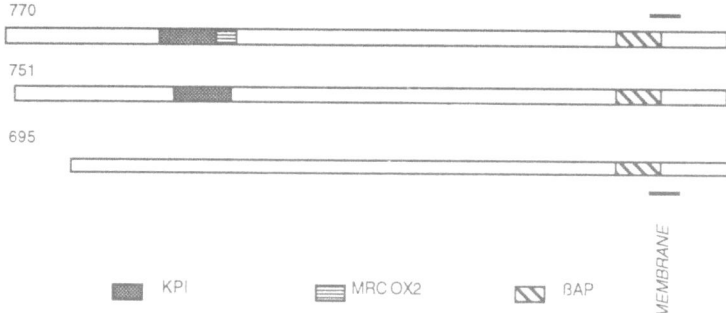

Fig. 1. Major βAPP isoforms containing Aβ (βAP)

contain the βAP, peptide. The other four βAPP mRNAs (Kitaguchi et al. 1988; Ponte et al. 1988; Tanzi et al. 1988; Golde et al. 1990), which encode proteins of 695, 714, 751, and 770 amino acids, are produced through alternative splicing of two adjacent exons. One of these exons encodes a 56-amino acid domain that is highly homologous to the Kunitz family of serine protease inhibitors; the other encodes a 19-amino acid domain with homology to the MRC OX-2 antigen found on the surface of neurons and thymocytes. βAPP_{714} is produced in trace amounts only (Golde et al. 1990). In each of the three major βAPP mRNAs (Fig. 1), the 43 residue Aβ is encoded as an internal peptide beginning 99 residues from the carboxyl terminus of the βAPP and extending from the extracellular/intraluminal region (28 amino acids) into the putative membrane-spanning domain (15 amino acids; Kang et al. 1987; Dyrks et al. 1988). It appears, therefore, that proteolytic cleavage of the βAPP on both the amino and carboxyl sides of the Aβ is necessary to generate the Aβ found in amyloid deposits.

The Pathologic Cascade that Produces AD: A Working Hypothesis Based on the Genetic Forms of AD (trisomy 21 and Familial AD)

The central question with respect to amyloid deposition in AD has been whether amyloid deposition triggers the complex pathology observed in AD or is an endstage product of that pathology. The genetic forms of AD have been particularly helpful in resolving this issue. If amyloid deposition triggers the development of AD pathology, then the genetic defects that produce AD should be related to amyloid deposition. This has, so far, proven to be the case.

Individuals with Down's syndrome (DS, trisomy 21) who are over the age of 40 invariably develop central nervous system pathology that is essentially identical to that seen in AD (Ropper and Williams 1980; Mann et al. 1986). This observation is significant because it indicates that increased dosage of one or more of the loci on chromosome 21 is sufficient to cause AD. The finding that the βAPP gene is located on chromosome 21 immediately indicates that the βAPP gene is likely to be the locus (or at least one of the loci) that is responsible for the AD pathology that develops in DS. This proposal is supported by the observation that, in DS brains, deposits labeled with antisera to the βAP are observed before other aspects of AD pathology develop.

In rare families, AD is inherited as an autosomal dominant trait. Analysis of a large number of familial AD (FAD) kindreds (St George-Hyslop et al. 1990) has shown them to be genetically heterogeneous. Some families with early onset of symptoms show linkage to chromosome 21 (St George-Hyslop et al. 1990; Pericak-Vance et al. 1988); whereas other early onset families (St George-Hyslop et al. 1990; Schellenberg et al. 1988; Goate et al. 1989) and late onset families (St George-Hyslop et al. 1990; Pericak-Vance et al. 1988) do not. A number of FAD kindreds have now been identified in which point mutations at βAPP$_{717}$ (resulting in substitution of isoleucine, phenylalanine, or glycine for valine$_{717}$ in βAPP$_{770}$) cosegregate with the disease (Goate et al. 1991; Naruse et al. 1991; Yoshioka et al. 1991; Hardy 1991; Murrell et al. 1991; Chartier-Harlin et al. 1991). These mutations have been identified in many unrelated families on different continents, and they have not been detected in any controls despite exhaustive analysis. Thus there is excellent evidence that this mutation in the βAPP gene causes AD. Recently, another βAPP mutation has been shown to cosegregate with the AD phenotype in two large Swedish kindreds (Mullan et al. 1992a). In this case, the defect is a double mutation that converts the lysine-methionine located immediately amino to $A\beta_1$ (lys$_{670}$–met$_{671}$ in βAPP$_{770}$) to asparagine-leucine. The location of these mutations in close proximity to the amino and carboxyl ends of $A\beta$ (Fig. 2) immediately suggests that they cause AD by altering βAPP processing in a way that is amyloidogenic.

On the basis of this genetic evidence it is reasonable to propose, as a working hypothesis, that AD is a heterogeneous disorder in which multiple initiating mechanisms alter βAPP processing in a way that results in amyloid deposition which, in turn, produces the complex pathology that characterizes this disorder.

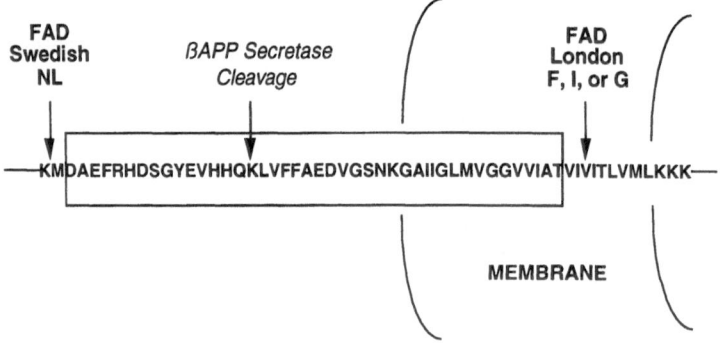

Fig. 2. $A\beta$ domain of βAPP molecule (box) showing mutations associated with FAD

Recently mutations on chromosome 14 (Schellenberg et al. 1992; Van Broeck-hoven et al. 1992; Mullan et al. 1992b; St George Hyslop et al. 1992) and 19 (Pericak-Vance et al. 1991) have been linked to FAD. These mutations are obviously not in the βAPP gene, but the affected genes may well encode proteins (e.g., proteases or protease inhibitors) that alter βAPP processing in a way that is amyloidogenic. Identifying these and other mutated genes that are linked to FAD and determining whether they alter βAPP processing in a way that is amyloidogenic is, therefore, an important way to continue to test the hypothesis that amyloid deposition plays a central role in the development of AD.

Normal βAPP Processing Produces a Complex Set of Carboxyl-Terminal Derivatives

It is well established that the βAPP is normally processed by a secretase in a constitutive secretory pathway. This processing cleaves full length βAPP at $A\beta_{16}$ to generate a secreted derivative and an ~ 8.7 kD carboxyl-terminal fragment that cannot produce amyloid because neither contains the entire $A\beta$ (Fig. 3). Recently we have shown that normal processing also generates a complex set of carboxyl-terminal derivatives (Fig. 3) that include a potentially amyloidogenic ~ 11.4 kD form with $A\beta$ at its amino terminus (Estus 1992; Golde et al. 1992).

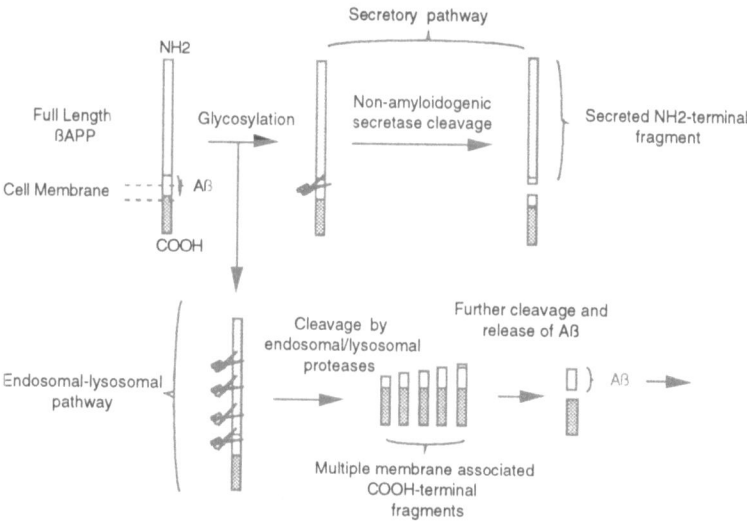

Fig. 3. Schematic diagram of βAPP processing (note that the cellular origin of $A\beta$ is uncertain)

Normal βAPP Processing Produces and Releases 4 kD Aβ

To determine whether Aβ can be produced from Aβ-bearing carboxyl-terminal βAPP derivatives (Shoji et al. 1992), we stably transfected human mononuclear leukemic (K562) cells with LC_{99}, a construct that begins with the 17 amino acid βAPP signal peptide, continues with the leucine that normally follows the βAPP signal peptide, and ends with the 99 amino acids at the carboxyl end of the βAPP, a sequence that begins with the Aβ. To detect Aβ released from K562-LC_{99} cells, we used SGY2134, a rabbit antiserum raised to synthetic $Aβ_{1-40}$ that recognizes primarily $Aβ_{1-16}$, to immunoprecipitate the protein in medium conditioned with K562-LC_{99} cells. The immunoprecipitated protein was separated on 10/16% tris/tricine gels, transferred to immobilon P, and labeled with 4G8, a mouse monoclonal antibody to $Aβ_{17-24}$. As a control, synthetic $Aβ_{1-40}$ was added to culture medium and analyzed identically. Using this approach, a 4 kD protein that comigrated with synthetic $Aβ_{1-40}$ was identified in medium conditioned with K562-LC_{99} cells but not in medium conditioned with K562 cells transfected with vector alone. This 4 kD protein was definitively identified as Aβ by isolating it from a large volume of culture medium and directly sequencing it. Thus cells transfected with a model Aβ-bearing carboxyl-terminal derivative process that derivative to release Aβ into the medium.

The same assay used to detect synthetic $Aβ_{1-40}$ and the Aβ released from K562-LC_{99} cells was employed to determine whether Aβ is also released into human CSF and by cultured cells expressing full length βAPP (Shoji et al. 1992). In our initial experiment on CSF, we analyzed 3-ml samples obtained at autopsy from seven AD patients and seven controls. Strong signals were obtained in five of the seven autopsy-confirmed AD cases, but considerable Aβ was also present in three of the seven controls. We also examined 3-ml samples of CSF from living patients, five from patients with probable AD and five from age-matched, non-AD patients. Again, there was considerable overlap in the amount of Aβ observed in the AD and non-AD group. Thus our initial survey indicates that there is 1) readily detectable Aβ in the CSF of AD and control patients, 2) considerable apparent interindividual variation in the amount of Aβ in CSF, and 3) no obvious correlation between AD and the amount of Aβ in CSF. Additional studies are needed, however, to determine whether the measurement of Aβ in CSF will be useful in the diagnosis or management of AD patients and to determine, in particular, if high levels of Aβ are a significant risk factor in the development of AD.

To determine whether Aβ is released by cultured cells expressing full length βAPP, we analyzed medium conditioned with human neuroblastoma (M17) cells stably transfected with a $βAPP_{695}$ expression construct. In our initial experiments, the transfected M17 cells were differentiated for seven days with retinoic acid to induce the formation of long neurites. These differentiated M17-$βAPP_{695}$ cells released readily detectable levels of a 4 kDa protein, and subsequent experiments showed the same to be true for undifferentiated M17 cells. The 4 kD Aβ released by these cells was definitively identified as Aβ by metabolically labeling them with [^{3}H]-phenylalanine, isolating the 4 kD protein released into the culture medium. and radiosequencing it to demonstrate phenylalanine at the predicted 4, 19, and 20 positions. Remarkably, some 4 kD Aβ was even detected in the medium of M17 cells expressing only endogenous βAPP.

Essentially identical results have been reported by Haass et al. (1992) and Seubert et al. (1992) in their studies of a variety of transfected cells and mixed human fetal brain cultures. Significantly, Seubert et al. (1992) showed by mass spectrometry that at least some of the 4 kD Aβ released by cultured cells is Aβ_{1-40}.

Taken together, the analyses of human CSF and transfected cells performed by our group (Shoji et al. 1992) and two others (Haass et al. 1992; Seubert et al. 1992) provide compelling evidence that normal cellular processing of the βAPP produces significant amounts of a soluble extracellular 4 kD derivative essentially identical to the Aβ that forms amyloid in AD. Thus it now appears that amyloid deposition in human brain depends on 1) the rate at which soluble Aβ is produced and released into the extracellular fluid, 2) the rate at which soluble, extracellular Aβ is removed from the extracellular fluid, and 3) the rate at which soluble, extracellular Aβ is converted into insoluble amyloid deposits.

Processing of FAD-Linked Mutant βAPPs

To evaluate production of Aβ and Aβ-bearing COOH-terminal derivatives in cells expressing the FAD-linked mutant βAPPs, we compared human neuro-blastoma (M17) cells stably transfected with mutant (ΔI, ΔNL) or wild type (WT) βAPP$_{694}$ (Cai et al. 1993). In our initial experiment, two ΔNL lines, a ΔI line, a WT line, and a line transfected with vector alone (CEP4β) were metabolically labeled with [^{35}S]-methionine for 20 min to assess βAPP synthesis, and for 12 hours to analyze the COOH-terminal βAPP derivatives accumulating in cells and the Aβ released into the medium. After 12 hours of continuous labeling, the WT and ΔI lines were similar with respect to the COOH-terminal βAPP derivatives that accumulated and the Aβ that was released. In contrast, the 8–12 kD COOH-terminal derivatives accumulating in the two ΔNL lines were completely different, showing a marked increase in the relative amount of the 11.4 kD derivative, a derivative that has Aβ at its amino terminus. In addition, the medium conditioned by the two ΔNL lines contained, on average, 15-fold more 4 kD Aβ than the medium conditioned by the WT and ΔI lines. After pulse labeling for 20 min, the two 695ΔNL lines contained five fold more full length βAPP than the WT and ΔI lines, but this increased expression did not account for the 15-fold increase in Aβ.

To pursue this observation, we retransfected M17 cells producing new stably transfected 695WT, 695ΔI, and 695ΔNL lines. During pulse labeling for 20 min, the three new ΔI and the three new ΔNL lines accumulated comparable amounts of full-length βAPP, but the three new WT lines accumulated 3.3-fold more βAPP, indicating that expression was 3.3-fold higher in these lines. Despite βAPP expression less than one third that of the WT lines, the ΔNL lines accumulated considerably more of the 11.4 kD Aβ-bearing COOH-terminal derivative after eight hours of continuous labeling, and medium conditioned with the ΔNL lines contained considerably more 4 kD Aβ. Quantitative analysis of these results using phosphorimaging technology showed that, in cells pulse labeled for eight hours, the ratio of the 11.4 to 8.7 kD cell-associated derivatives was over five-fold higher in the ΔNL as compared to the WT or ΔI lines. When the amount of Aβ in medium was normalized to the full-length βAPP present after pulse labeling for 20 min, Aβ was over six times higher in the ΔNL than in the ΔI or WT lines. Recently, Citron and colleagues (1992) have reported that 293 cells expressing βAPP$_{ΔNL}$ show a similar increase in Aβ release.

The observation that M17 cells expressing βAPP$_{ΔNL}$ show a marked increase in Aβ-bearing COOH-terminal derivatives and release increased amounts of 4 kD Aβ provides strong evidence that βAPP$_{ΔNL}$ causes AD because its processing is altered in a way that releases increased amounts of Aβ, thereby fostering amyloid deposition. More generally, the linkage of this form of FAD to a βAPP$_{ΔNL}$ mutation demonstrated to increase Aβ production in cultured cells 1) provides strong evidence that the pathway producing Aβ in cultured cells is highly relevant to AD and 2) greatly strengthens the hypothesis that amyloid deposition plays a central role in the development of all forms of AD.

If amyloid deposition is invariably pivotal in the development of AD, then one would also expect the βAPP$_{717}$ mutations (ΔI, ΔF, and ΔG) to alter βAPP processing in a way that is amyloidogenic. Our data provide no indication, however, that the processing of βAPP$_{ΔI}$ in M17 cells is altered in a way that would obviously promote amyloidogenesis. In fact, our data suggest that, if anything, M17 cells expressing βAPP$_{ΔI}$ produce less secreted 4 kD Aβ than those producing wild type βAPP. Isolation of Aβ from AD amyloid has revealed COOH-terminal heterogeneity with Aβs ranging in size from Aβ$_{1-39}$ to Aβ$_{1-43}$ (Tanzi et al. 1988; Jacobsen et al. 1991; De Sauvage and Octave 1989; Golde et al. 1990; Dyrks et al. 1988). Although some secreted 4 kD Aβ is Aβ$_{1-40}$ (Seubert et al. 1992), our working hypothesis is that the Aβ normally secreted by cultured cells shows COOH-terminal heterogeneity similar to that observed in AD amyloid. Our data indicate that the ΔNL mutation increases Aβ production by augmenting cleavage at the site of mutation on the amino side of Aβ, and we propose that this mutation increases all Aβ in a way that does not alter the specific site(s) of COOH-terminal cleavage. Although the βAPP$_{717}$ mutations do not increase overall Aβ production, our working hypothesis is that these mutations on the COOH-side of Aβ shift cleavage to favor generation of longer Aβs such as Aβ$_{1-42}$ or Aβ$_{1-43}$, forms that are specifically associated with senile plaque amyloid and not with vascular amyloid (Prelli et al. 1988; Masters et al. 1985; Selkoe et al. 1986; Kang et al. 1987). Since these longer Aβs have biophysical properties that favor amyloid deposition (Burdick et al. 1992; Hilbich et al. 1991), shifting the site of cleavage could result in amyloid deposition without increasing the overall amount of Aβ produced.

References

Burdick D, Soreghan B, Kwon M, Kosmoski J, Knauer M, Henshen A, Yates J, Cotman C, Glabe C (1992) Assembly and aggregation properties of synthetic Alzheimer's A4/beta amyloid peptides analogs. J Biol Chem 267:546–554

Cai XD, Golde TE, Younkin SG (1993) Release of excess amyloid β protein from a mutant amyloid β protein precursor. Science 259:514–516

Chartier-Harlin M-C, Crawford F, Houlden H, Warren A, Hugues D, Fidani L, Goate A, Rossor M, Roques P, Hardy J, Mullan M (1991) Early onset Alzheimer's disease caused by mutation at codon 71 of the β-amyloid precursor gene. Nature 353:844–846

Citron M, Oltersdorf T, Haass C, McConlogue L, Hung AY, Seubert P, Vigo-Pelfrey C, Lieberburg I, Selkoe DJ (1992) Mutations of the β amyloid precursor protein in familial Alzheimer's disease increase β protein production. Nature 360:672–674

De Sauvage F, Octave J-N (1989) A novel mRNA of the A4 amyloid precursor gene coding for a possibly secreted protein. Science 245:651–653

Dyrks T, Weidemann A, Multhaup G, Salbaum JM, Lemaire HG, Kang J, Muller-Hill B, Masters CL, Beyreuther K (1988) Identification, transmembrane orientation and biogenesis of the amyloid A4 precursor of Alzheimer's disease. EMBO J 7:949–957

Estus S, Golde TE, Kunishita T, Blades D, Lowery D, Eisen M, Usiak M, Qu XM, Tabira T, Greenberg BD, Younkin S (1992) Potentially amyloidogenic, carboxyl-terminal derivatives of the amyloid protein precursor. Science 255:726–728

Glenner GG (1983) Alzheimer's disease: multiple cerebral amyloidosis. In: Katzman R (ed) Banbury Report 15: Biological aspects of Alzheimer's disease. Cold Spring Harbor Laboratory, New York, pp 137–144

Glenner GG, Wong CW (1984) Alzheimer's Disease and Down's syndrome: sharing of a unique cerebrovascular amyloid fibril tangles. Biochem Biophys Res Commun 122:1131–1135

Goate AM, Haynes AR, Owen MJ, Farrall M, James LA, Lai LY, Mullan MJ, Roques P, Rossor MN, Williamson R, Hardy JA (1989) Predisposing locus for Alzheimer's disease on chromosome 21. Lancet 1:352–355

Goate A, Chartier-Harlin M-C, Mullan M, Brown J, Crawford F, Fidani L, Giuffra L, Haynes A, Irving N, James L, Mant R, Newton P, Rooke K, Roques P, Talbot C, Pericak-Vance M, Roses A, Williamson R, Rossor M, Owen M, Hardy J (1991) Segregation of a missense mutation in the amyloid precursor protein gene with familial Alzheimer's disease. Nature 34:704–706

Golde TE, Estus SG, Usiak M, Younkin LH, Younkin SG (1990) Expression of β Amyloid protein precursor mRNAs: recognition of a novel alternatively spliced form and quantitation in Alzheimer's disease using PCR. Neuron 4:253–267

Golde TE, Estus S, Younkin LH, Selkoe DJ, Younkin SG (1992) Processing of the amyloid protein precursor to potentially amyloidogenic derivatives. Science 255:728–730

Goldgaber D, Lerman MI, McBride OW, Saffiotti U, Gajdusek DC (1987) Characterization and chromosomal localization of a cDNA encoding brain amyloid of Alzheimer's disease. Science 235:877–880

Haass C, Schlossmacher MG, Hung AY, Vigo-Pelfrey C, Mellon A, Ostaszewski BL, Lieberburg I, Koo EH, Schenk D, Teplow DB, Selkoe DJ (1992) Amyloid β peptide is produced by cultured cells during normal metabolism. Nature 359:322–325

Hardy J, Mullan M, Chartier-Harlin M-C, Brown J, Goate A, Rossor M, Collinge J, Roberts G, Luthert P, Lantos P, Naruse S, Kaneko K, Tsuji S, Miyatake T, Shimizu T, Kojima T, Nakano I, Yoshioka K, Sakaki Y, Miki T, Katsuya T, Ogihara T, Roses A, Pericak-Vance M, Haan J, Roos R, Lucotte G, David F (1991) Molecular classification of Alzheimer's disease. Lancet 337:1342–1343

Hilbich C, Kisters-Woike B, Reed J, Masters CL, Beyreuther K (1991) Aggregation and secondary structure of synthetic amyloid β A4 peptides of Alzheimer's disease. J Mol Biol 218:149–163

Jacobsen JS, Muerkel HA, Blume AJ, Vitek MP (1991) A novel species-specific RNA related to alternatively spliced amyloid precursor protein mRNAs. Neurobiol Aging 12:575–583

Kang, J, LeMaire HG, Unterbeck A, Salbaum JM, Masters CL, Grzeschik K-H, Multhaup G, Beyreuther K, Müller-Hill B (1987) The precursor of Alzheimer's disease amyloid A4 protein resembles a cell-surface receptor. Nature 325:733–736

Kitaguchi N, Takahashi Y, Tokushima Y, Shiojiri S, Ito H (1988) Novel precursor of Alzheimer's disease amyloid protein shows protease inhibitory activity. Nature 331:530–532

Mann DMA, Yates PO, Marcyniuk B, Ravindra CR (1986) The topography of plaques and tangles in Down's Syndrome patients of different ages. Neuropath Appl Neurobiol 12:447–457

Masters CL, Simms G, Weinman NA, Multhaup G, McDonald BL, Beyreuther K (1985) Amyloid plaque core protein in Alzheimer disease and Down syndrome. Proc Natl Acad Sci USA 82:4245–4249

Mori H, Takio K, Ogawara M, Selkoe DJ (1992) Mass spectrometry of purified amyloid β protein in Alzheimer's disease. J Biol Chem 267:17082–17086

Mullan M, Crawford F, Axelman K, Houlden H, Lilius L, Winblad B, Lannfeld L (1992a) A pathogenic mutation for probable Alzheimer's disease in the APP gene at the N-terminus of β-amyloid. Nature Genet 1:345–347

Mullan M, Houlden H, Windelspelcht M, Fidani L, Lombardi C, Diaz P, Rossor M, Crook R, Hardy J, Duff K, Crawford F (1992b) A locus for familial early-onset Alzheimer's disease on the long arm of chromosome 14, proximal to the α1-antichymotrypsin gene. Nature Genet 2:340–342

Murrell J, Farlow M, Ghetti B, Benson MD (1991) A mutation in the amyloid precursor protein associated with hereditary Alzheimer's disease. Science 254:97–99

Naruse S, Igarashi S, Kobayashi H, Aoki K, Inuzuka T, Kaneko K, Shimizu T, Iihara K, Kojima T, Miyatake T, Tsuji S (1991) Mis-sense mutation Val → Ile in exon 17 of amyloid precursor protein gene in Japanese familial Alzheimer's disease (letter) Lancet 337:978–979

Pericak-Vance MA, Yamakoa LH, Haynes CS, Speer MC, Haines JL, Gaskell PC, Hung WY, Clark CM, Heyman AL, Trofatter JA, Eisenmenger JP, Gilbert JR, Lee JE, Alberts MJ, Dawson DV, Bartlett RJ, Earl NL, Siddique T, Vance JM, Conneally PM, Roses AD (1988) Genetic linkage studies in Alzheimer's disease families. Expl Neurol 102:271–279

Pericak-Vance MA, Bebout JL, Gaskell PC Jr, Yamakoa LH, Hung WY, Alberts MJ, Walker AP, Bartlett RJ, Haynes CA, Welsh KA (1991) Linkage studies in familial Alzheimer's disease: evidence for chromosome 19 linkage. Am J Human Genet 48:1034–1050

Ponte G, Gonzales-De Whitt P, Schilling J, Miller J, Hsu D, Greenberg B, Davis K, Wallace W, Lieberburg I, Fuller F, Cordell B (1988) A new A4 amyloid mRNA contains a domain homologous to serine protease inhibitors. Nature 331:525–527

Prelli F, Castano E, Glenner GG, Frangione BJ (1988) Differences between vascular and plaque core amyloid in Alzheimer's Disease. Neurochemistry 51:648–651

Robakis NK, Wisniewski HM, Jenkins EC, Devine-Gage EA, Houck GE, Yao XL, Ramakrishna N, Wolfe G, Silverman WP, Brown WT (1987) Chromosome 21q21 sublocalisation of gene encoding beta-amyloid peptide in cerebral vessels and neuritic (senile) plaques of people with Alzheimer disease and Down syndrome. Lancet 1:384–385

Ropper AH, Williams RS (1980) Relationship between plaques, tangles and dementia in Down syndrome. Neurology 30:639–644

Schellenberg GD, Bird TD, Wijsman EM, Moore DK, Boehnke M, Bryant EM, Lampe TH, Nochlin D, Sumi SM, Deeb SS, Beyreuther K, Martin GM (1988) Absence of linkage of chromosome 21q21 markers to familial Alzheimer's disease. Science 241:1507–1510

Schellenberg GD, Bird TD, Wijsman EM, Orr HT, Anderson L, Nemens E, White JA, Bonnycastle L, Weber JL, Alonso ME (1992) Genetic linkage evidence for a familial Alzheimer's disease locus on chromosome 14. Science 258:668–671

Selkoe DJ, Abraham CR, Podlisny MB, Duffy LK (1986) Isolation of low-molecular-weight proteins from amyloid plaque fibers in Alzheimer's disease. J Neurochem 46:1820–1834

Seubert P, Vigo-Pelfrey C, Esch F, Lee M, Dovey H, Davis D, Sinha S, Schlossmacher M, Whaley J, Swindlehurst C, McCormack, R, Wolfert R, Selkoe D, Liebenburg I, Schenk D (1992) Isolation and quantification of soluble Alzheimer's β peptide from biological fluids. Nature 359:325–327

Shoji M, Golde TE, Ghiso J, Cheung TT, Estus S, Shaffer LM, Cai XD, McKay DM, Tintner R, Frangione B, Younkin SG (1992) Production of the Alzheimer amyloid β protein by normal proteolytic processing. Science 258:126–129

St George-Hyslop PH, Haines JL, Farrer LA, Polinsky R, van Broeckhoven C, Goate A, Crapper McLachlan DR, Orr H, Bruni AC, Sorbi S, Rainero I, Foncin J-F, Pollen D, Cantu JM, Tupler R, Voskersenskaya N, Mayeux R, Growdon J, Fried VA, Myers RH, Nee L, Backhoven H, Martin JJ, Rossor M, Owen MJ, Mullan M, Percy ME, Karlinski H, Rich S, Heston L, Montesi M, Mortilla M, Nacmias N, Gusella JF, Hardy JA (1990) Genetic linkage studies suggest that Alzheimer's disease is not a single homogeneous disorder. Nature 347:194–197

St George-Hyslop P, Haines J, Rogaev E, Mortilla M, Vaula G, Pericak-Vance M, Foncin J-F, Montesi M, Bruni A, Sorbi S, Rainero I, Pinessi L, Pollen D, Polinski R, Nee L, Kennedy J, Macciardi F, Rogaeva E, Liang Y, Alexandrova N, Lukiw W, Schlumpf K, Tanzi R, Tsuda T, Farrer L, Cantu J-M, Duara R, Amaducci L, Bergamini L, Gusella J, Roses A, Crapper McLachlan D (1992) Genetic evidence for a novel familial Alzheimer's disease locus on chromosome 14. Nature Genet 2:330–334

Tanzi RE, Gusella JF, Watkins PC, Bruns GAP, St George-Hyslop P, Van Keuren ML, Patterson D, Pagan S, Kurmit DN, Neve RI (1987) Amyloid β-protein gene: cDNA, mRNA distribution and genetic linkage near the Alzheimer locus. Science 235:880–884

Tanzi RE, McClatchey AI, Lamperti ED, Villa-Komaroff L, Gusella JF, Neve RL (1988) Protease inhibitor domain encoded by an amyloid protein precursor mRNA associated with Alzheimer's disease. Nature 331:528–530

Terry RD (1985) Alzheimer's disease. In: Davis RL, Robertson DM (eds) Textbook of neuropathology. Williams & Wilkins, Baltimore, pp 824–841

Van Broeckhoven C, Backhovens H, Cruts M, De Winter G, Bruyland, Cras P, Martin J-J (1992) Mapping a gene predisposing to early-onset Alzheimer's disease to chromosome 14q24.3. Nature Genet 2:335–339

Yoshioka K, Miki T, Katsuya T, Ogihara T, Sakaki Y (1991) The 717Val → Ile substitution in amyloid precursor protein is associated with familial Alzheimer's disease regardless of ethnic groups. Biochem Biophys Res Commun 178:1141–1146

Mechanism of Cerebral Amyloidosis in Alzheimer's Disease

D. Allsop*, A. Clements, H. Kennedy, D. Walsh, and C. Williams

Summary

The detailed molecular mechanisms involved in the release of the $\beta/A4$ peptide from its precursor (APP), and the particular isoform(s) of APP involved, are still unclear. Western blots of secreted APP from CSF and brain have suggested that $\beta/A4$ may be derived from the brain-specific APP-695 isoform. Antibodies to the initial part of $\beta/A4$ detected only those bands that reacted with antisera to the Kunitz-type protease inhibitor (KPI). Thus, secreted forms of APP with KPI seemed to retain the initial part (residues 1–15) of the $\beta/A4$ sequence, whereas those of APP-695 did not. This may be due to a potentially amyloidogenic cleavage of APP-695 on the N-terminal side of $\beta/A4$. It has been reported recently that secreted APP lacking the $\beta/A4$ sequence (predominantly APP-695) is released by primary cultures of brain tissue. Evidence was presented for cleavage of the Met–Asp bond on the immediate N-terminal side of $\beta/A4$.

Despite a plethora of studies, little is known about the enzymes involved in APP processing. Since these are a potential target for therapeutic intervention, they remain an area of great interest.

Several mutations in the APP gene have been found to segregate with familial Alzheimer's disease or cerebrovascular amyloidosis. One likely effect of pathogenic mutations *within* the amyloid region is to promote aggregation of the $\beta/A4$ peptide after its release from APP. We have examined the fibrillogenic properties of synthetic peptides corresponding to residues 13–26 of $\beta/A4$ containing the normal sequence, or the mutations E^{22} to Q (Q22) or A^{21} to G (G21). All of the peptides formed fibrils in solution at 37 °C and pH 7.4, but the peptide with the Q22 mutation showed greatly accelerated fibril formation compared to the other two. The results suggest that the Q22 mutation confers increased amyloidogenic properties on the $\beta/A4$ peptide, whereas the G21 mutation acts by a different pathogenic mechanism.

* Smith Kline Beecham Pharmaceuticals, Department of Molecular Neuropathology, Coldharbour Road, The Pinnacles, Harlow, Essex CM19 5AD, UK, and Division of Biochemistry, The Queen's University of Belfast, Medical Biology Centre, 97 Lisburn Road, Belfast BT9 7BL, Northern Ireland, UK

C.L. Masters et al. (Eds.)
Amyloid Protein Precursor in Development,
Aging and Alzheimer's Disease
© Springer-Verlag Berlin Heidelberg 1994

Introduction

The 39–43 residue peptide referred to here as β/A4 is the major constituent of senile plaque and vascular amyloid in the brain in Alzheimer's disease (AD) (for reviews see Hardy and Allsop 1991; Multhaup et al. 1993). This peptide does not appear to be an integral component of paired helical filaments (PHF), although amyloid-like fibrils composed of β/A4 can be deposited on the surface of PHF in extracellular "ghost" tangles (Allsop et al. 1990; Yamaguchi et al. 1991). The β/A4 peptide is thought to be derived by proteolysis from its membrane-spanning precursor, APP (Kang et al. 1987). Multiple isoforms of APP are produced by alternative mRNA splicing from a single gene on human chromosome 21, and some of these contain a Kunitz-type protease inhibitor (KPI) sequence (Multhaup et al. 1993). The most abundant form of APP mRNA in brain encodes APP-695 (Kang and Müller-Hill 1990) which lacks KPI. However, the predominance of APP-695 mRNA in brain is not necessarily reflected at the protein level (Van Nostrand et al. 1991). The recent discovery of several presumed pathogenic APP gene mutations in familial forms of AD or cerebrovascular amyloidosis has highlighted the central role played by amyloid in the pathogenesis of these conditions (Hardy and Allsop 1991). This chapter is concerned with the molecular mechanisms responsible for amyloid formation, the particular isoform(s) of APP involved, and the pathogenic effects of the various APP gene mutations, all of which require considerable further clarification.

Proteolytic Processing of APP
and Release of the β/A4 Peptide

Soluble, secretory derivatives of APP have been detected in cerebrospinal fluid (CSF; Palmert et al. 1989a), brain (Moir et al. 1992), and serum (Bush et al. 1990; Podlisny et al. 1990), and in the conditioned media of various cells in culture (Weidemann et al. 1989). In early studies on the proteolytic processing of APP by cultured cells, a large N-terminal fragment was found to be released by an unknown APP "α-secretase" acting at the Lys^{16}–Leu^{17} bond in the middle of the β/A4 sequence (Esch et al. 1990; Anderson et al. 1991). Palmert et al. (1989b) reported the presence of two different secretory APP derivatives in brain and CSF with molecular masses of approximately 125 and 105 kDa (with and without KPI, respectively), both of which reacted with antibodies to residues 1–13, 1–15, or 1–17 of β/A4. It was concluded that APP in brain is invariably cleaved at the Lys^{16}–Leu^{17} site, thus precluding the secretory pathway as a route to amyloid formation.

The first indication that the situation may not be as simple as this came from the finding that brain tissue contains not one, but several small, membrane-bound, C-terminal fragments of APP, some of which encompass the entire β/A4

Table 1. Summary of immunoreactivities of 93–123 k bands in cerebrospinal fluid

Region of APP used for anti-peptide antisera		Extracellular domain	Kunitz-type inhibitor	Initial part of β/A4	Z31
123 k		+	+	+	+
105–112 k	top	+	+	+	+
	middle	+	faint	−	+
	bottom	+	smear	−	+
97 k		+	−	−	−
93 k		+	−	−	−

For further details of antibodies see Kennedy et al. (1992) and Allsop et al. (1993). Anti-Z31 reacts with residues 577–596 of APP-695 (immediately prior to the β/A4 sequence) and was a gift from Dr Yamaguchi. + strongly positive; − negative.

sequence (Estus et al. 1992). Formation of these potentially amyloidogenic fragments was initially attributed to the re-uptake and lysosomal degradation of intact APP (Golde et al. 1992; Haass et al. 1992) rather than any alternative cleavages at the cell surface. However, our own work points to a different interpretation (Kennedy et al. 1992; Allsop et al. 1993; Kametani et al. 1993). We have examined normal, orthopaedic CSF by Western blotting using a wide range of antibodies of various parts of APP, and have obtained clear evidence for six immunoreactive bands of molecular mass 123 kDa, 105–112 kDa (triplet) and 93–97 kDa (doublet; Kennedy et al. 1992). We reconcile our results with those of Palmert et al. (1989b) by suggesting that the broad 105 k band described by these authors actually contains more than one component. In our experiments, several different antibodies to the initial part of β/A4 detected only those bands (123 and 112 k) that were found to react unambiguously with antisera to KPI (Table 1). The other APP-immunoreactive bands were not detected by anti-KPI or anti-β/A4 antibodies. Immunoreactive polypeptides with the same molecular weights were found in soluble extracts of human brain tissue. In this case the identity of the 105–112 k and 93–97 k components was confirmed by N-terminal amino acid sequencing (Kametani et al. 1993). This pattern of bands looks identical to that described by Moir et al. (1992) for soluble APP purified from brain. The immunoreactivities of the 105–112 k triplet components in CSF and brain did appear to be slightly different (Kametani et al. 1993), but in each case we could find no clear evidence for a secreted form of APP-695 retaining residues 1–15 of β/A4. Thus we postulated that this isoform might be secreted predominantly by cleavage on the N-terminal side of β/A4, and not at Lys^{16}–Leu^{17} (Kennedy et al. 1992). This would leave the whole of the amyloid sequence behind on a small, membrane-bound fragment, which could be further processed to release the β/A4 peptide. This could explain the location of amyloid fibrils only in brain, since significant amounts of APP-695 are not found in other tissues throughout the body (Spillantini et al. 1989). However, an alternative possibility remains, namely that following the action of the α-secretase, residues

1–15 of β/A4 are selectively removed from secreted APP-695 by limited proteolysis at the C-terminal end.

Recently, a group at Athena Neurosciences has confirmed that C-terminally truncated forms of secreted APP, lacking the β/A4 sequence, are indeed present in CSF (Seubert et al. 1993). Furthermore, these truncated forms were also found to be released by primary cultures of human foetal brain tissue, apparently via a putative "β-secretase" acting at the Met–Asp bond on the immediate N-terminal side of β/A4. This was demonstrated by immunoreaction of secreted APP with antibody "92" which appears to detect residues 591–596 of APP (695 numbering) only in the presence of a free carboxy-terminal methionine. Within the brain itself, the relative proportions of the various APP isoforms that are processed at the α- and β-secretase sites has not been established. With primary brain cultures, Seubert reported that "the alternative processing of KPI-containing APP forms to produce antibody 92-reactive material is less apparent . . . ." Embryonic 293 kidney cells transfected with APP-695 or APP-751 both secreted small amounts of 92-reactive material (Seubert et al. 1993). However, this may not reflect the actual situation in the brain itself (see "Concluding Comments" below). We have found that the 92 antibody (kindly supplied by Athena Neurosciences) detects only a single band in cerebrospinal fluid with a molecular mass of 108 kDa (Kennedy and Allsop, unpublished observation). This band migrates at the centre of the 105–112 k triplet (Kennedy et al. 1992), but it is not clear yet whether it is a KPI-containing form or not. However, if both APP-695 and APP-751/770 are processed at the β-secretase site in brain, and both of the secreted derivatives are reasonably stable, then the 92 antibody should have revealed two corresponding immunoreactive bands in CSF. Obviously, it will be very important for an understanding of APP processing in brain to determine the nature of this 92-reactive protein.

Recently it has been found that transfected cells overexpressing APP secrete β/A4 into the culture medium (Shoji et al. 1992; Busciglio et al. 1993). This fact, together with the presence of β/A4 in the CSF of individuals without AD (Seubert et al. 1992; Shoji et al. 1992), suggests that this peptide is a normal product of APP processing. Two alternative pathways for the production of β/A4 have been put forward: 1) the re-uptake of intact cell-surface APP and its degradation in lysosomes (Golde et al. 1992; Haass et al. 1992); and 2) cleavage of APP, at or en route to the cell surface, by the putative β-secretase (Seubert et al. 1993) followed by further processing to remove the C-terminal tail. The lack of effect of the lysosomal inhibitors chloroquine, ammonium chloride, and leupeptin on the secretion of β/A4 by transfected cells (Busciglio et al. 1993) favours the latter as the correct explanation, although the mechanism of cleavage within the membrane at the C-terminal end of β/A4 remains difficult to explain. Busciglio et al. (1993) found that human astrocyte primary cultures produced larger amounts of β/A4 than primary neuronal cultures. Astrocytes in primary cultures from rat brain apparently produce mainly APP subtypes which lack KPI (Berkenbosch et al. 1990). These results are compatible with the derivation of brain amyloid predominantly from APP-695 (Kennedy et al. 1992).

Transfected cells also secrete N-terminally extended forms of β/A4 commencing 3 or 6 residues prior to the usual N-terminal aspartate (Busciglio et al. 1993). Thus, further corresponding APP secretory cleavage sites may remain to be discovered.

Proteolytic Enzymes Involved in APP Processing

The identity of neither α- nor β-secretase has been determined unequivocally. A number of proteolytic enzyme activities have been shown to cleave appropriate short synthetic peptide substrates at the correct position (Abraham et al. 1991; Ishiura 1991; McDermott et al. 1992; McDermott and Gibson 1991; Razzaboni et al. 1992; Small et al. 1991), but demonstrating physiologically relevant cleavage of intact APP at the same peptide bond has been a much more difficult proposition.

It has been claimed that α-secretase has an unusually broad specificity (Sisodia 1992). This enzyme activity does not appear to be inhibited by the addition of general inhibitors of serine-, aspartyl- or cysteine-proteinases to the media of differentiated PC-12 cells (Walsh et al. 1993), suggesting that it may be a metalloproteinase. Indeed, the most recent candidate for α-secretase is the metalloproteinase gelatinase A (Miyazaki et al. 1993). This enzyme cleaves synthetic β/A4 10–20 at the Lys^{16}–Leu^{17} bond and is also inhibited by secretory forms of APP. These observations raise the intriguing possibility that APP processing could be subject to autoregulation via the putative APP inhibitory domain for gelatinase A. Miyazaki et al. (1993) could find no homology between APP and other naturally occurring inhibitors of collagenases/gelatinases known as TIMPS (tissue inhibitors of metalloproteinases), but we have noticed a small homologous motif between residues 407–417 of APP-695 and Cys^3–Cys^{13} of TIMP (Fig. 1). The latter region has been implicated as being important for the inhibitory properties of TIMP (O'Shea et al. 1992). This potential inhibitory sequence in the APP molecule deserves further investigation. However, as noted above, gelatinase A cannot be considered a strong contender for being α-secretase until it has been shown to cleave full-length, membrane-bound APP at the β/A4 Lys^{16}–Leu^{17} bond.

There are presently no strong candidates for β-secretase.

```
          3                       13
TIMP -C-V-P-P-H-P-Q-T-A-F-C-

APP  -A-V-P-P-R-P-R-M-V-F-N-
       407                     417
```

Fig. 1. Close homology between APP (695 numbering) and a small region of TIMP (O'Shea et al. 1992) thought to be important for the inhibition of gelatinases. Five of the nine amino acids between the two Cys residues in TIMP are identical in the APP sequence. Of the remaining four residues, only one (R^{413}) is non-conservative

Pathogenic Effects of APP Gene Mutations

In familial AD, APP mutations *outside* of the β/A4 sequence include the KM to NL double mutation on the immediate N-terminal side of β/A4 (Mullan et al. 1992) and the V to I, G or F point mutations on the C-terminal side of β/A4 (Goate et al. 1991; Chartier-Harlin et al. 1991; Murrell et al. 1991). Kidney or neuroblastoma cells transfected with APP-695 containing the former double mutation produce 6- to 8- fold more β/A4 than cells transfected with the normal sequence, suggesting that the mutant APP is more susceptible to cleavage at the β-secretase site (Citron et al. 1992: Cai et al. 1993). The pathogenic effects of the V to I, G or F point mutations are unknown. One hypothesis has been that they destabilize the stem of a putative iron-responsive element in exon 17 of the APP mRNA (Tanzi and Hyman 1991). However, the finding of a silent, but non-pathogenic mutation that should also disrupt this same stem loop structure makes this unlikely (Zubenko et al. 1992) Another possible effect of these mutations is to enhance cleavage of APP at the C-terminal end of the amyloid peptide, but there is no evidence to support this idea. A more remote possibility is that the mutant amyloid is extended beyond the normal 39–43 residues so that the substituted amino acid is included. If this extended mutant form of β/A4 is a highly amyloidogenic intermediate in the proteolytic processing of APP, then the first pathogenic mechanism described below would be feasible.

Additional APP mutations found *within* the amyloid region include E^{22} to Q (Q22) in Dutch cerebral amyloid angiopathy, and A^{21} to G (G21) in a Dutch family with a history of cerebrovascular amyloidosis and AD (Hendriks et al. 1992; Levy et al. 1990). These mutations might act by a number of additional mechanisms, including: 1) an increased propensity of the mutant β/A4 peptide to aggregate into amyloid (Wisniewski et al. 1991); 2) increased stability of amyloid formed from the mutant peptide (Fraser et al. 1992); 3) a decrease in the rate of cleavage at the α-secretase site, diverting more APP through an alternative amyloid-forming pathway; and 4) reduced susceptibility of the mutant β/A4 peptide to proteolytic degradation. Since the β/A4 peptide presumably has some important physiological function in the brain, it is probable that specific proteolytic mechanisms exist to inactivate it. If the mutations conferred increased resistance to such proteolysis, amyloid fibril formation might be enhanced.

Synthetic peptides corresponding to the full-length sequence and also smaller fragments of β/A4 are known to aggregate *in vitro* to produce fibrils with similar ultrastructural and Congo red tinctorial properties as native amyloid (see for example Castano et al. 1986; Kirschner et al. 1987). The C-terminal hydrophobic region of β/A4 is thought to be important in promoting fibrillogenesis (Burdick et al. 1992; Halverson et al. 1990). However, Wisniewski et al. (1991) showed that short peptides lacking this region will still aggregate. Moreover, those containing the Q22 mutation formed fibrils much more readily than the corresponding normal sequences. This could be due to their increased β-pleated sheet content (Fabian et al. 1993) and supports mechanism 1 (above) for the pathogenic effects of this mutation.

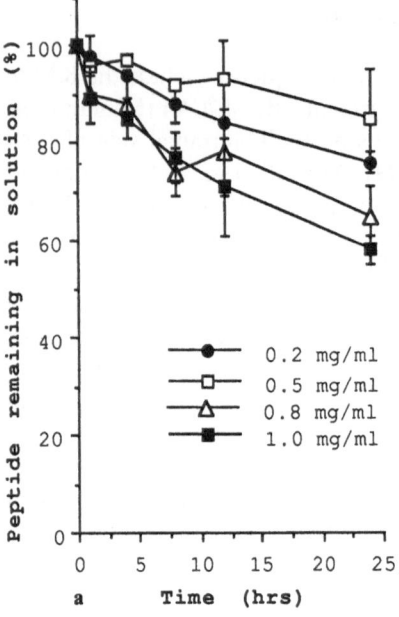

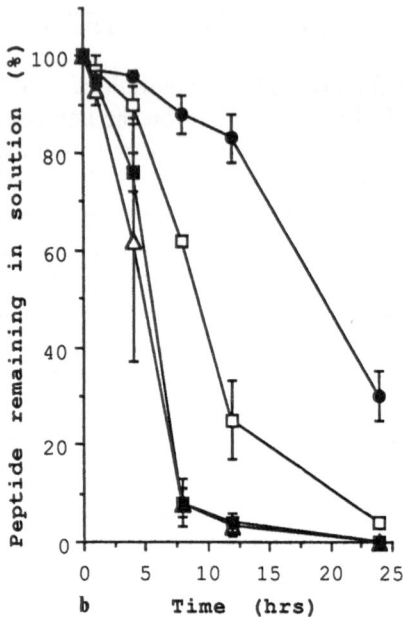

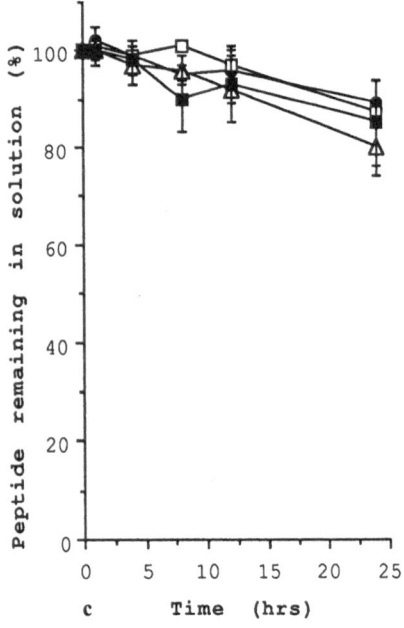

Fig. 2. Effects of concentration on the kinetics of aggregation of (**a**) β_{13-26}, (**b**) β_{13-26} Q22 and (**c**) β_{13-26} G21. Peptide solutions (200–300 μl) were incubated at 37 °C and centrifuged (17,500 × g for 10 min) after 1, 4, 8, 12 and 24 hr. Samples (10 μl) of each supernatant were analysed by reverse phase HPLC. The amount of peptide remaining in solution was calculated from peak areas. Three independent experiments were carried out (results show mean ± SD)

We assessed the fibrillogenic properties of synthetic peptides corresponding to residues 13–26 of β/A4, containing either the normal sequence (β_{13-36}) or each of the mutations Q22 and G21 (peptides β_{13-36} Q22 and β_{13-36} G21, respectively; Clements et al. 1993). The aggregation of the peptides was monitored at different time points over a period of 24 hours. This was achieved by centrifugation to remove insoluble fibrils, followed by reverse-phase HPLC analysis of the amount of peptide remaining in solution. The rates of aggregation of the three peptides at concentrations of 0.2–1 mg/ml in 50mM Tris-HCl, pH 7.4 at 37 °C are shown in Figure 2. At an initial concentration of 1 mg/ml, approximately 60% of β_{13-26} and 75% of β_{13-26} G21 remained in solution after 24 hours, whereas by this time β_{13-26} Q22 has completely aggregated. In marked contrast to the behaviour of the other two peptides, the aggregation of β_{13-26} Q22 accelerated considerably as the initial concentration was increased from 0.2–0.8 mg/ml.

The pellets obtained at the end of each of the 24-hour incubations were transferred to carbon-coated formvar grids and observed by negative stain electron microscopy (Fig. 3). Fibrils closely resembling amyloid were formed by

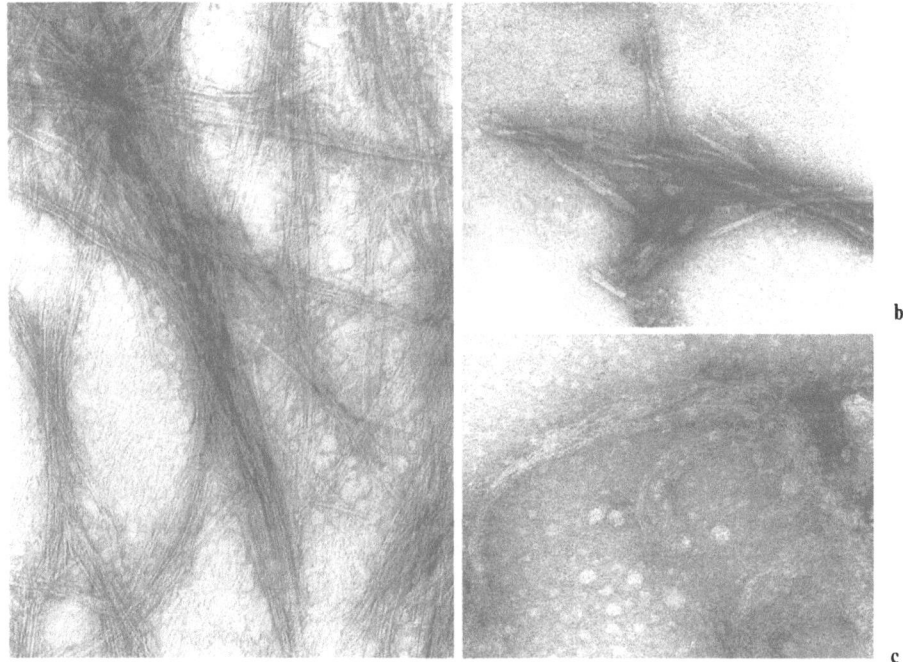

a

b

c

Fig. 3. Negative-stain electron micrographs of fibrils formed by (**a**) β_{13-26}, (**b**) β_{13-26} Q22 and (**c**) β_{13-26} G21. Pellets obtained after 24-hr incubations at 1 mg/ml were resuspended in distilled water, applied to carbon-coated formvar grids, and stained for 2 min with 2% (aq.) uranyl acetate. In each case magnification = 100,000

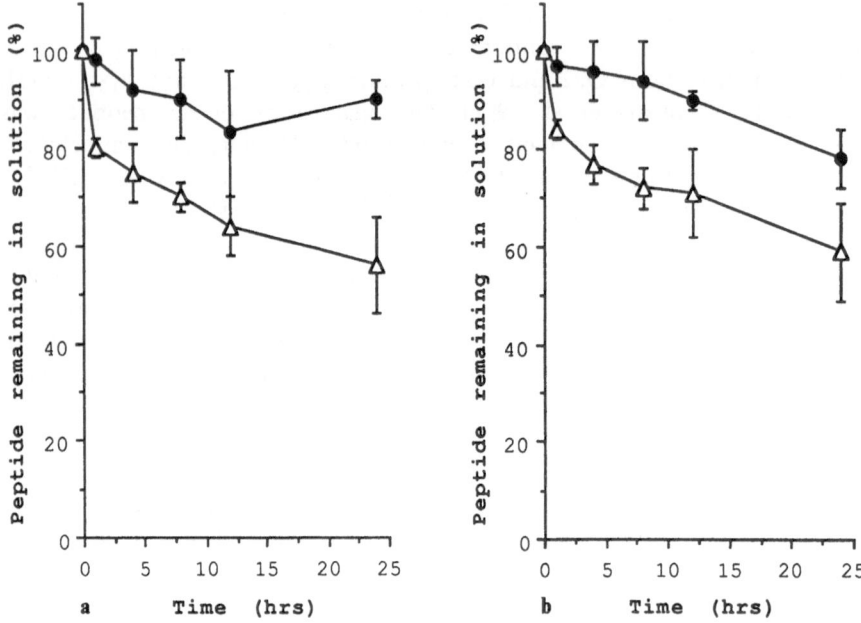

Fig. 4. Results with mixtures of two peptides (0.5 mg/ml β_{13-26} + 0.5 mg/ml β_{13-26} Q22 or β_{13-26} G21). (a) Effects of β_{13-26} Q22 (triangles) or β_{13-26} G21 (circles) on the aggregation of β_{13-26} (b) Effect of β_{13-26} on the aggregation of β_{13-26} Q22 (triangles) or β_{13-26} G21 (circles conditions as for Fig. 2)

the peptides β_{13-26} and β_{13-26} G21. Although the β_{13-26} Q22 peptide assemblies were of similar diameter (7–15 nm) to fibrils from the other peptides, they were shorter in length and showed more evidence of clumping. When stained with Congo red, the fibril pellets all exhibited the characteristic green-red birefringence of amyloid.

Both of the Q22 and G21 mutations exhibit autosomal dominance, so affected individuals will usually be heterozygous and produce both normal and mutant forms of APP. Furthermore, in the case of Q22, both the normal and mutant sequences have been identified in the deposited amyloid (Prelli et al. 1990). It is important, therefore, to study potential interactions between normal and mutant peptides during aggregation. A mixture of β_{13-26} and β_{13-26} Q22 (0.5 mg/ml of each in 50mM Tris-HCl; pH 7.4) was incubated at 37 °C and the rate of fibril formation was followed by HPLC as before (Fig. 4). The two peptides were clearly resolved, allowing them to be monitored separately. Each peptide disappeared from solution at an almost identical rate. This rate was much slower than that observed with 1.0 mg/ml of β_{13-26} Q22 on its own, but marginally faster (only evident at the earlier time points) than that obtained with 1.0 mg/ml of β_{13-26} on its own. These results demonstrate that the two peptides do interact with each other, the most notable effect being the decreased rate of aggregation of β_{13-26} Q22 in the presence of β_{13-26}. Under these circumstances, fibrillogenesis might proceed via formation of an oligomeric intermediate (possibly a heterodimer) containing both normal and mutant peptide molecules.

A mixture of 0.5 mg/ml β_{13-26} and 0.5 mg/ml β_{13-26} G21 was also examined (Fig. 3). For each peptide, the rate of aggregation remained low, showing that even if the β_{13-26} and β_{13-26} G21 peptides interact in some way, this does not increase the rate of fibril formation.

Our observations support the findings of Wisniewski et al. (1991) that peptides with the Q22 mutation show increased fibrillogenic properties, although the experiments with the peptide mixtures do not fully support this as a mechanism of accelerated amyloid formation in heterozygous individuals. We failed to find accelerated fibril formation for the more recently described G21 mutation, suggesting that it operates by a different pathogenic mechanism (possibly mechanisms 2, 3, or 4, above).

Concluding Comments

While great advances in understanding the processing of both normal and mutant APP have undoubtedly been made, many fundamental questions remain unanswered, such as the identity of the α-and β-secretases. Experiments with cultured cells (especially cells transfected with APP) have produced much valuable information on APP processing, but it should be stressed that caution is required in applying these results to the brain itself. There is evidence that overexpression of APP in transfected cells can lead to alterations in its proteolytic processing (Fukuchi et al. 1992). Also Lahiri (1993) has reported that APP is processed differently in various cell types. It would not be surprising, therefore, if transfected kidney cells (which have been widely used to study APP processing) do not turn out to be a good model for the brain. APP processing in brain is almost certainly regulated by complex physiological control mechanisms (possibly involving interactions between neurons and glia) that cannot operate in homogeneous cell cultures. For example, it is perfectly possible that in the brain cell-surface APP is produced by one type of cell and cleaved by an enzyme produced by another. We believe that future studies should concentrate more on APP processing in the brain itself and/or primary cultures derived from brain, and less on monocell cultures of permanent cell lines.

Acknowledgements. We wish to thank The Medical Research Council, the Wellcome Trust, Research Into Ageing and The British Council for supporting our research. AC is also grateful to The Department of Education for Northern Ireland for a Postgraduate Studentship.

References

Abraham CR, Driscoll J, Potter H, Van Nostrand WE, Tempst P (1991) A calcium-activated protease from Alzheimer's disease brain cleaves at the N-terminus of the amyloid β-protein. Biochem Biophys Res Commun 174:790–796

Allsop D, Haga S, Bruton C, Ishii T. Roberts GW (1990) Neurofibrillary tangles in some cases of dementia pugilistica share antigens with amyloid β-protein of Alzheimer's disease. Am J Pathol 136:255–260

Allsop D, Kennedy HE, Kametani F (1993) Secretory derivatives of Alzheimer's amyloid precursor protein in cerebrospinal fluid and brain: Only Kunitz-containing forms show amyloid immunoreactivity. In: Corain B, Iqbal K, Nicoli M, Winblad B, Wisniewski H, Zatta P (eds) Alzheimer's disease: Advances in clinical and basic research. John Wiley, Chichester, pp 421–429

Anderson JP, Esch FS, Keim PS, Sambamurti K, Lieberberg I., Robakis NK (1991) Exact cleavage site of Alzheimer amyloid precursor in neuronal PC-12 cells. Neurosci Lett 128:126–128

Berkenbosch F, Refolo LM, Friedrich VL, Casper D, Blum M, Robakis NK (1990) The Alzheimer's amyloid precursor protein is produced by type 1 astrocytes in primary cultures of rat neuroglia. J Neurosci Res 25:431–440

Burdick D, Soreghan B, Kwon M, Kosmoski J, Knauer M, Henschen A, Yates J, Cotman C, Glabe, C (1992) Assembly and aggregation properties of synthetic Alzheimer's A4/β amyloid peptide analogs. J Biol Chem 267:546–554

Busciglio J, Gabuzda DH, Matsudaira P, Yankner BA (1993) Generation of β-amyloid in the secretory pathway in neuronal and nonneuronal cells. Proc Natl Acad Sci USA 90:2092–2096

Bush AI, Martins RN, Rumble B, Moir R, Fuller S, Milward E, Currie J, Ames D, Weidemann A, Fischer P, Multhaup G, Beyreuther K, Masters CL (1990) The amyloid precursor of Alzheimer's disease is released by human platelets. J Biol Chem 265:15977–15983

Cai X-D, Golde TE, Younkin SG (1993) Release of excess amyloid β protein from a mutant amyloid β protein precursor. Science 259:514–516

Castano EM, Ghiso J, Prelli F, Gorevic PD, Migheli A, Frangione, B (1986) In vitro formation of amyloid fibrils from two synthetic peptides of different lengths homologous to Alzheimer's disease β-protein. Biochem Biophys Res Commun 141:782–789

Chartier-Harlin M-C, Crawford F, Houlden H, Warren A, Hughes D., Fidani L, Goate A, Rossor M, Roques P, Hardy J, Mullan M (1991) Mutations at codon 717 of the β-amyloid precursor protein gene cause Alzheimer's disease. Nature 353:844–846

Citron M, Oltersdorf T, Haass C, McConlogue L, Hung AY, Seubert P, Vigo-Pelfrey C, Lieberburg I, Selkoe, DJ (1992) Mutation of the β-amyloid precursor protein in familial Alzheimer's disease increases β-protein production. Nature 360:672–674

Clements A, Walsh DM, Williams CH, Allsop D (1993) Effects of the mutations Glu22 to Gln and Ala21 to Gly on the aggregation of a synthetic fragment of the Alzheimer's amyloid β/A4 peptide. Neurosci Lett 161:17–20

Esch FS, Keim PS, Beattie EC, Blacher RW, Culwell AR, Oltersdorf T, McClure D, Ward PI (1990) Cleavage of amyloid β peptide during constitutive processing of its precursor. Science 248:1122–1124

Estus S, Golde TE, Kunishita T, Blades D, Lowery D, Eisen M, Usiak M, Qu X, Tabira T, Greenberg BD, Younkin SG (1992) Potentially amyloidogenic, carboxy-terminal derivatives of the amyloid protein precursor. Science 225:726–728

Fabian H, Szendrei GI, Mantsch HH, Otvos L (1993) Comparative analysis of human and Dutch-type Alzheimer β-amyloid peptides by infrared spectroscopy and circular dichroism. Biochem Biophys Res Commun 191:232–239

Fraser PE, Nguyen JT, Inouye H, Surewicz WK, Selkoe DJ, Podlisny MB, Kirschner DA (1992) Fibril formation by primate, rodent, and Dutch-hemorrhagic analogues of Alzheimer amyloid β-protein. Biochemistry 31:10716–10723

Fukuchi K, Kamino KI, Deeb SS, Furlong CE, Sundstrom JA, Smith AC, Martin GM (1992) Expression of a carboxy-terminal region of the β-amyloid precursor protein in a heterogeneous culture of neuroblastoma cells: evidence for altered processing and selective neurotoxicity. Molec Brain Res 16:37–46

Goate A, Chartier-Harlin M-C, Mullan M, Brown J, Crawford F, Fidani L, Giuffra L, Haynes A, Irving N, James L, Mant R, Newton P, Rooke K, Roques, P, Talbot, C, Williamson R, Rossor M, Owen M, Hardy J (1991) Segregation of a missense mutation in the amyloid precursor protein gene with familial Alzheimer's disease. Nature 349:383–388

Golde TE, Estus S, Younkin LH, Selkoe DJ, Younkin SG (1992) Processing of the amyloid protein precursor to potentially amyloidogenic derivatives. Science 225:728–730

Haass C, Koo EH, Mellon A, Hung AY, Selkoe DJ (1992) Targeting of cell-surface β-amyloid precursor protein to lysosomes: alternative processing into amyloid-bearing fragments. 357:500–503

Halverson K, Fraser PE, Kirschner DA, Lansbury PT (1990) Molecular determinants of amyloid deposition in Alzheimer's disease: conformational studies of synthetic β-protein fragments. Biochemistry 29:2639–2644

Hardy J, Allsop D (1991) Amyloid deposition as the central event in the aetiology of Alzheimer's disease. Trends Pharmacol Sci 12:383–388

Hendriks L, van Duijn CM, Cras P, Cruts M, van Hul W, van Harskamp F, Warren A, McInnis MG, Antonarakis SE, Martin J-J, Hofman A, van Broeckhoven C (1992) Presenile dementia and cerebral haemorrhage linked to a mutation at codon 692 of the β-amyloid precursor protein gene. Nature Genet 1:218–221

Ishiura S (1991) Proteolytic cleavage of the Alzheimer's disease amyloid A4 precursor protein. J Neurochem 56, 363–369

Kametani F, Tanaka K, Ishii T, Ikeda S, Kennedy HE, Allsop D (1993) Secretory form of Alzheimer amyloid precursor protein 695 in human brain lacks β/A4 amyloid immunoreactivity. Biochem Biophys Res Commun 191:392–398

Kang J, Müller-Hill B (1990) Differential splicing of Alzheimer's disease amyloid A4 protein precursor RNA in rat tissues: preA4$_{695}$ mRNA is predominantly produced in rat and human brain. Biochem Biophys Res Commun 166:1192–1200

Kang J, Lemaire HG, Unterbeck A, Salbaum JM, Masters CL, Grzeschik KH, Multhaup G, Beyreuther K, Müller-Hill B (1987) The precursor of Alzheimer's disease amyloid A4 protein resembles a cell-surface receptor. Nature 341:144–147

Kennedy HE. Kametani F, Allsop D (1992) Only Kunitz-inhibitor-containing isoforms of secreted Alzheimer amyloid precursor protein show amyloid immunoreactivity in normal cerebrospinal fluid. Neurodegen 1:59–64

Kirschner DA, Inouye H, Duffy LK, Sinclair A, Lind M, Selkoe, DJ (1987) Synthetic peptides homologous to β protein from Alzheimer disease forms amyloid-like fibrils *in vitro*. Proc Natl Acad Sci USA 84:6953–6957

Lahiri DK (1993) The stability of β-amyloid precursor protein in nine different cell lines. Biochem Mol Biol Int 29:849–858

Levy E, Carman MD, Fernandez-Madrid IJ, Power MD, Lieberburg I, van Duinen SG, Bots GTAM, Luyendijk W, Frangione D (1990) Mutation of the Alzheimer's disease amyloid gene in hereditary cerebral hemorrhage, Dutch type. Science 248:1124–1126

McDermott JR, Gibson AM (1991) The processing of Alzheimer A4/β-amyloid precursor: Identification of a human brain metallopeptidase which cleaves Lys–Leu in a model peptide. Biochem Biophys Res Commun 179:1148–1154

McDermott JR, Biggins JA, Gibson AM (1992) Human brain peptidase activity with the specificity to generate the N-terminus of the Alzheimer β-amyloid protein from its precursor. Biochem Biophys Res Commun 185:746–751

Miyazaki K, Hasegawa M, Funahashi K, Umeda M (1993) A metalloproteinase inhibitor domain in Alzheimer amyloid protein precursor. Nature 362:839–841

Moir RD, Martins RN, Bush AI, Small DH, Milward EA, Rumble BA, Multhaup G, Beyreuther K, Masters CL (1992) Human brain βA4 amyloid protein precursor of Alzheimer's disease: Purification and partial characterisation. J Neurochem 59:1490–1498

Mullan M, Crawford F, Axelman K, Houlden H, Lilius L, Winblad B, Lannfelt L (1992) A pathogenic mutation for probable Alzheimer's disease in the APP gene at the N-terminus of β-amyloid. Nature Genet 1:345–347

Multhaup G, Masters CL, Beyreuther K (1993) A molecular approach to Alzheimer's disease. Biol Chem Hoppe-Seyler 374:1–8

Murrell J, Farlow M, Ghetti B, Benson MB (1991) A mutation in the amyloid precursor protein associated with hereditary Alzheimer's disease. Science 245:97–99

O'Shea M, Willenbrock F, Williamson RA, Cockett M, Freedman RB, Reynolds JJ, Docherty AJP and Murphy G (1992) Site-ditected mutations that alter the inhibitory activity of the tissue inhibitor of metalloproteinases-1: Importance of the N-terminal region between Cysteine 3 and Cysteine 13. Biochemistry 31:10146–10152

Palmert MR, Podlisny MB, Witker DS, Oltersdorf T, Younkin LH, Selkoe DJ, Younkin SG (1989a) The β-amyloid protein precursor of Alzheimer disease has soluble derivatives found in human brain and cerebrospinal fluid. Proc Natl Acad Sci USA 86:6338–6342

Palmert MR, Siedlak SL, Podlisny MB, Greenberg B, Shelton ER, Chan HW, Usiak M, Selkoe DJ, Perry G, Younkin SG (1989b) Soluble derivatives of the β amyloid protein precursor of Alzheimer's disease are labelled by antisera to the β amyloid protein. Biochem Biophys Res Commun 165, 182–188

Podlisny MB, Mammen AL, Schlossmacher MG, Palmert MR, Younkin SG, Selkoe DJ (1990) Detection of soluble forms of the β-amyloid precursor protein in human plasma. Biochem Biophys Res Commun 167:1094–1101

Prelli F, Levy E, van Duinen SG, Bots GTAM, Luyendijk W, Frangione B (1990) Expression of a normal and variant Alzheimer's beta-protein gene in amyloid of hereditary cerebral hemorrhage, Dutch type: DNA and protein diagnostic assays. Biochem Biophys Res Commun 170:301–317

Razzaboni BL, Papastoitsis G, Koo EH, Abraham CR (1992) A calcium-stimulated serine protease from monkey brain degrades the β-amyloid precursor protein. Brain Res 589:207–216

Seubert P, Vigo-Pelfrey C, Esch F, Lee M, Dovey H, Davis D, Sinha S, Schlossmacher M, Whaley J, Swindlehurst C, McCormack R, Wolfert R, Selkoe DJ, Lieberburg I, Schenk D (1992) Isolation and quantification of soluble Alzheimer's β-peptide from biological fluids. Nature 359:325–327

Seubert P, Oltersdorf T, Lee MG, Barbour R, Blomquist C, Davis DL, Bryant K, Fritz LC, Galasko D, Thal LJ, Lieberburg I, Schenk DB (1993) Secretion of β-amyloid precursor protein cleaved at the amino terminus of the β-amyloid peptide. Nature 361:260–263

Shoji M, Golde TE, Ghiso J, Cheung TT, Estus S, Shaffer LM, Cai X-D, McKay DM, Tintner R, Frangione B, Younkin SG (1992) Production of the Alzheimer amyloid β-protein by normal proteolytic processing. Science 258:126–129

Sisodia SS (1992) β-amyloid precursor protein cleavage by a membrane-bound protease. Proc Natl Acad Sci USA 89:6075–6079

Small DH, Moir RD, Fuller SJ, Michaelson S, Bush AI, Li Q-X, Milward E, Hilbich C, Weidemann A, Beyreuther K, Masters CL (1991) A protease activity associated with acetylcholinesterase releases the membrane-bound form of the amyloid protein precursor of Alzheimer's disease. Biochem 30:10795–10799

Spillantini MG, Hunt SP, Ulrich J, Goedert M (1989) Expression and cellular localization of amyloid β-protein precursor transcripts in normal human brain and in Alzheimer's disease. Molec Brain Res 6:143–150

Tanzi RE, Hyman BT (1991) Alzheimer's mutation. Nature 350:564

Van Nostrand WE, Farrow JS, Wagner SL, Bhasin R, Goldgaber D, Cotman CW, Cunningham DD (1991) The predominant form of the amyloid β-protein precursor in human brain is protease nexin 2. Proc Natl Acad Sci USA 88:10302–10306

Walsh DM, Williams CH, Kennedy HE, Allsop D (1993) An investigation into the proteolytic processing of Alzheimer amyloid precursor protein in PC-12 cells. Biochem Soc Trans 22, 14S

Weidemann A, Konig G, Bunke D, Fischer P, Salbaum JM, Masters CL, Beyreuther K (1989) Identification, biogenesis, and localisation of precursors of Alzheimer's disease A4 amyloid protein. Cell 57:115–126

Wisniewski T, Ghiso J, Frangione B (1991) Peptides homologous to the amyloid protein of Alzheimer's disease containing a glutamine for glutamic acid substitution have accelerated amyloid fibril formation. Biochem Biophys Res Commun 179:1247–1254

Yamaguchi H, Nakazato Y, Shoji M, Okamoto K, Ihara Y, Morimatsu, M, Hirai S (1991) Secondary deposition of beta amyloid within extracellular neurofibrillary tangles in Alzheimer-type dementia. Am J Pathol 138:699–705

Zubenko GS, Farr J, Scoot Stiffler J, Hughes HB, Kaplan BB (1992) Clinically-silent mutation in the putative iron-responsive element in exon 17 of the β-amyloid precursor protein gene. J Neuropathol Exp Neurol 51:459–463

Effects of Fragments of the β-Amyloid Protein on Hippocampal Neurons in Young and Aged Rats: An Electrophysiological Study

B. Potier*, P. Dutar, and Y. Lamour

Introduction

The deposition of the polypeptide β-amyloid protein (βAP or A4), the primary constituent of the dense core of senile plaques and cerebro-vascular deposits in Alzheimer's disease and Down's syndrome (Masters et al. 1985, Selkoe 1991; Hardy and Higgins 1992), plays an important role in Alzheimer's disease pathogenesis (Hardy and Allsop 1991; Yankner et al. 1990). A number of studies of the possible toxicity of β-amyloid protein (β-AP) fragments are available in the literature, but their conclusions are generally conflicting.

Neurotrophic (Whitson et al. 1989, 1990; Yankner et al. 1989) as well as neurotoxic (Pike et al. 1991, 1992; Yankner et al. 1989, 1990) effects of βAP have been reported on neurons (especially hippocampal neurons) main-tained in monolayer culture. *In vivo* experiments have also showed a neuro-toxic effect of βAP fragments (Kowall et al. 1991, 1992). However, recent reports could not demonstrate a neurotoxic effect of βAP after incubation with rat hippocampal neurons in slices cultures (Malouf 1992) or after direct infusion of the peptide in rat hippocampus or cortex *in vivo* (Frautschy et al. 1991; Games et al. 1992; Stein-Behrens et al. 1992; Clemens and Stephenson 1992) or in rhesus monkey cortex (Podlisny et al. 1992). The methods used to test βAP effects (cell cultures versus *in vivo* applications), the structure studied (hippocampus, cortex, etc.) and the species used (rodent, primates) were different. In light of these different results it is difficult to draw definite conclusions about β-AP action.

We used a different approach, searching for an early effect which could predict βAP neurotoxicity. For instance, if β-AP induces a change in neuronal calcium homeostasis (Mattson et al. 1992), some early modifications in calcium-dependent events must occur and should be recorded using electrophysiological techniques such as intracellular recordings.

* Laboratoire de Physiopharmacologie du Système Nerveux, INSERM U 161, 2 rue d'Alésia, 75014 Paris, France

C.L. Masters et al. (Eds.)
Amyloid Protein Precursor in Development,
Aging and Alzheimer's Disease
© Springer-Verlag Berlin Heidelberg 1994

Protocol

The protocol we used was the following:

1) Intracellular recordings were obtained from CA1 pyramidal neurons in the rat *in vitro* hippocampal slice. We tested two fragments of the protein, $\beta1-28$ and $\beta25-35$, since these two fragments may have different properties. The $\beta1-28$ fragment is a portion of the extracellular domain of the amyloid precursor; it has neurotrophic rather than neurotoxic activity (Whitson et al. 1989). In contrast, the $\beta25-35$ fragment includes an extracellular and a transmembrane hydrophobic sequence (Pike et al. 1993) and is supposed to be neurotoxic (Yankner et al. 1990).

2) Two different modes of application were used. In the first set of experiments, $\beta1-28$ or $\beta25-35$ (1–10 μM) was applied in the superfusion bath during intracellular recordings (applications for up to two hours). Neuronal properties were studied before, during and after application of βAP. In the second set of experiments, slices from hippocampus were incubated for 10 to 16 hours in a solution of Ringer containing $\beta25-35$ (5–30 μM). The properties of the neurons were compared to those of control neurons incubated in a solution of Ringer plus DMSO.

3) We also hypothesized that neurons from aged animals might be more sensitive to the effect of βAP than neurons of young animals. Therefore, the effects of βAP were compared in young (3- to 4-month-old) and aged (25- to 32-month-old) male Sprague-Dawley rats.

4) In some experiments, electrophysiological techniques were combined with an immunohistochemical approach to study the effect of β-AP on the distribution of the calcium-binding protein calbindin (CaBP). It has been suggested that the distribution of CaBP in hippocampus depends on the intracellular Ca^{2+} concentration (see Dutar et al. 1991 for experimental details).

5) Electrophysiological events recorded include: a) the membrane input resistance, defined as the value of the slope of the regression line of the current-voltage curve, measured at resting membrane potential, in its linear portion; b) the amplitude and duration of the Na^+ spike; c) the after-hyperpolarization (AHP), driven by the activation of a Ca-dependent potassium conductance, induced by applying a depolarizing pulse to the neuron through the recording electrode; d) the calcium spike, induced by applying a depolarizing pulse into the neuron (100–120 ms) in the presence of the voltage-dependent Na^+ channel blocker TTX and the K^+ channel blocker TEA; and e) the synaptic events elicited by electrical stimulation of the Schaffer collateral/commissural fibers which reflect the release of endogenous neurotransmitters. These include the fast EPSP, due to the release of excitatory amino-acids, and the biphasic IPSP following the fast EPSP, due to the action of GABA which acts on $GABA_A$ and $GABA_B$ receptors to induce the fast and the slow IPSP, respectively.

Additional details are given elsewhere (Dutar et al., in press).

Effect of β-AP in Neurons from Young Rats

Electrophysiology

Peptides β1–28 or β25–35 (1–10 μM) were applied in the superfusion medium during intracellular recordings of CA1 pyramidal neurons. Membrane potential, membrane resistance, spike amplitude and duration, after-hyperpolarization, and synaptic events (EPSPs and IPSPs) were not significantly modified by the application of βAP (up to two-hour applications).

We hypothesized that a two-hour application may be too short to modify membrane parameters. Therefore, we incubated hippocampal slices for eight to 16 hours in a solution of Ringer containing β25–35 (5–30 μM). The properties of the neurons were compared to those of control neurons incubated in a solution of Ringer plus DMSO. The same parameters as above, and the calcium spike, were studied. We observed a decrease in the spike and EPSP amplitudes and a decrease in the IPSP duration. However, the differences were only marginally significant ($p = 0.05$). The amplitude and duration of calcium spikes were not statistically different in control and incubated slices (Table 1).

Immunohistochemistry

The distribution pattern of calbindin D-28k immunoreactivity (CaBP-IR) in hippocampal neurons is dependent on intracellular Ca^{2+} concentration (Dutar et al. 1991). We tested the hypothesis that β25–35 could modify the intracellular Ca^{2+} concentration and as a consequence, could change CaBP-IR distribution. In young rats, dendritic alterations in the CA1 field were observed in sections incubated in β25–35 for eight to 16 hours. The main morphological alteration was the presence of beaded, swollen varicose profiles and a fragmentation of the CaBP-IR dendrites in stratum radiatum. The number of slices having such dendritic alterations was low in control slices from young rats (seven slices

Table 1. Changes in CA1 hippocampal pyramidal neuron properties induced by β25–35 application

	Young	Aged
Membrane potential and resistance	nc[a]	nc
After-hyperpolarization (AHP)	nc	nc
Sodium spike	↘ (amplitude)	nc
EPSPs	↘ (amplitude)	nc
IPSPs	↘ (duration)	nc
Calcium spike	nc	nc
Dystrophic dendrites	↗ (+ +)	↗ (+)

[a] nc, no change.

among 90 studied; 7.7%), but the proportion rose to 34% in the presence of β25–35. The difference between control and incubated slices was statistically significant ($p < 0.05$, t-test).

Effects of β-AP on Neurons from Aged Rats

Electrophysiology

The same protocol was applied to the aged rats. No changes in electrophysiological parameters were observed in neurons from aged rats following application of β25–35 or β1–28, whatever the mode of application (short-term application or long-term incubation).

Immunohistochemistry

In aged rats, the proportion of slices having "dystrophic" dendrites was 22% in control, non-incubated slices and 39% in slices incubated in the presence of β25–35 (55 slices among 143). However, the difference was not statistically significant.

Conclusion

No consistent, short-term modifications of the membrane properties of CA1 hippocampal neurons were observed following β1–28 or β25–35 application. Spike duration and synaptic events were only slightly altered in young rats. If βAP had a neurotoxic effect through an increased calcium entry into the cell, one would expect an effect on the calcium-dependent events within a few minutes or hours. This was not the case, even after 16-hour applications of βAP. Immunohistochemical studies of slices after βAP incubation revealed alterations of CA1 pyramidal cells dendrites immunoreactivity. We observed swollen varicosities and fragmentation of dendrites more frequently in stratum radiatum after 8–16 hours incubation in the presence of β25–35. Interestingly, these morphological alterations seemed to occur spontaneously in aged rats since a larger proportion of control slices in the aged rat displayed an altered dendritic morphology. Thus, if toxic effects occur in those cells they are probably limited to dendrites of CA1 neurons and spare the cell bodies, whose membrane properties seem unaltered. However, the changes in dendritic CaBP-IR do not imply a toxic effect and could be simply due to changes in CaBP distribution within the dendrites. We also hypothesized that neurons in the aged rat could be more sensitive to the effect of βAP than in the young rat, since amyloid deposits are observed in aged brains even during "physiological" aging. However, in our experimental conditions, neurons from aged rats do not appear more sensitive to βAP than neurons from young rats.

Acknowledgment. This study was supported by a grant from Bayer Pharma France.

References

Clemens JA, Stephenson DT (1992) Implants containing β-amyloid protein are not neurotoxic to young and old rat brain. Neurobiol Aging 13:581–586

Dutar P, Potier B, Lamour Y, Emson PC, Senut MC (1991) Loss of calbindin-28k immunoreactivity in hippocampal slices from aged rats: A role for calcium? Eur J Neurosci 9: 839–849

Dutar P, Potier B, Laman Y (1994) Short term effect of beta-amyloid protein on CA1 hippocampal neurons in young and aged rats: a study of calcium-dependent events. Neurodegeneration, in press

Frautschy SA, Baird A, Cole GM (1991) Effects of injected Alzheimer β-amyloid cores in rat brain. Proc Natl Acad Sci USA 88:8362–8366

Games D, Khan KM, Soriano FG, Keim PS, Davis DL, Bryant K, Lieberburg I (1992) Lack of Alzheimer pathology after β-amyloid protein injections in rat brain. Neurobiol Aging 13:569–576

Hardy JA, Allsop D (1991) Amyloid deposition as the central event in the aetiology of Alzheimer's disease. Trends Pharmacol Sci 12:383–388

Hardy JA, Higgins GA (1992) Alzheimer's disease: the amyloid cascade hypothesis. Science 256: 184–185

Kowall NW, Beal MF, Busciglio J, Duffy LK, Yankner BA (1991) An in vivo model for the neurodegenerative effects of β-amyloid and protection by substance P. Proc Natl Acad Sci USA 88:7247–7251

Kowall NW, McKee AC, Yankner BA, Beal MF (1992) In vivo neurotoxicity of beta amyloid [β(1–40)] and the β(25–35) fragment. Neurobiol Aging 13:537–542

Malouf AT (1992) Effect of beta amyloid peptides on neurons in hippocampal slice cultures. Neurobiol. Aging 13:543–551

Masters CL, Simms G, Weinman NA, Multhaup G, McDonald BL, Beyreuther K (1985) Amyloid plaque core protein in Alzheimer disease and Down syndrome. Proc Natl Sci USA 82:4245–4249

Mattson MP, Cheng B, Davies D, Bryant K, Lieberburg, I, Rydel R (1992) β-Amyloid peptides render human cortical neurons vulnerable to glutamate neurotoxicity by destabilizing calcium homeostasis. J Neurosci 12:376–389

Pike CJ, Walencewicz AJ, Glabe CG, Cotman CW (1991) *In vitro* aging of β-amyloid protein causes peptides aggregation and neurotoxicity. Brain Res 563:311–314

Pike CJ, Cummings BJ, Cotman CW (1992) β-Amyloid induces neuritic dystrophy *in vitro*: similarities with Alzheimer pathology. NeuroReport 3:769–772

Pike CJ, Burdick D, Walencewicz AJ, Glabe CG, Cotman CW (1993) Neurodegeneration induced by β-amyloid peptides in vitro: the role of peptide assembly state. J Neurosci 13:1676–1687

Podlisny MB, Stephenson DT, Frosch MP, Leiberburg I, Clemens JA, Selkoe DJ (1992) Synthetic amyloid β-protein fails to produce specific neurotoxicity in monkey cerebral cortex. Neurobiol Aging 13:561–567

Selkoe DJ (1991) The molecular pathology of Alzheimer's disease. Neuron 6:487–498

Stein-Behrens B, Adams K, Yeh M, Sapolsky R (1992) Failure of beta-amyloid protein fragment 25–35 to cause hippocampal damage in the rat. Neurobiol Aging 13:577–579

Whitson JS, Selkoe DJ, Cotman CW (1989) Amyloid β protein enhances the survival of hippocampal neurons in vitro. Science 243:1488–1490

Whitson JS, Glabe CG, Shintani E, Abcar A, Cotman CW (1990) Beta-amyloid protein promotes neuritic branching in hippocampal cultures. Neurosci Lett 110:319–324

Yankner BA, Dawes LR, Fisher S, Villa-Komaroff L, Oster-Granite ML, Neve RL (1989) Neurotoxicity of a fragment of the amyloid precursor associated with Alzheimer's disease. Science 245:417–420

Yankner BA, Duffy LK, Kirschner DA (1990) Neurotrophic and neurotoxic effects of amyloid β protein: Reversal by tachykinin neuropeptides. Science 250:279–282

The Role of the Extracellular Matrix in Regulating the Function of the Amyloid Protein Precursor of Alzheimer's Disease

D. H. Small*, V. Nurcombe, G. Reed, H. Clarris, K. Beyreuther, and
C. L. Masters

Summary

Studies on rare autosomal dominant mutations affecting the amyloid protein precursor (APP) gene have highlighted the importance of APP in the pathogenesis of Alzheimer's disease (AD). However, the link between the observed changes in APP processing and the pathogenic mechanism remains unclear. We have examined the possibility that disruption of the normal function of APP may underlie the neurodegenerative changes. The presence of APP in cells important for tissue repair following injury (platelets and fibroblasts) and the observation that APP expression is increased during early development suggest that APP has a function in cell growth and regeneration. We have found that APP promotes neurite outgrowth from PC12 cells when added directly to the cell growth medium. APP was also found to stimulate neurite outgrowth from primary cultures of central and peripheral neurons. The effect of APP on neurite outgrowth from primary cultures was most marked when APP was in substratum-bound form, and was dependent upon the presence of heparan sulphate proteoglycans (HSPGs). The binding of APP to HSPGs *in vitro* may mimic certain aspects of the binding of APP to the extracellular matrix (ECM) *in vivo*. Thus the interaction of secreted APP with ECM may be an important step in the activation of APP. Basement membrane ECM regulates the guidance of neurites towards their targets in the developing nervous system. Major protein components of ECM include collagen, laminin and the HSPGs, which have all been reported to interact with APP. APP interacts with HSPGs by binding to the heparan sulphate moieties. APP also binds heparin, an analogue of heparan sulphate. Molecular modelling and site-directed mutagenesis experiments suggest that at least one heparin-binding site exists close to the N-terminus of APP between amino acid residues 96 and 110. A peptide homologous to this region of APP blocked the action of APP on neurite outgrowth.

Our data indicate that secreted APP acts as a neurite outgrowth-promoting factor and that it has important functions in regulating growth and development in the embryonic brain. It seems likely that APP binds to ECM components in

* Department of Pathology, University of Melbourne, and The Mental Health Research Institute, Parkville, Victoria 3052, Australia

C.L. Masters et al. (Eds.)
Amyloid Protein Precursor in Development,
Aging and Alzheimer's Disease
© Springer-Verlag Berlin Heidelberg 1994

the ageing brain as well. As ECM proteins undergo degenerative changes during ageing, a defective interaction of APP with the ECM (due to an alteration in APP or in an ECM component) may underlie the pathogenesis of Alzheimer's disease (AD). The synaptic loss that occurs in certain regions of the AD brain may be related to a loss of the neurite outgrowth-promoting action of APP.

Introduction

Studies on rare cases of familial AD (Levy et al. 1990; Goate et al. 1991; Chartier-Harlin et al. 1991; Mullan et al. 1992) have demonstrated that the amyloid protein precursor (APP) is directly involved in the pathogenic mechanism which causes Alzheimer's disease (AD). However, despite intensive research since APP was first cloned (Kang et al. 1987), the precise relationship between APP and AD has remained unexplained. Although amyloid has been reported to exacerbate the neurotoxic effects of glutamate (Mattson et al. 1992), and although the extent of the clinical deficit correlates roughly with the number of amyloid plaques found in the brain upon autopsy (Blessed et al. 1968), it is not known whether the production of amyloid plaques is the direct cause of AD. A defect in the normal function of APP might also contribute to the pathogenesis of AD (Fig. 1).

Several studies (DeKosky and Scheff 1990; Terry et al. 1991; Lassman et al. 1992) have demonstrated that the cognitive deficit in AD correlates better with the extent of synaptic loss than with the density of amyloid plaques. We have examined the possibility that this synaptic loss is a direct consequence of a disturbance in the normal function of APP.

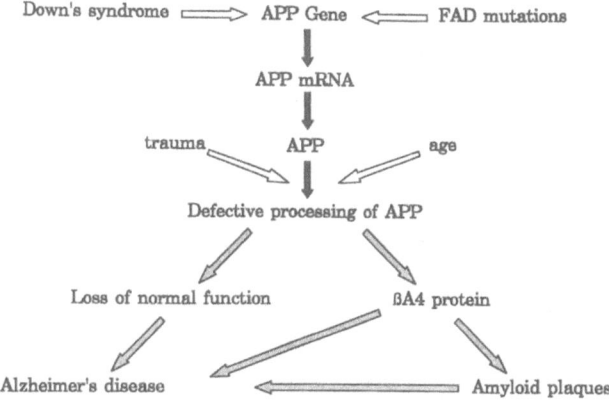

Fig. 1. Schematic representation of the etiology of AD. The figure shows the central importance of defective processing of APP in the pathogenic mechanism. Various risk or causative factors have already been identified (trisomy 21, familial AD (FAD) mutation, trauma, age). These factors can influence the processing of APP at various steps in the pathway. Defective processing of APP could cause AD either through the increased production of the βA4 protein or through the loss of a normal trophic function associated with APP

The Function of APP

Several lines of evidence indicate that APP may play a role in cell growth, repair or adhesion mechanisms. The expression of APP is high in cells associated with wound healing such as fibroblasts (Van Nostrand and Cunningham 1987) and platelets (Bush et al. 1990). APP is stored in the α-granules of platelets and is released in response to activating stimuli (Bush et al. 1990). Roch et al. (1992) found that APP has mitogenic actions on a fibroblast cell line (AG2804). This mitogenic effect has been localised to a domain close to the Kunitz protease inhibitor (KPI) region. Studies on hippocampal neurons suggest that APP can inhibit the excitotoxic effects of glutamate (Mattson et al. 1993). This protective activity has been localised to a domain close to the βA4 region.

The level of APP expressed in tissues correlates well with changes in cellular differentiation or growth. Studies by Abe et al. (1991) have shown that APP is increased in response to focal ischemia, an observation consistent with the presence of acute phase elements in the APP gene promoter (Salbaum et al. 1988). The expression of APP also correlates with the extent of cellular differentiation of SY5Y neuroblastoma cells after treatment with retinoic acid (König et al. 1990).

Role of APP in Neurite Outgrowth

There is strong evidence that APP is involved in regulating neurite outgrowth. First, the level of APP expression correlates with the extent of neurite outgrowth. In the developing chick brain, APP expression is increased precisely during the developmental period (E7–E10) when neurite outgrowth is maximal (Small et al. 1992). In PC12 cells, NGF concomitantly stimulates neurite outgrowth and APP expression (Refolo et al. 1989). In the central nervous system, the level of APP also correlates with NGF-stimulated neurite outgrowth. We have found that explants of E18 (but not P0) mouse hippocampus extend neurites in response to NGF (Clarris et al. 1994). Concomitant with its effects on hippocampal neurite outgrowth, NGF also increases the secretion of APP.

Several studies have shown direct effects of APP on neurite outgrowth. We have found that neurite outgrowth is increased when PC12 cells are grown in the presence of recombinant APP (Milward et al. 1991). Other groups have reached similar conclusions. Studies by Schubert et al. (1989), Whitson et al. (1989, 1990), and Breen et al. (1991) have implicated APP in neuronal adhesion and survival, while studies by Yankner et al. (1990) suggest that the βA4 region of APP may have direct effects on neurite outgrowth.

The effect of APP on neurite outgrowth from chick sympathetic or mouse hippocampal neurons can be greatly increased if the cells are cultured on a substrate of APP (Small et al. 1993, 1994). The effect of substratum-bound APP on neurite outgrowth is dependent upon the presence of heparan sulphate proteoglycan (HSPG), which must also be present as part of the substrate upon which the cells are grown. We have found that the type of HSPG is important. HSPG purified from P3 mouse brain (a developmental period during which neurite outgrowth occurs and the HSPG composition is complex) supports the effect on neurite outgrowth. However, HSPG from E10 mouse brain (prior to the major phase of neurite outgrowth) does not support the effect of APP. Therefore, we conclude that specific, developmentally regulated HSPGs may be important for the function of APP in neurite outgrowth.

APP Binds to Components of the Extracellular Matrix

The effect of substratum-bound APP on neurite outgrowth may mimic significant aspects of the interaction of APP with the extracellular matrix (ECM). APP can bind saturably and with high affinity to purified ECM (Small et al. 1992). APP can bind to heparin, an analogue of heparan sulphate, the carbohydrate component of HSPGs. Studies by Narindrasorasak et al. (1991) have shown that APP can bind with high affinity to a basement membrane form of HSPG. APP may also bind to other ECM components such as laminin (Narindrasorasak et al. 1992; Multhaup et al., in preparation) and collagen (Breen 1992; Multhaup et al., in preparation).

To determine which ECM proteins bind APP, we have purified ECM from cultures of embryonic chick brain neurons and have examined the effect of agents which disrupt ECM on the binding of ^{125}I-APP to purified ECM (Table 1). We found that APP binds less to ECM prepared from cells pre-treated

Table 1. Effect of pre-treatment with xyloside, chlorate and enzymes on the binding of ^{125}I-APP to chick brain ECM[a]

Treatment	Amount bound to ECM (cmp/well)	
	^{125}I-APP	^{125}I-basic FGF
Control	676 ± 34	1262 ± 113
Xyloside (1 mM)	136 ± 8*	519 ± 87*
Chlorate (10 mM)	126 ± 13*	642 ± 42*
Heparitinase (10 mIU/ml)	132 ± 24*	600 ± 52*
Collagenase (100 μg/ml)	842 ± 27*	1368 ± 94

[a] Adapted from Small et al. (1992). Chick brain neurons were cultured in 24-well dishes in the presence or absence of xyloside or chlorate. ECM was prepared from confluent cultures and then incubated with heparitinase or collagenase, followed by ^{125}I-labelled APP or ^{125}I-labelled basic FGF (1.0 nCi/well) for 1 hour as described (Small et al. 1992). The amount of bound radioactivity was then measured. Values are means ± SEM (n = 4). Asterisks, significantly different from controls (P < 0.05).

with xyloside, an inhibitor of proteoglycan biosynthesis. This suggests that APP binds to one or more proteoglycans in the ECM. The conclusion is supported by the observation that chlorate, an inhibitor of proteoglycan sulphation, and heparitinase, an enzyme which digests the heparan sulphate moieties of HSPG, both decreased the number of APP binding sites on the ECM. The relative amount of APP bound to the ECM after each treatment was found to be similar to that of basic fibroblast growth factor (FGF), which is known to bind principally to HSPG. In contrast, incubation of ECM with collagenase increased the total number of APP binding sites. This finding suggests that APP does not bind to collagen in intact ECM.

There is increasing evidence to suggest that the ECM plays a complex role in regulating neurite outgrowth during early development. The ECM protects growth factors from proteolytic digestion (Saskela et al. 1988) and provides a storage compartment for factors, which can be rapidly mobilised by the action of specific ECM-degrading proteases (Saskela and Rifkin 1990). The ECM also regulates the binding of molecules to specific high affinity cell surface receptors (Klagsbrun and Baird 1991). ECM proteins such as laminin and fibronectin have neurite outgrowth-promoting effects (Lander 1987). Although HSPGs have an important function in acting as an intermolecular "glue" between ECM components (Reichardt and Tomaselli 1991), specific developmentally regulated HSPG may also be involved in the activation of ECM-associated growth factors (Nurcombe et al. 1993).

A Heparin-Binding Domain of APP

Previous studies have demonstrated the importance of basic residues in heparin binding (Villanueva 1984; Cardin and Weintraub 1989; Jackson et al. 1991). APP possesses three regions within its extracellular domain which are rich in basic residues and which might therefore form heparin-binding domains. The regions of APP$_{695}$ include residues 99–110, residues 411–447, and a previously defined region encoded within exon 9 (residues 318–330; Multhaup et al., manuscript in preparation).

We have identified a domain close to the N-terminus of APP which proves to be necessary for the neurite outgrowth-promoting function of substratum-bound APP. Secondary structure prediction and molecular modelling studies suggest that a region of APP rich in basic amino acids (residues 96–110) could form a loop domain that is stabilised by a disulphide bond between two cysteine residues at positions 98 and 105 (Fig. 2). This domain has homology to the heparin-binding domains of other proteins, and contains the consensus sequence for heparin binding proposed by Cardin and Weintraub (1989; Table 2). The importance of this domain is also highlighted by the fact that its sequence is conserved in both rat and mouse APP. Interestingly, although the amino acid sequence is not highly conserved in other APP-like proteins such as the *Drosophila* APPL, APLP and APLP-2, a cluster of basic residues at

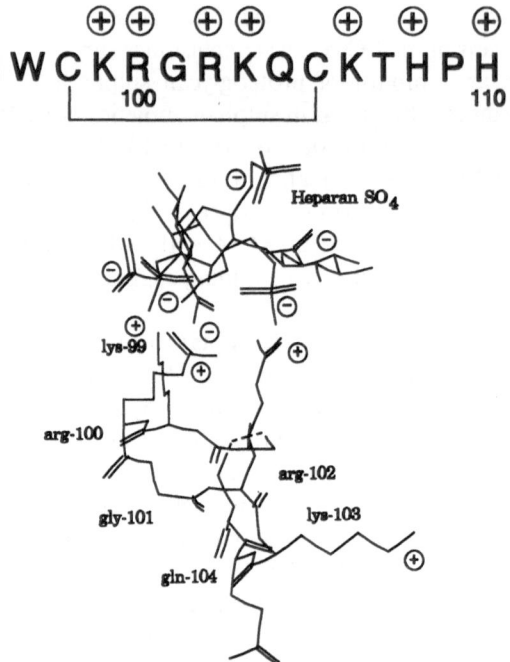

Fig. 2. Structure of a heparin-binding domain on APP. The amino acid sequence of the heparin-binding domain from residues 96–110 is represented by the standard one-letter code for amino acids. The domain contains seven positively charged basic amino acid residues. Based on a secondary structure prediction algorithm, a disulphide bond is predicted between the cysteine residues at positions 98 and 105. The figure also shows the results of computer-assisted molecular modelling of the heparin-binding domain. The polypeptide backbone and amino acid side chains are shown in this model as well as a disulphide bond between the two cysteine residues (dashed line). Three residues in particular (lysine-99, arginine-100 and arginine-102) are predicted to be critical for binding to heparan sulphate

approximately the same position is found in all sequences. The two cysteine residues predicted to be important for stabilising a loop domain are also conserved (Table 2).

Biochemical and cell culture studies demonstrate that this N-terminal loop domain is a heparin-binding site (Small et al., submitted for publication). A peptide homologous to the putative heparin-binding domain was found to bind heparin with an affinity similar to that of APP itself. Molecular modelling studies suggested that three amino acid residues of APP (lysine-99, arginine-100 and arginine-102) were important for the interaction of APP with heparin. Mutation of these residues using a PCR-based approach was found to decrease the affinity of APP for binding to heparin.

To determine whether the binding of APP to HSPG was necessary for the neurite outgrowth-promoting effect of APP, we tested the effect of the heparin-binding peptide on neurite outgrowth from dissociated cultures of chick

Table 2. Amino acid sequence of a heparin-binding domain of APP and other proteins

Protein	Amino acid sequence of heparin-binding domain
Consensus sequence	B B X B
	95 100 105 110 115
Human APP	Q N W C K R G - R K Q C K T H P H - F V I P Y R
Mouse APP	Q N W C K R G - R K Q C K T H T H - I V I P Y R
Rat APP	Q N W C K R G - R K Q C K T H T H - I V I P Y R
APLP-2	D N W C R R D - K K Q C K S R - - - F V T P F K
APLP	E R W C G G T - R S G R C A H P H H E V V P F H
APPL	G G W C R Q G A L N A K C K G S H R W I K P F R

Amino acid residues are shown using standard one-letter code. Spaces have been introduced in the sequences to obtain optimal alignment. Basic residues are shown underlined. Note the position of the conserved cysteine residues (C) shown in bold. Sequences: human APP (Kang et al. 1987), mouse APP (Yamada et al. 1987), rat APP (Shivers et al. 1988). APLP-2 (Sprecher et al. 1993), APLP (Wasco et al. 1992), and APPL (Rosen et al. 1989). Consensus sequence is from Cardin and Weintraub (1989).

sympathetic and mouse hippocampal neurons. The concentration of peptide (10^{-7} M) required to inhibit the neurite outgrowth-promoting effect was identical to the concentration required to inhibit the binding of APP to heparin.

Our studies demonstrate that APP is involved in the regulation of neurite outgrowth and that the binding of APP to HSPG is an important step in this process. A mechanism whereby APP may regulate neurite outgrowth is depicted (Fig. 3). APP may act similarly to other heparin-binding molecules which become activated when bound to heparin or HSPGs. For example, basic FGF must first bind to HSPG before it can bind to a specific high affinity cell surface receptor (Klagsbrun and Baird 1991; Rapraeger et al. 1991). Heparin-binding proteins such as glia-derived nexin (GDN) and antithrombin III are activated by binding to heparin (Craig et al. 1989; Wallace et al. 1989). Our studies suggest that a major site of ECM attachment is within the cysteine-rich region of APP. This domain was predicted to have a "receptor" function because of its highly folded conformation (Kang et al. 1987). The cell attachment domain associated with the neurite outgrowth effect in our studies has not yet been mapped. This domain could reside within a region previously characterised by Roch et al. (1992) or, alternatively, it could be associated with a domain close to the βA4 sequence, which several studies (Whitson et al. 1989, 1990; Yankner et al. 1990) have implicated in the regulation of neurite outgrowth.

The observation that, under certain culture conditions, APP stimulates neurite outgrowth but, under other conditions, is toxic to cells suggests that APP may have complex actions on cells. In this regard, APP may function like thrombospondin, another ECM-associated molecule, which has subtle modulatory roles in altering the total cellular environment (Sun et al. 1992).

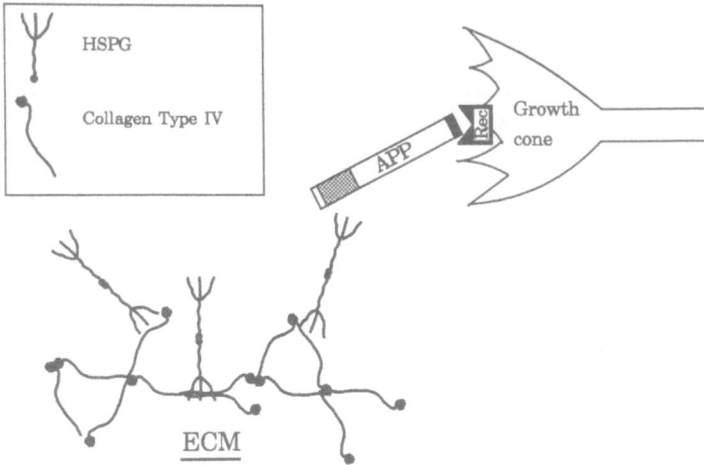

Fig. 3. Model of mechanism by which the binding of APP to ECM regulates neurite outgrowth. APP is anchored to HSPG through a heparin-binding site in the cysteine-rich region. The binding to HSPG sequesters APP and allows it to be delivered to a specific high affinity cell surface receptor (Rec) on the growing neurite. The binding of APP to this receptor triggers specific intracellular events which promote neurite outgrowth

A Role for APP in the Pathogenesis of AD

The interaction of APP with HSPG has implications for the pathogenesis of AD. HSPGs have been identified in amyloid plaques (Snow et al. 1988). The loss of synapses, known to occur in specific regions of the AD brain, could be related to the loss of the normal trophic or neuroprotective effect of APP (Mattson et al. 1993). It is well known that ECM proteins undergo changes during aging (Hall 1976). The localisation of ECM-associated proteins (HSPG, laminin, FGF, acetylcholinesterase) in amyloid plaques suggests that there may be a disturbance in the underlying ECM in the brain of patients with AD. Such a disturbance could lead to an alteration in APP function, perhaps resulting in an abnormal neuritic response around the plaque.

It would be worthwhile examining whether APP processed via an amyloidogenic pathway can exert the same trophic or neuroprotective influence on cells as forms of APP produced from the action of a normally functioning APP secretase. Altered interactions of APP with HSPGs might contribute to the biochemical or pathologic changes that occur in AD.

Acknowledgments. This work was supported by grants from the National Health and Medical Research Council of Australia, the Aluminium Development Corporation and the Victorian Health Promotion Foundation. K.B. is supported by the Deutsche Forschungsgemeinschaft and the Bundesministerium für Forschung und Technologie.

References

Abe K, Tanzi RE, Kogure K (1991) Selective induction of Kunitz-type protease inhibitor domain-containing amyloid precursor protein mRNA after persistent focal ischemia in rat cerebral cortex. Neurosci Lett 125:172–174

Blessed G, Tomlinson BE, Roth M (1968) The association between quantitative measures of dementia and of senile change in the cerebral grey matter of elderly subjects. Br J Psychiat 114:797–811

Breen KC (1992) APP-collagen interaction is mediated by a heparin bridge mechanism. Mol Chem Neuropathol 16:109–121

Breen KC, Bruce M, Anderton BH (1991) Beta amyloid precursor protein mediates neuronal cell-cell and cell-surface adhesion. J Neurosci Res 28:90–100

Bush AI, Martins RN, Rumble B, Moir R, Fuller S, Milward E, Currie J, Ames D, Weidemann A, Fischer P, Multhaup G, Beyreuther K, Masters CL (1990) The amyloid precursor protein of Alzheimer's disease is released by human platelets. J Biol Chem 265:15977–15983

Cardin AD, Weintraub HJR (1989) Molecular modeling of protein-glycosaminoglycan interactions. Arteriosclerosis 9:21–32

Chartier-Harlin M, Crawford F, Houlden H, Warren A, Hughes D, Fidani L, Goate A, Rossor M, Roques P, Hardy J, Mullan M (1991) Early-onset Alzheimer's disease caused by mutations at codon 717 of the β-amyloid precursor protein gene. Nature 353:844–846

Clarris H, Nurcombe V, Small DH, Beyreuther K, Masters CL (1994) Secretion of nerve growth factor from septum stimulates neurite outgrowth and release of the amyloid protein precursor of Alzheimer's disease from hippocampal explants. J Neurosci Res, in press

Craig PA, Olson ST, Shore JD (1989) Transient kinetics of heparin-catalyzed protease inactivation by antithrombin III. Characterization of assembly, product formation, and heparin dissociation steps in the factor Xa reaction. J Biol Chem 264:5452–5461

DeKosky ST, Scheff SW (1990) Synapse loss in frontal cortex biopsies in Alzheimer's disease: correlation with cognitive severity. Ann Neurol 27:457–464

Goate AM, Chartier-Harlin M, Mullan M, Brown J, Crawford F, Fidani L, Giuffra L, Haynes A, Irving N, James L, Mant R, Newton P, Rooke K, Roques P, Talbot C, Pericak-Vance M, Roses A, Williamson R, Rossor M, Owen M, Hardy J (1991) Segregation of a missense mutation in the amyloid precursor protein gene with familial Alzheimer's disease. Nature 349:704–706

Hall DA (1976) The ageing of connective tissues. Academic Press, London

Jackson RL, Busch SJ, Cardin AD (1991) Glycosaminoglycans: molecular properties, protein interactions, and role in physiological processes. Physiol Rev 71:481–539

Kang J, Lemaire H, Unterbeck A, Salbaum JM, Masters CL, Grzeschik K, Multhaup G, Beyreuther K, Müller-Hill B (1987) The precursor of Alzheimer's disease amyloid A4 protein resembles a cell-surface receptor. Nature 325:733–736

Klagsbrun M, Baird A (1991) A dual receptor system is required for basic fibroblast growth factor activity. Cell 67:229–231

König G, Masters CL, Beyreuther K (1990) Retinoic acid induced differentiated neuroblastoma cells show increased expression of the βA4 amyloid gene of Alzheimer's disease and an altered splicing pattern. FEBS Lett 269:305–310

Lander A (1987) Molecules that make axons grow. Mol Neurobiol 1:213–245

Lassman H, Weiler R, Fischer P, Bancher C, Jellinger K, Floor E, Danielczyk W, Seitelberger F, Winkler H (1992) Synaptic pathology in Alzheimer's disease: immunological data for markers of synaptic and large dense core vesicles. Neuroscience 46:1–8

Levy E, Carman MD, Fernandez-Madrid IJ, Power MD, Lieberburg I, van Duinen SG, Bots GTAM, Luyendijk W, Frangione B (1990) Mutation of the Alzheimer's disease amyloid gene in hereditary cerebral hemorrhage, Dutch type. Science 248:1124–1126

Mattson MP, Cheng B, Davis D, Bryant K, Lieberburg I, Rydel RE (1992) β-amyloid peptides destabilize calcium homeostasis and render human cortical neurons vulnerable to excitotoxicity. J Neurosci 12:376–389

Mattson MP, Cheng B, Culwell AR, Esch FS, Lieberburg I, Rydel RE (1993) Evidence for excitoprotective and intraneuronal calcium-regulating roles for secreted forms of the β-amyloid precursor protein. Neuron 10:243–254

Milward E, Papadopoulos R, Fuller SJ, Moir RD, Small D, Beyreuther K, Masters CL (1991) The amyloid protein precursor of Alzheimer's disease is a mediator of the effects of nerve growth factor on neurite outgrowth. Neuron 9:129–137

Mullan M, Crawford F, Axelman K, Houlden H, Lilius L, Winblad B, Lannfelt L (1992) A pathogenic mutation for probable Alzheimer's disease in the APP gene at the N-terminus of β-amyloid. Nature Genet 1:345–347

Narindrasorasak S, Lowery D, Gonzalez-DeWhitt P, Poorman RA, Greenberg B, Kisilevsky R (1991) High affinity interactions between the Alzheimer's β-amyloid precursor proteins and the basement membrane form of heparan sulfate proteoglycan. J Biol Chem 266:12878–12883

Narindrasorasak S, Lowery DE, Altman RA, Gonzalez-DeWhitt PA, Greenberg BD, Kisilevsky R (1992) Characterization of high affinity binding between laminin and Alzheimer's disease amyloid precursor proteins. Lab Invest 67:643–652

Nurcombe V, Ford MD, Wildschut JA, Bartlett PF (1993) Developmental regulation of neural response to FGF-1 and FGF-2 by heparan sulphate proteoglycan. Science 260:103–106

Rapraeger AC, Krufka A, Olwin BB (1991) Requirement of heparan sulphate for bFGF-mediated fibroblast growth and myoblast differentiation. Science 252:1705–1708

Refolo LM, Salton SRJ, Anderson JP, Mehta P, Robakis NK (1989) Nerve and epidermal growth factors induce the release of the Alzheimer amyloid precursor from PC12 cultures. Biochem Biophys Res Commun 164:664–670

Reichardt LF, Tomaselli KJ (1991) Extracellular matrix molecules and their receptors: functions in neural development. Ann Rev Neurosci 14:531–570

Roch J, Shapiro IP, Sundsmo MP, Otero DAC, Refolo LM, Robakis NK, Saitoh T (1992) Bacterial expression, purification, and functional mapping of the amyloid β/A4 protein precursor. J Biol Chem 267:2214–2221

Rosen DR, Martin-Morris L, Luo L, White K. (1989) A *Drosophila* gene encoding a protein resembling the human beta-amyloid protein precursor. Proc Natl Acad Sci USA 86:2478–2482

Salbaum JM, Weidemann A, Lemaire H, Masters CL, Beyreuther K (1988) The promoter of Alzheimer's disease amyloid A4 precursor gene. EMBO J 7:2807–2813

Saskela O, Rifkin DB (1990) Release of basic fibroblast growth factor-heparan sulfate complexes from endothelial cells by plasminogen activator-mediated proteolytic activity. J Cell Biol 110:767–775

Saskela O, Moscatelli D, Sommer A, Rifkin DB (1988) Endothelial cell-derived heparan sulfate binds basic fibroblast growth factor and protects it from proteolytic degradation. J Cell Biol 107:743–751

Schubert D, Jin LW, Saitoh T, Cole G (1989) The regulation of amyloid β protein precursor secretion and its modulatory role in cell adhesion. Neuron 3:689–694

Shivers BD, Hilbich C, Multhaup G, Salbaum M, Beyreuther K, Seeburg PH (1988) Alzheimer's disease amyloidogenic glycoprotein: expression pattern in rat brain suggests a role in cell contact. EMBO J 7:1365–1370

Small DH, Nurcombe V, Moir R, Michaelson S, Monard D, Beyreuther K, Masters CL (1992) Association and release of the amyloid protein precursor of Alzheimer's disease from chick brain extracellular matrix. J Neuroscience 12:4143–4150

Small DH, Nurcombe V, Clarris H, Beyreuther K, Masters CL (1993) The role of extracellular matrix in the processing of the amyloid protein precursor of Alzheimer's disease. In: Nitsch RM, Growdon JH, Corkin S, Wurtman RJ (eds) Alzheimer's disease: amyloid precursor proteins, signal transduction, and neural transplantation. Center for Brain Sciences and Metabolism Charitable Trust, Cambridge, pp 187–192

Small DH, Nurcombe V, Reed G, Clarris H, Moir R, Beyreuther K, Masters CL (1994) A heparin-binding domain the amyloid protein precursor is involved in the regulation of neurite outgrowth. J. Neurosci, in press

Snow, AD, Mar H, Nochlin D, Kimata K, Kato M, Suzuki S, Hassell J, Wight TN (1988) The presence of heparan sulphate proteoglycans in the neuritic plaques and congophilic angiopathy in Alzheimer's disease. Am J Pathol 133:456–463

Sprecher CA, Grant FJ, Grimm G, O'Hara PJ, Norris F, Norris K, Foster DC (1993) Molecular cloning of the cDNA for a human amyloid precursor protein homolog: evidence for a multigene family. Biochemistry 32:4481–4486

Sun X, Skorstengaard K, Mosher DF (1992) Disulfides modulate RGD-inhibitable cell adhesive activity of thrombospondin. J Cell Biol 118:693–701

Terry RD, Masliah E, Salmon DP, Butters N, DeTheresa R, Hill R, Hansen LA, Katzman R (1991) Physical basis of cognitive alterations in Alzheimer's disease: synaptic loss is the major correlate of cognitive impairment. Ann Neurol 30:572–580

Van Nostrand WE, Cunningham DD (1987) Purification of protease nexin II from human fibroblasts. J Biol Chem 262:8508–8514

Villanueva GB (1984) Predictions of the secondary structure of antithrombin III and the location of the heparin-binding site. J Biol Chem 259:2531–2536

Wallace A, Rovelli G, Hofsteenge J, Stone SR (1989) Effect of heparin on the glia-derived-nexin-thrombin interaction. Biochem J 257:191–196

Wasco W, Bupp K, Magendantz M, Gusella JF, Tanzi RE, Solomon F (1992) Identification of a mouse brain cDNA that encodes a protein related to the Alzheimer disease-associated amyloid β protein precursor. Proc Natl Acad Sci USA 89:10758–10762

Whitson JS, Selkoe DJ, Cotman CW (1989) Amyloid β protein enhances the survival of hippocampal neurons *in vitro*. Science 243:1488–1490

Whitson JS, Glabe CG, Shintani E, Abcar A, Cotman CW (1990) β-Amyloid protein promotes neuritic branching in hippocampal cultures. Neurosci lett 110:319–324

Yamada T, Sasaki H, Furuya H, Miyata T, Goto I, Sakaki Y (1987) Complementary DNA for the mouse homolog of the human amyloid beta protein. Biochem Biophys Res Commun 149:665–671

Yankner BA, Duffy LK, Kirschner DA (1990) Neurotrophic and neurotoxic effects of amyloid β protein: reversal by tachykinin neuropeptides. Science 250:279–282

Studies of the Amyloid Precursor Protein (APP) in Brain: Regulation of APP-Ligand Binding

G. Multhaup*

Summary

The specific binding of the amyloid precursor protein (APP) to glycosamino-glycans (GAG) suggests that APP is a cell adhesion molecule (CAM) and/or substrate adhesion molecule (SAM). In order to characterize this activity of APP in the brain at the molecular level, we have purified and characterized the major APP species from rat brain. The major isoform isolated was sequenced and found to be APP_{695}. In a solid-phase binding assay, the specificity of this brain-specific APP isoform-GAG interaction was assessed. The binding of APP to the glycosaminoglycan heparin was found to be time dependent and satur-able. A strong heparin binding site within a region conserved in rodent and human APP was identified. Saturable binding to heparin through this binding site was found to occur at nanomolar concentrations of APP. This putative high-affinity site was then located within a sequence of 22 amino acids in length corresponding to amino acids 316–337 of APP_{695}. This sequence is encoded by APP exon 9 and the first three codons of exon 10. Since all APP and L-APP isoforms so far described include these exons, the strong heparin binding site is a ubiquitous feature of all APP and L-APP isoforms, strongly suggesting that the brain-specific and neuronal as well as the non-neuronal and peripheral APPs and L-APPs do have CAM- and SAM-like activities.

Certain metal ions including zinc(II) have been proposed as risk factors in Alzheimer's disease (AD). Recently we showed that APP binds zinc(II) at higher nanomolar concentrations. We identified this zinc binding site to be located within the sequence of APP encoded by exon 5. Because zinc ions are involved in tissue repair and because of the CAM and SAM activity of APP, the mecha-nisms by which zinc(II) may exert an influence on the pathogenesis of AD were sought by studying the binding of APP to heparin in the presence of varying zinc(II) concentrations. We found that zinc(II) is a modulating factor for the CAM and SAM activity of APP that is exerted through the heparin-like GAG side-chains of heparan sulfate proteoglycans (HSPGs). Because the binding of APP to GAG in the presence of zinc(II) resembles an allosteric interaction, the

* Center for Molecular Biology, University of Heidelberg, Im Neuenheimer Feld 228, 69120 Heidelberg, Germany

C.L. Masters et al. (Eds.)
Amyloid Protein Precursor in Development,
Aging and Alzheimer's Disease
© Springer-Verlag Berlin Heidelberg 1994

proposed disturbance of zinc(II) homeostasis in AD may have an effect on conformation and stability of APP and thus influence the processes leading to amyloid βA4 protein generation.

Introduction

Alzheimer's disease (AD) is the most prevalent cause of dementia, affecting 5% of the population over the age of 65 (Terry and Katzman 1983). The structural lesions in the brain are characterized by several neuropathological changes, including neurofibrillary tangles, amyloid plaques and amyloid accumulation around blood vessels. Protein sequencing of amyloid from brains of patients with AD as well as Down's syndrome (DS) revealed the βA4 protein as the subunit of amyloid fibrils, having a length of up to 39 to 43 residues (Glenner and Wong 1984a,b; Masters et al. 1985a,b; Kang et al. 1987). The βA4 protein is derived by unidentified proteolytic processes from larger membrane-bound glycoproteins collectively known as the amyloid precursor proteins (APP; Glenner and Wong 1984b; Masters et al. 1985b; Kang et al. 1987; Sisodia et al. 1990a). This precursor of the amyloid βA4 protein is encoded by a single-copy gene on chromosome 21 (Kang et al. 1987; Goldgaber et al. 1987; Salbaum et al. 1988).

The APP gene gives rise to a range of APP products of various length. Alternative splicing of exons 7, 8 and 15 leads to primary translation products of 770, 752, 751, 733, 714, 696, 695 and 677 amino acids, respectively (for a review, see Multhaup et al. 1993a). The two largest isoforms contain a 56 amino acid domain, similar to the Kunitz family of proteinase inhibitors (KPI). In addition to APP which include the βA4 sequence, there exist amyloid precursor-related (APrP) and amyloid precursor-like proteins (APLP) with varying degrees of relatedness. APrP are derived by alternative splicing from the APP gene on chromosome 21 with 365 and 563-amino-acid products, whereas the APLP have been mapped to different chromosomes (Sprecher et al. 1993; Wasco et al. 1992). None of them contains the βA4 amyloidogenic region encoded within exons 16 and 17 of the APP gene.

After synthesis, APP undergoes post-translational modifications that include signal peptide removal, N-glycosylation, O-glycosylation, sulfation of tyrosine residues, phosphorylation and proteolytic cleavage (Ghiso et al. 1989; Buxbaum et al. 1990; Oltersdorf et al. 1990; Weidemann et al. 1989; Dyrks et al. 1988; Bunke et al. 1991). This proteolytic cleavage within the βA4 sequence prevents amyloid formation and dissects the extracellular domains of the APP from the transmembrane and cytoplasmic domains. Secreted forms of APP have been identified as protease nexin II, a serine protease inhibitor (Oltersdorf et al. 1989; Van Nostrand et al. 1989). The precise site of cleavage by α-secretase (Esch et al. 1990) was determined to be C-terminal to the βA4-lysine residue 16 (APP$_{695}$ residue 612). The two fragments produced are secreted APP and an 83-amino acid fragment that remains associated with the membrane (Weidemann et al. 1989; Esch et al. 1990; Sisodia et al. 1990b; Younkin 1991).

An alternative pathway, in contrast, generates N-terminal fragments of APP lacking βA4 and C-terminal peptides containing βA4 (Seubert et al. 1993; Estus et al. 1992). Additionally, soluble βA4-like peptides have been identified in cell cultures, cerebrospinal fluid and plasma obtained from normal and AD patients (Shoji et al. 1992; Haass et al. 1992; Seubert et al. 1992). Primary structure analysis indicated that this βA4-like peptide resembles the amyloid protein extracted from amyloid depositions around blood vessels, identified as βA4 1–40 (Prelli et al. 1988; Busciglio et al. 1993). The significance of soluble βA4-like peptides for an understanding of the mechanism and the pathogenesis of amyloid formation within the neuropil, the perikarya of neurons and their neuritic processes remains to be elucidated. At these sites the release of spontaneously aggregating βA4 from its precursor is likely to occur having a length of up to 39–43 residues. One proposed mechanism of amyloid deposition includes an as yet unidentified chymotrypsin-like mast cell protease that generates the N-terminus of βA4 as the initiating step (Nelson et al. 1993). After membrane damage a second proteolytic event yields the variable C-terminus of βA4 (Dyrks et al. 1988, 1992).

Until now, neither the processing of APP to βA4 nor the genesis of the amyloid deposits has been precisely defined, so that the characteristics and the risk factors affecting the deposition of βA4 remain key questions in the pathogenesis of AD. Compelling evidence for the central role that APP and its pathologic breakdown product βA4 must play in the pathogenesis of AD has been provided by mutations at different positions of the βA4 region. These pathogenic mutations in the APP locus cause familial AD (St George-Hyslop et al. 1987).

Functional Association Between APP and the Extracellular Matrix (ECM)

Because it has been suggested that APP is a cell surface receptor (Kang et al. 1987; Dyrks et al. 1988) involved in cell (CAM) and substrate adhesion (SAM; Schubert et al. 1991; Shivers et al. 1988), and thus crucial in the brain for neuronal plasticity, we began to analyze which part of APP might be responsible for this CAM and SAM activity.

The first binding site that we searched for was that for heparin because APP secreted from PC12 cells is able to bind to heparin. Since heparin and its functional equivalent heparan sulfate are quite similar, APP may be able to interact with heparin-like heparansulfateproteoglycans (HSPGs), a property common to adhesion molecules belonging to the CAM and SAM families (Schubert et al. 1989; Narindrasorasak et al. 1991). Before describing the experiments that led to the discovery of a very strong heparin binding site within the APP sequence, I will discuss why I consider this binding to be of interest in regard to APP function and AD.

First, the earliest and diffuse or amorphous βA4 amyloid depositions colocalize with heparan sulfate accumulations, suggesting an interation between HSPGs and βA4 or, more likely, between HSPGs and APP (Snow et al. 1990). APP-HSPG complexes in neuronal cell interactions would be expected to play an integral role in development of the nervous system, similar to laminin-HSPG complexes (Sandrock and Metthew 1987; Davies et al. 1987).

Second, heparin of HSPGs are obligatory for the activity of the heparin-binding fibroblast growth factor (FGF) family (Kan et al. 1993). Consistent with the function of binding of heparin of FGFs it could well be that the binding of proteoglycans protects APP from degradation (Damon et al. 1989). Moreover, binding to proteoglycan has been thought to be important in providing a matrix-bound or cell surface-bound reservoir of growth factors (Yayon et al. 1991). Additionally, binding to glycosaminoglycan might change the conformation of APP, resulting in binding to molecules that are not recognized in the absence of heparin, as has been previously reported for bFGF (Yayon et al. 1991).

Third, further evidence for the physiological importance of heparin binding is given by the demonstration that heparin or heparan sulfate regulate N-CAM-mediated cell–cell or cell–substratum interactions through a heparin binding domain (Cole and Glaser 1986; Cole et al. 1986; Kallapur and Akeson 1992). Specific and high affinity interactions between heparin binding domains of proteins and the matrix HSPG may regulate the anchoring of heparin binding proteins in the matrix (Heremans et al. 1990). In regard to APP, its involvement in the mediation of cell adhesion is supported by reports of treatment of primary cortical cell cultures with heparin; their cellular adhesiveness decreases while mRNA level for APP increases as a compensatory effect (Octave et al. 1989).

Fourth, APP has been localized to the extracellular matrix of R14 cells when examined by immunoelectron microscopic techniques (Klier et al. 1990). There is also increasing evidence that APP may be involved in the formation and maintenance of synapses (Schubert et al. 1991; Shivers et al. 1988; Doyle et al. 1990). In analogy to fibronectin, I postulate that one possible role of an APP interaction with heparin could be in mediating the transduction of the signals that neurites are able to bind free sites on HSPG components of the extracellular matrix (Doyle et al. 1990).

Identification of the Major APP Species
in Rat Brain as APP$_{695}$

To identify the major neuronal APP isoform, an efficient method to purify APP from rat brain was established. Affinity chromatography on heparin Sepharose CL6B and lentil lectin-Sepharose after differential centrifugation and ion exchange chromatography on DEAE-Sepharose represent the four-step procedure that was worked out to isolate sufficient amounts of homogeneous protein for

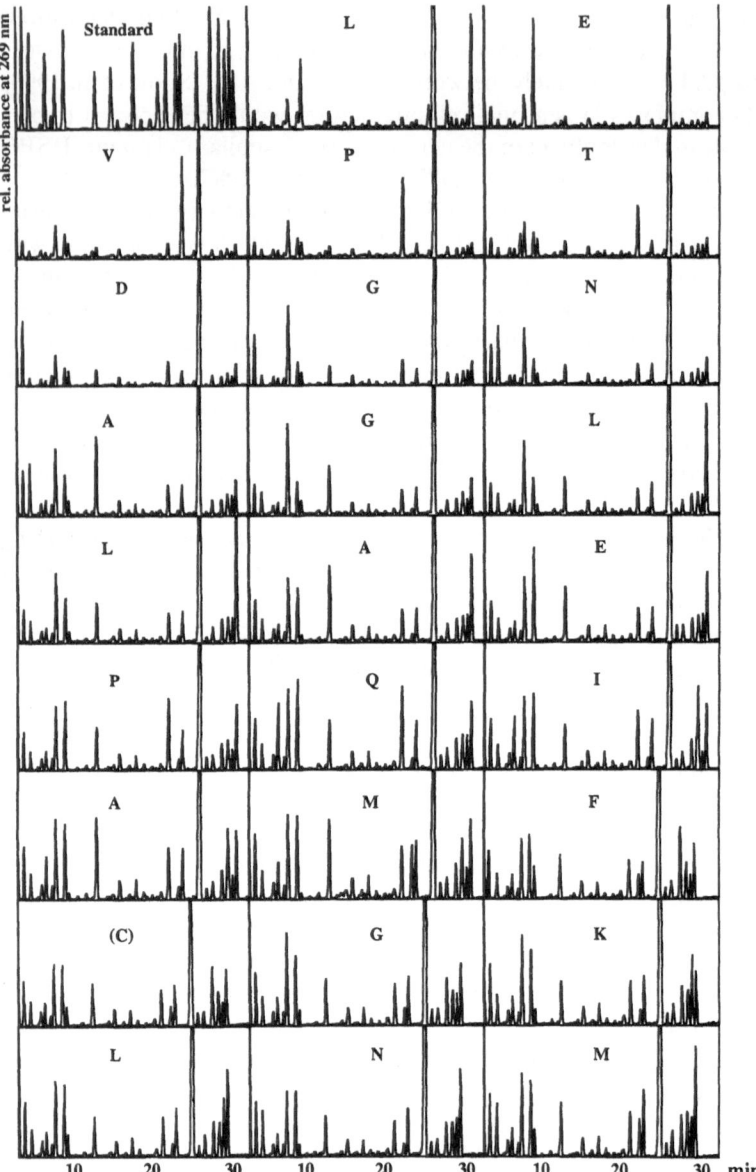

Fig. 1. N-terminal amino acid sequence analysis of APP purified from rat brain. HPLC chromatograms of the standard and the N-terminal 26 amino acid residues of APP represent 50 pmol of rat APP in Edman degradation in step 1. The cysteine in step 21 predicted by the c-DNA sequence (Kang et al. 1987) could not be detected under the conditions used

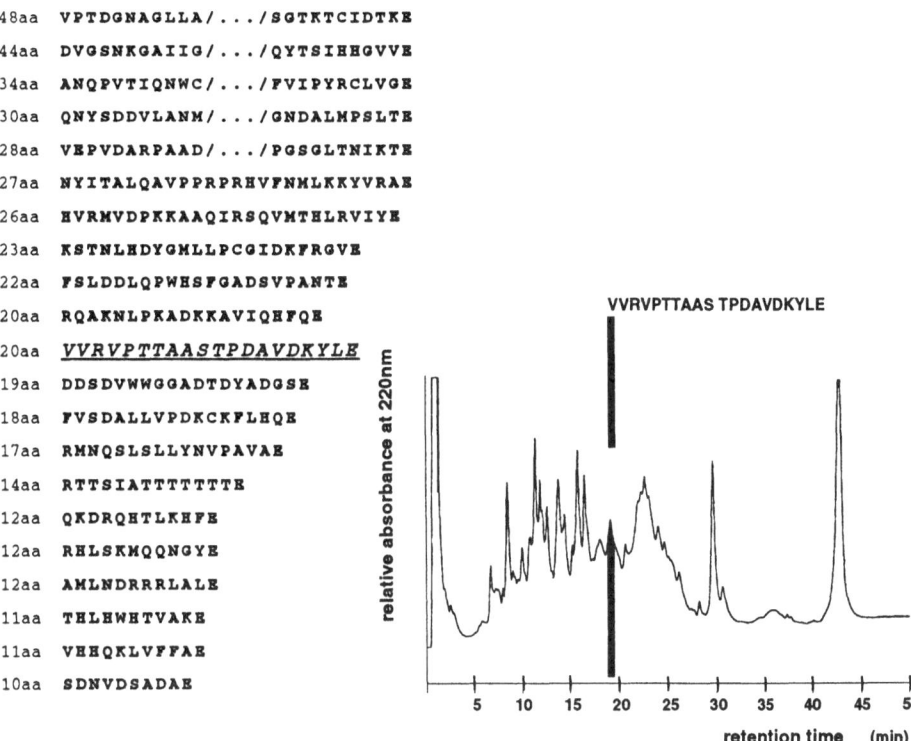

```
48aa  VPTDGNAGLLA/.../SGTKTCIDTKE
44aa  DVGSNKGAIIG/.../QYTSIHHGVVE
34aa  ANQPVTIQNWC/.../FVIPYRCLVGE
30aa  QNYSDDVLANM/.../GNDALMPSLTE
28aa  VEPVDARPAAD/.../PGSGLTNIKTE
27aa  NYITALQAVPPRPRHVFNMLKKYVRAE
26aa  EVRMVDPKKAAQIRSQVMTELRVIYE
23aa  KSTNLEDYGMLLPCGIDKFRGVE
22aa  FSLDDLQPWHSFGADSVPANTE
20aa  RQAKNLPKADKKAVIQHFQE
20aa  VVRVPTTAASTPDAVDKYLE
19aa  DDSDVWWGGADTDYADGSE
18aa  FVSDALLVPDKCKFLHQE
17aa  RMNQSLSLLYNVPAVAE
14aa  RTTSIATTTTTTTE
12aa  QKDRQHTLKEFE
12aa  RHLSKMQQNGYE
12aa  AMLNDRRRLALE
11aa  THLHWHTVAKE
11aa  VEEQKLVFFAE
10aa  SDNVDSADAE
```

VVRVPTTAAS TPDAVDKYLE

relative absorbance at 220nm

retention time   (min)

Fig. 2. Identification of the rat brain APP as APP$_{695}$ by sequence analysis of endo glu-C fragments. HPLC elution and sequence of the junction peptide representing APP$_{695}$ residues 286–305, with a list of theoretically expected endo glu-C fragments of APP$_{695}$ with more than 9 amino acids

amino acid sequence analyses, molecular weight determinations and binding study analyses subsequent to radio-iodination.

To document the purity of a typical preparation, the chromatograms of the N-terminal amino microsequence analysis of rat brain APP are shown in Figure 1. The apparent molecular weight of these transmembrane APP molecules was determined to be 105 kd.

The following experiments identified the purified rat brain APP as transmembrane APP$_{695}$. Sequencing of APP peptides obtained by digestion of purified rat brain APP with endo glu-C (Fig. 2) reveals the presence of a peptide (junction peptide) corresponding to residues 286–305 of APP$_{695}$, which is only expected to be generated from APP$_{695}$. Because this peptide, which can only be generated from APP$_{695}$ and not from APP$_{751}$ and APP$_{770}$, is found in roughly equal molar amounts to peptides derived from regions common to all known forms of APP, the majority of rat brain APP is likely to be APP$_{695}$.

This conclusion is also supported by the fact that we did not find peptides derived from the domains which are only present in APP$_{751}$ and APP$_{770}$ and are absent in APP$_{695}$. We were also able to isolate a tryptic peptide derived from

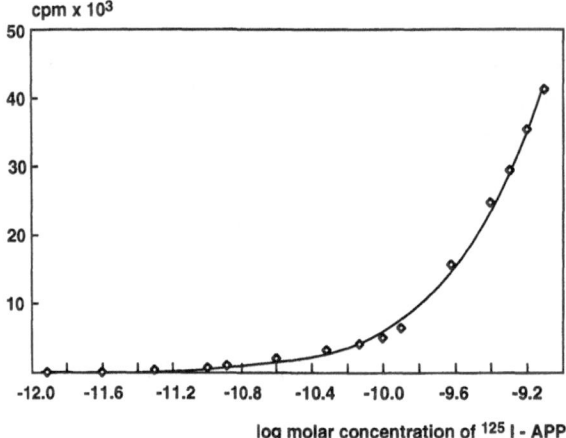

Fig. 3. Equilibrium measurement of binding of APP to heparin. Specific binding was determined by the incubation of increasing concentrations of radioiodinated APP with heparin-Sepharose. Values are corrected for non-specific binding to Sepharose CL-6B. Data represent mean values of independent experiments

the transmembrane domain starting with residue 625 of APP_{695}. Because this peptide was present in roughly equimolar amounts to the junction peptide, we conclude that the APP purified from rat brain corresponds to the transmembrane form of APP_{695}.

Characterization of a Strong Heparin Binding Site of APP_{695}

A solid phase binding assay based on heparin Sepharose was used to study the properties of heparin binding to APP. The binding occurs very rapidly with a half-life of about 8 minutes at 4 °C and maximal binding is reached after approximately 30 minutes. Equilibrium measurements of APP binding show a concentration dependency over a range of 10^{-9} to 10^{-11} M (Fig. 3).

The dissociation constant derived from Scatchard transformation is 3×10^{-10} M for heparin binding to APP. This is in good agreement with Kd values obtained by analysis of the binding of heparin to membranes isolated from LX-1 cells (Bilozur and Biswas 1990).

Based on the primary amino acid sequence of the heparin binding domain of N-CAM (Cole and Akeson 1989), a putative region of APP for heparin binding was identified in the carbohydrate domain of APP. The carbohydrate domain of APP corresponding to amino acid residues 290 to 596 of APP_{695} (Kang et al. 1987) includes a basic region of 22 amino acids (aa 316–337 in APP_{695}) with homology to the heparin binding site of NCAM. A synthetic peptide covering residues 316–337 of APP_{695} was prepared and named HP-1. This stretch of amino acids is conserved between human, mouse and rat APP and shares strong

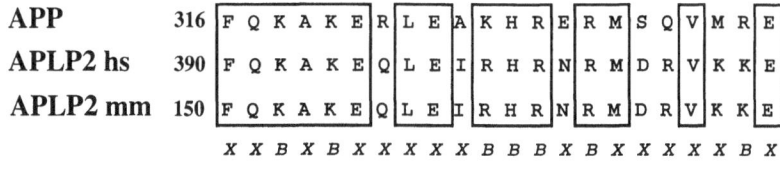

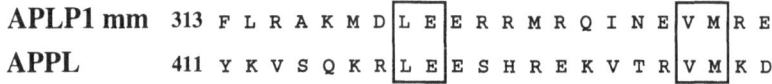

Fig. 4. Homology of the heparin binding region of APP. APP sequence is conserved between human (hs), mouse (mm) and rat. Residues 316–337 represent the heparin binding peptide in comparison to the homologous regions of the APLP1 and APLP2 sequences (Sprecher et al. 1993; Wasco et al. 1992; Vidal et al. 1992). Amino acid identity is boxed, and single letter abbreviations are used for the derived heparin binding consensus sequence (Cole and Akeson 1989), where *B* denotes the positively charged residues and *X* all others. APLP1 and Drosophila APPL might show less strong heparin binding because of the reduced homology to the consensus sequence

homology with human and mouse APLP2 (Kang et al. 1987; Sprecher et al. 1993; Shivers et al. 1988; Yamada et al. 1987; Vidal et al. 1992), but is only partially conserved in the APPL Drosophila homologue as residues 411–432 (Rosen et al. 1989) and in the APLP-1 mouse homologue as residues 313–334 (Wasco et al. 1992; Fig. 4).

Binding of [^{35}S] heparin to APP and HP-1 containing the putative binding site was demonstrated under isotonic conditions in dot blot assays. Heparin binding could be inhibited in the presence of a 50-fold molar excess of unlabelled heparin added prior to application of labelled heparin to the incubation buffer, as well as by adding the same molar excess of peptide HP-1 to the incubation buffer.

Zinc(II) Modulates Heparin Binding of APP$_{695}$

APP purified from rat brain was found to bind zinc(II) and a putative Zn^{2+} binding site was identified by endoproteinase Lys-C digestion of a fusion protein of APP expressed in *E. coli* (Multhaup et al. 1993b). The digestion fragment eluting from zinc(II) charged chelating Sepharose revealed that the zinc binding commenced at residue 179 of APP$_{695}$. Further studies of synthetic peptides showed the zinc binding site to be confined to amino acid residues 181–188 encoded by exon 5. This sequence represents one of the consensus patterns of amyloidogenic glycoprotein signatures given by the computer program "Prosite" (Bairoch 1992). It is highly evolutionary conserved among all members of the APP and APLP family.

One of the functional significances of zinc(II) binding was found to lie in the modulation of APP heparin affinity. Surface plasmon resonance revealed this

rel. RU

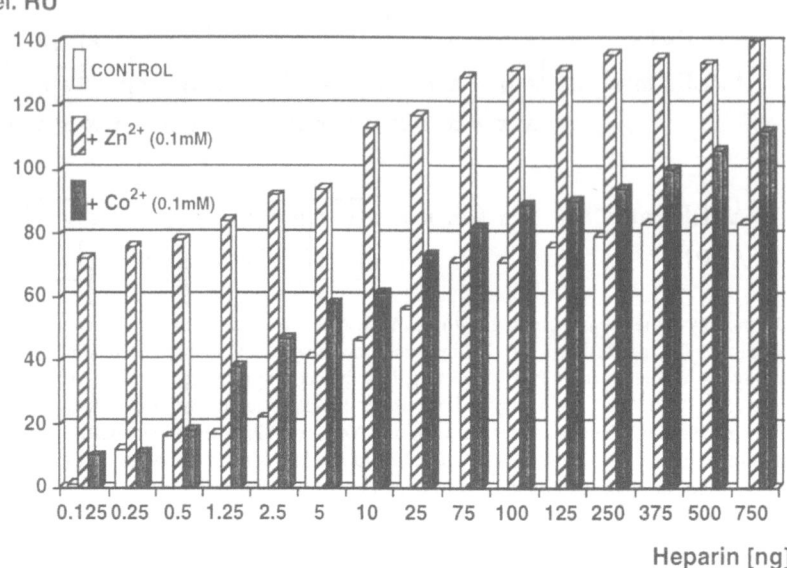

Fig. 5. Analysis of APP heparin binding by surface plasmon resonance (Malmquist 1993). Binding of increasing heparin concentrations was analyzed at fixed zinc (striped bars) and cobalt (black bars) concentrations. Results are expressed as an increase of relative response units (RU) in heparin binding upon addition of heparin and metal ions. The effect induced by calcium and magnesium did not result in an increase of response units in comparison to controls

effect to be specific for zinc compared to Ca^{2+}, Mg^{2+}, and Co^{2+} and was most evident at low heparin concentrations (Fig. 5).

Discussion

The described location of a heparin binding site of APP in an exposed hydrophilic domain with carbohydrate attachment sites is consistent with a role of APP in mediating the interaction of cells to matrix and between cells. Such a function for APP would be consistent with the biological effects of heparin, which include regulation of receptor function, regulation of growth and differentiation, regulation of proteinase and growth factors and modulation of cell–cell and cell–matrix adhesion (Ruoslahti 1988). Because structurally, heparin and heparan sulfate are components of glycosaminoglycan chains with proteoglycans which are present in cell membranes, extracellular matrices and basement membranes, binding of APP to heparin-like molecules would be expected to regulate APP bioavailability and distribution on these sites. Any alteration in this heparin binding could affect the biological activity of APP.

The functional significance of APP binding to heparin may therefore be related to the adhesion of the cell expressing APP to other cells and to glycosaminoglycans of the extracellular matrix. Because the extracellular matrix not only serves a mechanical role in supporting and maintaining tissue structure but also modulates a multitude of cell functions such as development, migration and proliferation, APP as a heparin-binding molecule may act as a mediator of these functions.

In brain, in the early stages of development, APP_{695} is predominant (Tanzi et al. 1987; Neve et al. 1988). While cell migration and neurite extension is taking place, one of the major functions of APP_{695} could be performed by the heparin binding site interacting with the extracellular matrix and membrane-bound heparan sulfate proteoglycans of target cells.

In regard to the amyloid pathology of AD, it is interesting that presence of immunoreactive markers for proteoglycans in deposits of amyloid $\beta A4$ protein (Snow et al. 1990) may suggest a disturbance of the cell–cell and cell–matrix adhesion events mediated through APP. Such a disturbance could result in a constitutive signal to neuronal cells towards, for example, neurite extension, which may contribute to amyloid formation if more APP is produced and transported to the site of amyloid deposition.

It has been shown that zinc(II) binding may influence APP processing (Bush et al. 1992). In this study, APP enriched by heparin affinity chromatography from plasma of patients with AD and controls was found to be more stable if isolated from the patients. Addition of zinc(II) removed the differences of the APP levels between the two groups (Bush et al. 1992). Because an abnormality of zinc(II) metabolism in AD and Down's syndrome has been reported (Franceschi et al. 1988; Napolitano et al. 1990), understanding the function of the zinc(II) binding site on APP may be of great importance to an understanding of the mechanism of amyloid formation in AD.

Recently, zinc, aluminium and iron have also been shown to promote the aggregation of the $\beta A4$ peptide *in vitro*, with zinc as the most effective ion under physiological conditions (Mantyh et al. 1993). These findings suggest that zinc could play a role *in vivo*, both by modulating the function of the $\beta A4$ amyloid protein precursor and by promoting the initial aggregation of $\beta A4$, which could accelerate the pathological process dramatically at an early step of amyloidogenesis.

References

Bairoch A, University of Geneva, Switzerland (1992) PC/Gene Release 6.7 InelliGenetics, Inc., Mountain View, CA 94040

Bilozur ME, Biswas C (1990) Identification and characterization of heparan sulfate-binding proteins from human lung carcinoma cells. J Biol Chem 265:19697–19703

Bunke D, Mönning U, Kypta RM, Courtneidge SA, Masters CL, Beyreuther K (1991) Tyrosine phosphorylation of the cytoplasmic domain of Alzheimer amyloid protein precursors. In: Iqbal K, McLachlan KDRC, Winblad B, Wisniewski, HM (eds.) Alzheimer's disease: basic mechanisms, diagnosis and therapeutic strategies. John Wiley Sons, New York, pp 229–235

Busciglio J, Gabuzda DH, Matsudaira P, Yankner BA (1993) Generation of beta-amyloid in the secretory pathway in neuronal and non-neuronal cells. Proc Natl Acad Sci USA 90: 2092–2096

Bush AI, Whyte S, Thomas LD, Williamson TG, Van-Tiggelen CJ, Currie J, Small DH, Moir RD, Li QX, Rumble B, Beyreuther K, Masters CL (1992) An abnormality of plasma amyloid protein precursor in Alzheimer's disease. Ann Neurol 32:57–65

Buxbaum JD, Gandy SE, Cicchetti P, Ehrlich ME, Czernik AJ, Fracasso RP, Ramabhadran TV, Unterbeck AJ, Greengard P (1990) Processing of Alzheimer beta/A4 amyloid precursor protein: modulation by agents that regulate protein phosphorylation. Proc Natl Acad Sci USA 87:6003–6006

Cole GJ, Glaser L (1986) A heparin-binding domain from NCAM is involved in neural cell-substratum adhesion. J Cell Biol 102:403–412

Cole GJ, Akeson R (1989) Identification of a heparin binding domain of the neural cell adhesion molecule N-CAM using synthetic peptides. Neuron 2:1157–1165

Cole GJ, Loewy A, Glaser L (1986) Neuronal cell–cell adhesion depends on interactions of NCAM with heparin-like molecules. Nature 320:445–447

Damon DH, Lobb RR, D'Amore PA, Wagner JA (1989) Heparin potentiates the action of acidic fibroblast growth factor by prolonging its biological half-life. J Cell Physiol 138:221–226

Davies GE, Klier FG, Engvall E, Cornbrooks C, Varon S, Manthorpe M (1987) Association of laminin with heparan and chondroitin sulfate-bearing proteoglycans in neurite-promoting factor complexes from rat Schwannoma cells. Neurochem Res 12:909–921

Doyle E, Bruce M, Breen KC, Smith DC, Anderton B, Regan CM (1990) Intraventricular infusion of antisera to the Alzheimer amyloid precursor protein impairs the acquisition of a passive avoidance paradigm in the rat. Neurosci Lett 11:97–102

Duncan MW, Marini AM, Watters R, Kopin IJ, Markey SP (1992) Zinc, a neurotoxin to cultured neurons, contaminates cycad flour prepared by traditional guamanian methods. J Neurosci 12:152315–152337

Dyrks T, Weidemann A, Multhaup G, Salbaum JM, Lemaire HG, Kang J, Müller-Hill B, Masters CL, Beyreuther K (1988) Identification, transmembrane orientation and biogenesis of the amyloid A4 Precursor of Alzheimer's disease. EMBO J 7:949–957

Dyrks T, Dyrks E, Hartmann T, Masters CL, Beyreuther K (1992) Amyloidogenicity of βA4 and βA4-bearing amyloid protein precursor fragments by metal-catalyzed oxidation. J Biol Chem 267:18210–18217

Esch GS, Keim PS, Beattie EC, Blacher RW, Culwell AR, Oltersdorf T, McClure D, Ward PJ (1990) Cleavage of amyloid β peptide during constitutive processing of its precursor. Science 248:1122–1124

Estus S, Golde TE, Kunishita T, Blades D, Lowery D, Eisen M, Usiak M, Qu XM, Tabira T, Greenberg BD, Younkin SG (1992) Potentially amyloidogenic, carboxyl-terminal derivatives of the amyloid protein precursor. Science 255:726–728

Franceschi C, Chiricolo M, Licastro F, Zannotti M, Masi M, Mocchegiani E, Fabris N (1988) Oral zinc supplementation in Down's syndrome: restoration of thymic endocrine activity and of some immune defects. J Mental Deficiency Res 32:169–181

Ghiso J, Tagliavini F, Timmers WF, Frangione B (1989) Alzheimer's disease amyloid precursor protein is present in senile plaques and cerebrospinal fluid: immunohistochemical and biochemical characterization. Biochem Biophys Res Commun 163:430–437

Glenner GG, Wong CW (1984a) Alzheimer's disease: initial report of the purification and characterization of a novel cerebrovascular amyloid protein. Biochem Biophys Res Commun 120:885–890

Glenner GG, Wong CW (1984b) Alzheimer's disease and Down's syndrome sharing of a unique cerebrovascular amyloid fibril protein. Biochem Biophys Res Commun 122:1131–1135

Goldgaber D, Lerman MI, McBride OW, Saffiotti U, Gajdusek DC (1987) Characterization and chromosomal localization of a cDNA encoding brain amyloid of Alzheimer's disease. Science 235:877–880

Haass C, Schlossmacher MG, Hung AY, Vigo-Pelfrey C, Mellon A, Ostaszewski BL, Lieberburg I, Koo EH, Schenk D, Teplow DB, Selkoe D (1992) Amyloid β-peptide is produced by cultured cells during normal metabolism. Nature 359:322–325

Heremans A, De Cock B, Cassiman JJ, Van den Berghe H, David G (1990) The core protein of the matrix-associated heparan sulfate proteoglycan binds to fibronectin. J Biol Chem 265:8716–8724

Kallapur SG, Akeson RA (1992) The neural cell adhesion molecule (NCAM) heparin binding domain binds to cell surfate heparan sulfate proteoglycans. J Neurosci Res 33:538–548

Kan M, Wang F, Xu J, Crabb JW, Hou J, McKeehan WL (1993) An essential heparin-binding domain in the fibroblast growth factor receptor kinase. Science 259:1918–1921

Kang J, Lemaire H-G, Unterbeck A, Salbaum JM, Masters CL, Grzeschik K-H, Multhaup G, Beyreuther K, Müller-Hill B (1987) The precursor of Alzheimer's disease amyloid A4 protein resembles a cell surface receptor. Nature 325:733–736

Klier FG, Cole G, Stallup W, Schubert D (1990) Amyloid beta-protein precursor is associated with extracellular matrix. Brain Res 515:336–342

Malmquist M (1993) Biospecific interaction analysis using biosensor technology. Nature 361:186–187

Mantyh PW, Ghilardi JR, Rogers S, Demaster E, Allen CJ, Stimson ER, Maggio JE (1993) Aluminium, iron, and zinc ions promote aggregation of physiological concentrations of β-amyloid peptide. J Neurochem 61:1171–1174

Masters CL, Multhaup G, Simms G, Pottgiesser J, Martins RN, Beyreuther K (1985a) Neuronal origin of a cerebral amyloid: neurofibrillary tangles of Alzheimer's disease contain the same protein as the amyloid of plaque cores and blood vessels. EMBO J 4:2757–2763

Masters CL, Simms G, Weinman NA, Multhaup G, McDonald BL, Beyreuther K (1985b) Amyloid plaque core protein in Alzheimer disease and Down syndrome. Proc Natl Acad Sci 82:4245–4249

Multhaup G, Masters CL, Beyreuther K (1993a) A molecular approach to Alzheimer's disease. Biol Chem Hoppe-Seyler 374:1–8

Multhaup G, Bush AI, Moir R, Williamson TG, Small DH, Rumble B, Pollwein P, Beyreuther K, Masters CL (1993b) A novel Zinc(II) binding site modulates the function of the βA4 amyloid protein precursor of Alzheimer's disease. J Biol Chem 268:16109–16112

Napolitano G, Palka G, Grimaldi S, Giuliani C, Laglia G, Calabrese G, Satta MA, Neri G, Monaco F (1990) Growth delay in Down syndrome and zinc sulphate supplementation. Am J Med Genet Suppl 7:63–65

Narindrasorasak S, Lowery D, Gonzales-DeWhitt P, Poorman RA, Greenberg B, Kisilevsky R (1991) High affinity interactions between the Alzheimer's β-amyloid precursor proteins and the basement membrane forms of heparan sulfate proteoglycan. J Biol Chem 266: 12878–12883

Nelson RB, Siman R, Iqbal MA, Huntington P (1993) Identification of a chymotrypsin-like mast cell protease in rat brain capable of generating the N-terminus of the Alzheimer amyloid β-protein. J Neurochem 61:567–577

Neve RL, Finch EA, Dawes LR (1988) Expression of the Alzheimer amyloid precursor gene transcripts in the human brain. Neuron 1:669–677

Octave JN, deSauvage F, Maloteaux JM (1989) Modification of neuronal cell adhesion affects the genetic expression of the A4 amyloid peptide precursor. Brain Res 486:369–371

Oltersdorf T, Fritz LC, Schenk DB, Lieberburg I, Johnson-Wood KL, Beatti EC, Ward PJ, Blacher RW, Dovey HF, Sinha S (1989) The secreted form of the Alzheimer's amyloid precursor protein with the Kunitz domain is protease nexin-II. Nature 341:144–147

Oltersdorf T, Ward PJ, Henriksson T, Beattie EC, Neve R, Lieberburg I, Fritz LC (1990) The Alzheimer amyloid precursor protein. Identification of a stable intermediate in the biosynthetic/degradative pathway. J Biol Chem 265:4492–4497

Prelli F, Castano E, Glenner GG, Frangione B (1988) Differences between vascular and plaque core amyloid in Alzheimer's disease. J Neurochem 51:648–651

Rosen DR, Martin-Morris L, Luo L, White K (1989) A Drosophila gene encoding a protein resembling the human beta-amyloid protein precursor. Proc Natl Acad Sci USA 86:2478–2482

Ruoslahti E (1988) Structure and biology of proteoglycans. Annu Rev Cell Biol 4:229–255

Sandrock AW Jr, Metthew WD (1987) Identification of a peripheral nerve neurite growth-promoting activity by development and use of an *in vitro* bioassay. Proc Natl Acad Sci USA 84:6934–6938

Salbaum JM, Weidemann A, Lemaire H-G, Masters CL, Beyreuther K (1988) The promoter of Alzheimer's disease amyloid A4 precursor gene. EMBO J 7:2807–2813

Schubert D, LaCorbiere M, Saitoh T, Cole G (1989) Characterization of an amyloid beta precursor protein that binds heparin and contains tyrosine sulfate. Proc Natl Acad Sci USA 86:2066–2069

Schubert W, Prior R, Weidemann A, Dircksen H, Multhaup G, Masters CL, Beyreuther K (1991) Localization of Alzheimer βA4 amyloid precursor protein at central and peripheral synaptic sites. Brain Res 563:184–194

Seubert P, Vigo-Pelfrey C, Esch F, Lee M, Dovey H, Davies D, Sinha S, Schlossmacher M, Whaley J, Swindlehurst C, McCormack R, Wolfert R, Selkoe D, Lieberburg I, Schenk D (1992) Isolation and quantification of soluble Alzheimer's β-peptide from biological fluids. Nature 359:325–327

Seubert P, Oltersdorf T, Lee MG, Barbour R, Blomquist C, Davies DL, Bryant K, Fritz LC, Galasko D, Thal LJ, Lieberburg I, Schenk D (1993) Secretion of β-amyloid precursor cleaved at the amino terminus of the β-amyloid peptide. Nature 361:260–263

Shivers BD, Hilbich C, Multhaup G, Salbaum M, Beyreuther K, Seeburg PH (1988) Alzheimer's disease amyloidogenic glycoprotein: Expression pattern in rat brain suggests role in cell contact. EMBO J 7:1365–1370

Shoji M, Golde TE, Ghiso J, Cheung TT, Estus S, Shaffer LM, Cai X-D, McKay DM, Tintner R, Frangione B, Younkin, SG (1992) Production of the Alzheimer β protein by normal proteolytic processing. Science 258:126–129

Sisodia SS, Koo EH, Beyreuther K, Unterbeck A, Price DL (1990a) Evidence that β-amyloid protein in Alzheimer's disease is not derived by normal processing. Science 248:492–495

Sisodia SS, Koo EH, Beyreuther K, Unterbeck A, Price DL (1990b) Evidence that β-amyloid protein in Alzheimer's disease is not derived by normal processing. Science 248:492–495

Snow AD, Mar H, Nochlin D, Sekiguchi RT, Kimata K, Koike Y, Wight TN (1990) Early accumulation of heparan sulfate in neurons and in the beta-amyloid protein-containing lesions of Alzheimer's disease and Down's syndrome. Am J Pathol 137:1253–1270

Snow AD, Mar H, Nochlin D, Sekiguchi K, Kimata Y, Koike TN, Wight TN (1990) Early accumulation of heparan sulfate in neurons and in the β-amyloid protein containing lesions of Alzheimer's disease and Down's syndrome. Neurobiol Aging 11:211

Sprecher CA, Grant FJ, Grimm G, O'Hara PJ, Norris F, Norris K, Foster DC (1993) Molecular cloning of the cDNA for a human amyloid precursor protein homolog: evidence for a multigene family. Biochem 32:4481–4486

St. George-Hyslop PH, Tanzi RE, Polinsky RJ, Haines JL, Nee L, Watkins PC, Myers RH, Feldman RG, Pollen D, Drachman D, Growdon J, Bruni A, Foncin J-F, Salmon D, Frommelt P, Amaducci L, Sorbi S, Piacenti S, Stewart GD, Hobbs WJ, Conneally PM, Gusella JF (1987) The genetic defect causing familial Alzheimer's disease maps on chromosome 21. Science 235:885–890

Tanzi RE, Gusella JF, Watkins PC, Burns GAP, St.George-Hyslop P, vanKeuren ML, Patterson D, Pagan S, Kurnit DM, Neve RL (1987) Amyloid beta protein gene: cDNA, mRNA distribution, and genetic linkage near the Alzheimer's locus. Science 235:880–884

Terry RD, Katzman R (1983) Senile dementia of the Alzheimer type. Ann Neurol 114:497–506

Van Nostrand WE, Wagner SL, Suzuki M, Choi BH, Farrow JS, Geddes JW, Cotman CW, Cunningham DD (1989) Protease nexin-II, a potent antichymotrypsin, shows identity to amyloid β-protein precursor. Nature 341:546–549

Vidal F, Blangy A, Rassoulzadegan M, Cuzin F (1992) A murine sequence-specific DNA binding protein shows extensive local similarities to the amyloid precursor protein. Biochem Biophys Res Commun 189:1336–1341

Wasco W, Bupp K, Magendantz M, Gusella JF, Tanzi RE, Solomon F (1992) Identification of a mouse brain cDNA that encodes a protein related to the Alzheimer disease-associated amyloid beta protein precursor. Proc Natl Acad Sci USA 89:10758–10762

Weidemann A, König G, Bunke D, Fischer P, Salbaum JM, Masters CL, Beyreuther K (1989) Identification, biogenesis and localization of precursors of Alzheimer's disease A4 amyloid protein. Cell 57:115–126

Yamada T, Sasaki H, Furuya H, Miyata T, Goto I, Sakaki Y (1987) Complementary DNA for the mouse homolog of the human amyloid beta protein precursor. Biochem Biophys Res Commun 149:665–671

Yayon A, Klagsbrun M, Esko JD, Leder P, Ornitz DM (1991) Cell-surface, heparin-like molecules are required for binding of basic fibroblast growth factor to its high affinity receptor. Cell 64:841–848

Younkin SG (1991) Processing of the Alzheimer's disease βA4 amyloid protein precursor (APP). Brain Pathol 1:253–262

The Biological Function
of Amyloid β/A4 Protein Precursor

T. Saitoh*, J.-M. Roch, L.-W. Jin, H. Ninomiya, D. A. C. Otero,
K. Yamamoto, and *E. Masliah*

Abstract

Amyloid β/A4 protein precursor (APP) is secreted into medium by most cultured cells and can function as an autocrine factor. To study the biological function of secreted forms of APP (sAPP) on neurons, we used a clonal CNS neuronal line B103 which synthesizes no detectable levels of APP. When B103 cells were plated at a low density in a defined serum-free medium, neurite outgrowth was promoted by the conditioned medium of APP-695 over-producing cells and by the bacteria-produced sAPP-695 (named KB75). A series of peptides having sequences between Ala-319 and Met-335 of APP-695 also stimulated neurite outgrowth of B103 cells. The sequence of five amino acids, RERMS (APP 328-332) within this stretch of sequence, was the shortest active peptide. Binding assay using ^{125}l-labeled APP 17-mer peptide corresponding to Ala-319 to Met-335 of APP-695 as a ligand demonstrated specific and saturable cell-surface binding sites which are extractable with detergent. These data indicate that sAPP induces neurite extension through a cell surface binding and that the RERMS domain represents the active site responsible for this function. The RERMS-containing APP peptide also exhibited neuronal survival activity on rat primary cortical neuronal culture. In addition, the infusion of the trophic APP peptide into rat brain ventricles increased the synaptic density in the frontoparietal cortex and enhanced the memory retention. These results firmly establish the neurotrophic properties of sAPP and raise the possibility that small APP peptides or non-peptidic compounds mimicking their activity may be used therapeutically for the improvement of memory performance.

Introduction

The amyloid β/A4 protein (Aβ) is the major component of both cerebrovascular and plaque amyloid deposits (Glenner and Wong 1984; Masters et al. 1985; Selkoe et al. 1986) found in the brain tissue of patients afflicted with Alzheimer's

* Department of Neurosciences, 0624, School of Medicine and Center for Molecular Genetics, University of California, San Diego, La Jolla, CA 92093, USA

C.L. Masters et al. (Eds.)
Amyloid Protein Precursor in Development,
Aging and Alzheimer's Disease
© Springer-Verlag Berlin Heidelberg 1994

disease (AD). The protein is derived from a membrane-spanning protein, amyloid β/A4 protein precursor (APP; Kang et al. 1987; Tanzi et al. 1987; Robakis et al. 1987; Goldgaber et al. 1987), of which at least five different forms of primary transcription products are now known. Three forms (APP-563, -751 and -770) contain a domain showing a strong homology with the protease inhibitors of the Kunitz type (KPI; Ponte et al. 1988; Tanzi et al. 1988; Kitaguchi et al. 1988; De Sauvage and Octave 1989), whereas the other forms (APP-695 and -714) do not (Kang et al. 1987; Goldgaber et al. 1987; Robakis et al. 1987; Tanzi et al. 1987; Golde et al. 1990). Subsequent studies have shown the existence of secreted forms of APP (sAPP), either in medium of cultured cells such as PC12 and fibroblasts (Schubert et al. 1989; Uéda et al. 1989; Weidemann et al. 1989) or in cerebral spinal fluid (Palmert et al. 1989; Weidemann et al. 1989; Kitaguchi et al. 1990). Since the identification of sAPP with KPI domain as protease nexin II (Van Nostrand et al. 1989; Oltersdorf et al. 1989), many reports have described biological functions for the secreted forms of APP which contain the KPI domain. These include the regulation of neurite extension (Robakis et al. 1990), a role in the blood coagulation process (Cole et al. 1990; Van Nostrand et al. 1990; Smith et al. 1990) and a role in the wound-healing process (Cunningham and Van Nostrand 1991). Little is known, however, about the physiological function of sAPP-695 which lacks KPI domain, in spite of evidence indicating that APP-695 is found almost exclusively in the brain (Neve et al. 1988; Ponte et al. 1988; Tanaka et al. 1988; König et al. 1991).

Considering that APP-695 is a brain-specific isoform of APP, one can speculate that the secreted form of APP-695 (sAPP-695) is a key molecule involved in some brain-specific mechanisms. It has been reported that the relative mRNA proportion of APP-695 to the KPI-containing forms of APP is reduced in AD (Johnson et al. 1990, Tanaka et al. 1988; Neve et al. 1990) and in behaviorally impaired aged animals (Higgins et al. 1990), although contradicting data have been reported by another group (Golde et al. 1990). Using a battery of different antibodies to various regions of APP, Cole et al. (1991) and Joachim et al. (1991) have shown that N-terminal as well as C-terminal fragments of APP accumulate in the periphery of the senile plaques. This finding probably indicates the presence of full-length APP in the swollen neurites surrounding the plaque core, which is consistent with the finding that APP undergoes fast anterograde axonal transport (Koo et al. 1989). These findings raise the possibility that N-terminal fragments of APP play a significant role in the aberrant sprouting reaction observed in the vicinity of the plaques. APP has been shown to colocalize with GAP-43 both in neuritic plaques (Masliah et al. 1992a) and growth cones (Masliah et al. 1992b), and it is proposed to be ultimately expressed at the synapses. If APP has a trophic or maintenance function in the synapses, an alteration in the processing of APP, and consequently an alteration of the concentration of secreted APP-695 in the synapses, could lead to synapse loss and neuronal death, as observed in AD. On the other hand, APP might be involved in the sprouting reactions of remaining neurons, which is also observed in AD. To determine whether or not this is the case, a full understanding of the physiological functions of APP is necessary.

As an initial attempt to study the physiological functions of APP, we used a human lung fibroblast cell line (AG2804) and applied an antisense RNA strategy to create a new cell line (A-1) that produces extremely low levels of APP and depends on the addition of exogeneous APP for a normal growth rate (Saitoh et al. 1989; Bhasin et al. 1991). This cell line A-1 was an essential tool in the functional mapping of APP. Using both APP fragments made in bacteria and chemically synthesized APP peptides, we showed that the only site of sAPP-695 involved in the stimulation of fibroblasts growth is around the RERMS sequence (APP 328-332, Kang sequence; Roch et al. 1992; Ninomiya et al. 1993). Recent studies in our laboratory have revealed that the target of the biological activity of this domain of sAPP is not limited to this particular cell line; the addition of synthetic peptides corresponding to this domain in the culture media caused significant morphological changes in rat CNS neuronal cells or primary cortical neurons from rats. Consistent with this trophic activity, APP treatment protected neurons from hypoxia-induced cell death (Mattson et al. 1993) and protected animals from ischemic damage on the spinal cord (Bowes et al. 1992). We also detected specific binding sites for the iodinated sAPP-695 fragment on rat CNS neuronal cells, presumably representing the receptor molecules for sAPP-695. Furthermore, we have evidence that *in vivo* administration of the active APP peptide into the rat brain causes significant changes in memory performance.

Results

The secreted form of APP-695 which lacks protease inhibitor domain exerts its effects on target neurons through receptor-mediated intracellular signal transduction system(s) and regulates neuronal and synaptic activity. We have developed the following assay systems to study the biological activity of APP fragments and have identified the trophic domain of sAPP-695 (Fig. 1).

Bioassay on a Fibroblast Cell Line A-1

We have established a fibroblast cell line A-1, transfected with a plasmid expressing an antisense APP RNA (Saitoh et al. 1989). This cell line produces very low levels of APP mRNA and its translation products, resulting in a slow growth rate. The growth of A-1 cells can be restored to the level of parent fibroblasts (AG2804) by addition of exogenous APP. The dependence of the growth of the cells on exogenous APP provided us with a rather simple bioassay to study the functional mapping of APP (Roch et al. 1992). Testing the activity of a series of sAPP-695 fragments obtained from our bacterial expression system on this bioassay, we have shown that at least one of the active sites of sAPP-695

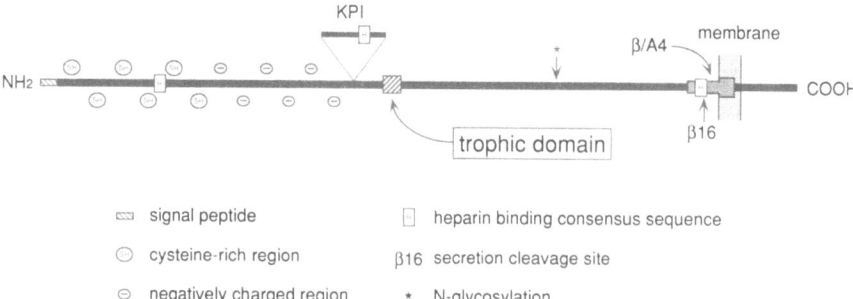

Fig. 1. Schematic presentation of APP. APP contains several important domains. The trophic domain is located in the center of the secreted N-terminal fragment. Neither putative heparine binding domains, Kunitz type protease inhibitor (KPI) domain, β/A4-protein domain, nor N-glycosylation are required for the trophic activity of APP

was localized within the 40-mer sequence (APP296-335; Roch et al. 1992). Further analyses have shown that the only active site is the pentamer sequence RERMS (APP 328-332; Ninomiya et al. 1993).

Bioassay on a Rat CNS Neuronal Cell Line B103

We found that a rat CNS neuronal cell line B103, expressing no detectable levels of APP, responds to sAPP by extending neurites. This was evaluated by blind quantification of the neurite number and length using a computer-assisted morphometric analysis. We have shown that the activity of sAPP-695 on this cell line was localized within the same pentamer sequence which was also active as a growth promoter on the A-1 fibroblast.

Bioassay on Primary Cortical Neuronal Cells from Rats

The biological activity of APP-fragments described above is not confined to specific cell lines. We found that the active peptide 17-mer (APP319-335) containing the aforementioned pentamer enhanced the survival of primary cortical neurons from rats. However, the RERMS site was necessary but not sufficient for this survival activity. Furthermore, the promoting effect of 17-mer on neurite extension, as observed for B103 cells, was also found on primary neuronal cultures.

Radioligand Binding Assay on B103 Cell Monolayer

We have been successful in finding binding sites for the iodinated APP peptide on the neuronal cell B103. The binding of [125]I-17-mer to B103 cell layer was time-dependent and saturable with a Kd value of 20 ± 5 nM and Bmax value of 80 ± 8 fmol/10^6 cells (means $\pm$ SEM of four determinations each done in triplicate). The binding was sequence-specific because unlabeled 17-mer but not reverse-sequence 17-mer could displace the binding. The bacteria-produced sAPP fragment without the active 17-mer sequence (named KB75δ) did not compete with ^{125}I-labeled 17-mer for binding or stimulated neurite extension. A peptide of sequence RMSQ (APP330-333), which partially overlaps the active sequence RERMS, at higher concentrations, could block the neurotrophic effects of both KB75 and 17-mer, although it showed no neurite extending activity in our bioassays. APP 17-mer was also found to induce the accumulation of inositol polyphosphates, suggesting that its effects are through activation of inositol phospholipid signal transduction systems.

Behavioral Assay on Water Maze

It is well established that some animals become behaviorally impaired with aging. We used old rats to evaluate the biological activity of 17-mer. Animals were trained to locate a hidden platform to escape from a water pool. After determination of behavioral performance, either the 17-mer peptide, the reverse sequence peptide or artificial cerebrospinal fluid was infused directly into ventricles (0.5 μl/hr of 1 mM solution) for two weeks, and animals were then tested in the water maze. For the test, the location of the hidden platform was changed (reverse learning paradigm). Thus, animals might remember the original position and go to the original position, or forget the original position while learning a new location. In non-impaired animals, 17-mer treatment caused the animals to go to the original position, thus prolonging the time for animals to find a new location. This 17-mer effect was not found in impaired animals. In addition, confocal microscopy study demonstrated that 17-mer increased the synaptic density in the neocortex.

How May APP be Involved in AD Pathogenesis?

The above results firmly establish the neurotrophic activity of sAPP, as well as its potential involvement in memory. What might be the significance of this activity in the pathophysiology of AD? The currently predominant hypothesis for the etiology of AD is that Aβ toxicity is responsible for neurodegeneration in this disease (Yankner et al. 1989, 1990a, 1990b; Joachim and Selkoe 1992; Kosik 1992; Hardy and Higgins 1992; Mattson et al. 1992; Citron et al. 1992; Cai et al. 1993; Pike et al. 1993). Although this is possible, for the sake of argument we would like to promote the idea that Aβ per se might not be the primary cause of the neuronal death, and hence of the dementia. It must be kept in mind that Aβ is found not only in AD patients but is also produced in normal individuals, and by the normal metabolism of cultured cells. Furthermore, in AD patients, Aβ

protein is found not only in the brain but also in peripheral tissue, although the neurodegeneration is confined to the CNS. The best evidence to date for an involvement of APP (or one of its breakdown products such as Aβ protein) in the development of AD stems from genetic data showing that some mutations in the APP gene cosegregate with the disease in some families struck by the disease (Goate et al. 1991; Murrell et al. 1991; Chartier-Harlin et al. 1991; Naruse et al. 1991; Yoshioka et al. 1991; Hendriks et al. 1992; Mullan et al. 1992). One of these mutations has been shown to result in a six-fold increase of Aβ secretion in cultured cells (Citron et al. 1992; Cai et al. 1993). However, this finding cannot account for all AD cases. In fact, some of the other mutations have been shown to result in a decrease of Aβ secretion, yet the people carrying the mutation do get AD. Therefore, the neurotoxic role of Aβ in the development of AD may not be sufficient. The release of Aβ protein by cultured cells under normal physiological conditions raises the question of how and why the Aβ peptide adopts the β-pleated amyloid conformation only in AD brains. In this respect, the interaction of the Aβ with other molecules might yield crucial information. In addition to apolipoprotein E (Strittmatter et al. 1993), one of the molecules that interact with Aβ is APP itself (Goldgaber et al. 1993). Hence, the possibility arises that trophic APP activity might be affected by the Aβ peptide. The secreted form of APP is involved in several biological mechanisms, like protease inhibition (Van Nostrand et al. 1989; Oltersdorf et al. 1989), blood coagulation (Cole et al. 1990; Van Nostrand et al. 1990; Smith et al. 1990), cell growth (Saitoh et al. 1989; Bhasin et al. 1991; Roch et al. 1992; Ninomiya et al. 1993), neurite extension (Robakis et al. 1990; Jin et al. 1992; Araki et al. 1991; Milward et al. 1992), regulation of intracellular calcium levels (Mattson et al. 1992), the memory process (Roch et al. 1993), synapse formation (Masliah et al. 1993; Roch et al. 1993) and finally neuronal survival (Bowes et al. 1992; Mattson et al. 1993). All these activities could be influenced by the binding of the Aβ peptide to the N-terminal region of APP. In spite of the six-fold increase of Aβ secretion resulting from the Swedish mutation, it is not clear how the other mutations can lead to dementia. There is no direct evidence for an obvious alteration of APP metabolism in AD. In particular, the balance between the two major pathways of APP, one leading to the "physiological" secretion of the N-terminal portion and the other leading to the secretion of the Aβ peptide, does not show a gross alteration in AD. Therefore, it is possible that other factors mediating APP activity and compartmentalization might be important in the development of AD. At this point, it has to be kept in mind that the best linkage to AD is a marker on chromosome 14, whereas the APP mutation is rather rare (Crawford et al. 1991; Schellenberg et al. 1991; Tanzi et al. 1992). In brief, APP and the Aβ protein play key roles in AD pathology, although they might not be the primary and direct cause of the neurodegeneration. While the Aβ peptide might be neurotoxic when deposited in the amyloid form, an alteration of the neurotrophic activity of the secreted form of its precursor might also be considered as an event potentially leading to dementia. Thus, our working hypothesis on the role of APP in the pathogenesis of AD is the following: APP is an important protein involved in the regulation of synaptic function and neuronal homeostasis. In AD patients, abnormal metabolism and compartmentalization of APP lead to an important alteration in the maintenance of synapses and the homeostasis of neurons. This, in turn, could lead to the massive neuronal loss and reactive sprouting observed in AD brains.

In conclusion, APP is a neurotrophic protein whose activity is represented by a small stretch of fragment in the middle portion of secreted aminoterminus of APP. There is a possibility that this neurotrophic activity of APP is not properly expressed in AD. It is an attractive possibility that a non-peptide drug may be designed based on the short APP fragment and used therapeutically to reduce the memory dysfunction and neuronal atrophy found in AD.

Acknowledgments. We are grateful to Ms. I. Hafner for help in preparing this paper. This research was supported by the Research grant from the National Institutes of Health (AG05131) and the generous support of Taisho Pharmaceutical Co., Ltd.

References

Araki W, Kitaguchi N, Tokushima Y, Ishii K, Aratake H, Shimohama S, Nakamura S, Kimura J (1991) Trophic effect of β-amyloid precursor protein on cerebral cortical neurons in culture. Biochem Biophys Res Commun 181:265–271

Bhasin R, Van Nostrand WE, Saitoh T, Donets MA, Barnes EA, Quitschke WW, Goldgaber D (1991) Expression of active secreted forms of human amyloid β-protein precursor by recombinant baculovirus-infected insect cells. Proc Natl Acad Sci USA 88:10307–10311

Bowes MP, Saitoh T, Zivin JA, Roch J-M, Uéda K (1992) A 17-mer peptide segment of the amyloid β/A4-protein (APP) reduces neurologic damage in a rabbit spinal cord ischemia model. Soc Neurosci Abstr 18:1437

Cai XD, Golde TE, Younkin SG (1993) Release of excess amyloid beta protein from a mutant amyloid beta protein precursor. Science 259:514–516

Chartier-Harlin M-C, Crawford F, Houlden H, Warren A, Hughes D, Fidani L, Goate A, Rossor M, Roques P, Hardy J, Mullan M (1991) Early-onset Alzheimer's disease caused by mutations at codon 717 of the β-amyloid precursor protein. Nature 353:844–846

Citron M, Oltersdorf T, Haass C, McConlogue L, Hung AY, Seubert P, Vigo-Pelfrey C, Lieberburg I, Selkoe DJ (1992) Mutation of the beta-amyloid precursor protein in familial Alzheimer's disease increases beta-protein production. Nature 360:672–674

Cole GM, Galasko D, Shapiro IP, Saitoh T (1990) Stimulated platelets release amyloid β-protein precursor. Biochem Biophys Res Commun 170:288–295

Cole GM, Masliah E, Shelton ER, Chan HW, Terry RD, Saitoh T (1991) Accumulation of amyloid precursor fragment of Alzheimer plaques. Neurobiol. Aging 12:85–91

Crawford F, Hardy J, Mullan M, Goate A, Hughes D, Fidani L, Roques P, Rossor M, Chartier-Harlin MC (1991) Sequencing of exons 16 and 17 of the beta-amyloid precursor protein gene in 14 families with early onset of Alzheimer's disease fails to reveal mutations in the beta-amyloid sequence. Neurosci Lett 133:1–2

Cunningham DD, Van Nostrand WE (1991) Protease nexin-2/amyloid β-protein precursor may function in wound repair. In: Regulation and genetic control of brain amyloid. Brain Res Rev 16:95–96

De Sauvage F, Octave JN (1989) A novel mRNA of the A4 amyloid precursor gene coding for a possibly secreted protein. Science 245: 651–653

Glenner GG, Wong CW (1984) Alzheimer's disease and Down's syndrome: sharing a unique cerebrovascular amyloid fibril protein. Biochem Biophys Res Commun 122: 1131–1135

Goate A, Chartier-Harlin M-C, Mullan M, Brown J, Crawford F, Fidani L, Giuffra L, Haynes A, Irving N, James L, Mant R, Newton P, Rooke K, Roques P, Talbot C, Pericak-Vance M, Roses A, Williamson R, Rossor M, Owen M, Hardy J (1991) Segregation of a missense mutation in the amyloid precursor protein gene with familial Alzheimer's disease. Nature 349: 704–706

Golde TE, Estus S, Usiak M, Younkin LH, Younkin SG (1990) Expression of β amyloid protein precursor mRNAs: recognition of a novel alternatively spliced form and quantitation in Alzheimer's disease using PCR. Neuron 4: 253–267

Goldgaber D, Lerman MI, McBride OW, Saffiotti U, Gajdusek DC (1987) Characterization and chromosomal localization of a cDNA encoding brain amyloid of Alzheimer's disease. Science 235: 877–880

Goldgaber D, Schwarzman AI, Bhasin R, Gregori L, Schmechel D, Saunders AM, Roses AD, Strittmatter WJ (1993) Sequestration of amyloid β peptide. Ann NY Acad Sci 695: 139–143

Hardy JA, Higgins GA (1992) Alzheimer's disease: The amyloid cascade hypothesis. Science 256: 184–185

Hendriks L, van Duijn CM, Cras P, Cruts M, Hul VW, van Harskamp F, Warren A, McInnis MG, Antonarakis SE, Martin J-J, Hofman A, Van Broeckhoven C (1992) Presenile dementia and cerebral haemorrhage linked to a mutation at codon 692 of the β-amyloid precursor protein gene. Nature Genet 1: 218–221

Higgins GA, Oyler GA, Neve RL, Chen KS, Gage FH (1990) Altered levels of amyloid protein precursor transcripts in the basal forebrain of behaviorally impaired aged rats. Proc Natl Acad Sci USA 87: 3032–3036

Jin L-W, Masliah E, Ninomiya H, Roch J-M, Otero DAC, Schubert D, Saitoh T (1992) Biological activity of the amyloid β/A4-protein precursor II: Neurotrophic effect of an APP peptide on a rat brain neuroblastoma cell line. Soc Neurosci Abstr 18: 1466

Joachim CL, Selkoe DJ (1992) The seminal role of beta-amyloid in the pathogenesis of Alzheimer disease. Alzheimer's Disease Assoc Disorders. 6: 7–34

Joachim CL, Games D, Morris J, Ward P, Frenkel D, Selkoe D (1991) Antibodies to non-beta regions of the beta-amyloid precursor protein detect a subset of senile plaques. Am J Pathol 138: 373 384

Johnson SA, McNeill T, Cordell B, Finch CE (1990) Relation of neuronal APP-751/APP-695 mRNA ratio and neuritic plaque density in Alzheimer's disease. Science 248: 854–857

Kang J, Lemaire HG, Unterbeck A, Salbaum JM, Masters CL, Grzeschik KH, Multhaup G, Beyreuther K, Müller-Hill B (1987) The precursor of Alzheimer's disease amyloid A4 protein resembles a cell-surface receptor. Nature 325: 733–736

Kitaguchi N, Takahashi Y, Tokushima Y, Shiojiri S, Ito H (1988) Novel precursor of Alzheimer's disease amyloid protein shows protease inhibitory activity. Nature 331: 530–532

Kitaguchi N, Tokushima Y, Oishi K, Takahashi Y, Shiojiri S, Nakamura S, Tanaka S, Kodaira R, Ito H (1990) Determination of amyloid β protein precursors harboring active form of proteinase inhibitors in cerebrospinal fluid of Alzheimer's disease patients by trypsin-antibody sandwich ELISA. Biochem Biophys Res Commun 166: 1453–1459

König G, Salbaum JM, Wiestler O, Lang W, Schmitt HP, Masters CL, Beyreuther K (1991) Alternative splicing of the βA4 amyloid gene of Alzheimer's disease in cortex of control and Alzheimer's disease patients. Mol Brain Res 9: 259–262

Koo EH, Sisodia SS, Archer DR, Martin LJ, Weidemann A, Beyreuther K, Fischer P, Masters CL, Price DL (1989) Precursor of amyloid protein in Alzheimer disease undergoes fast anterograde axonal transport. Proc Natl Acad Sci USA 87: 1561–1565

Kosik KS (1992) Alzheimer's disease: a cell biological perspective. Science 256: 780–783

Masliah E, Mallory M, Hansen L, Alford M, DeTeresa R, Terry R, Baudier J, Saitoh T (1992a) Localization of amyloid precursor protein in GAP43-immunoreactive aberrant sprouting neurites in Alzheimer's disease. Brain Res 574: 312–316

Masliah E, Mallory M, Ge N, Saitoh T (1992b) Amyloid precursor protein is localized in growing neurites of neonatal rat brain. Brain Res 593:323–328

Masliah E, Abraham C, Johnson W, Forss-Petter S, Mallory M, Terry R, Mucke L (1993) Synaptic alterations in the cortex of APP transgenic mice. J Neuropathol Exp Neurol 52:178

Masters CL, Multhaup G, Simms G, Pottgiesser J, Martins RN, Beyreuther K (1985) Neuronal origin of a cerebral amyloid: Neurofibrillary tangles of Alzheimer's disease contain the same protein as the amyloid plaque cores and blood vessels. EMBO J 4:2757–2763

Mattson MP, Cheng B, Davis D, Bryant K, Lieberburg I, Rydel RE (1992) β-amyloid peptides destabilize calcium homeostasis and render human cortical neurons vulnerable to excitotoxicity. J Neurosci 12:376–389

Mattson MP, Cheng B, Culwell AR, Esch FS, Lieberburg I, Rydel RE (1993) Evidence for excitoprotective and intraneuronal calcium-regulating roles for secreted forms of the beta-amyloid precursor protein. Neuron 10:243–254

Milward EA, Papadopoulos R, Fuller SJ, Moir RD, Small D, Beyreuther K, Masters CL (1992) The amyloid protein precursor of Alzheimer's disease is a mediator of the effects of nerve growth factor on neurite outgrowth. Neuron 9:129–137

Mullan M, Crawford F, Axelman K, Houlden H, Lilius L, Winblad, Lannfelt L (1992) A pathogenic mutation for probable Alzheimer's disease in the APP gene at the N-terminus of β-amyloid. Nature Genet 1:345–347

Murrell J, Farlow M, Ghetti B, Benson MD (1991) A mutation in the amyloid precursor protein associated with hereditary Alzheimer's disease. Science 14:26–28

Naruse S, Igarashi S, Kobayashi H, Aoki K, Inuzuka T, Kaneko K, Shimizu T, Iihara K, Kojima T, Miyatake T, Tsuki S (1991) Mis-sense mutation Val-lle in exon 17 of amyloid precursor protein gene in Japanese familial Alzheimer's disease. Lancet 337:978–979

Neve RL, Finch EA, Dawes LR (1988) Expression of the Alzheimer amyloid precursor gene transcripts in the human brain. Neuron 1:669–677

Neve RL, Rogers J, Higgins GA (1990) The Alzheimer amyloid precursor related transcript lacking the β/A4 sequence is specifically increased in Alzheimer's disease brain. Neuron 5:329–338

Ninomiya H, Roch J-M, Sundsmo MP, Otero DAC, Saitoh T (1993) Amino acid sequence RERMS represents the active domain of amyloid β/A4 protein precursor that promotes growth. J Cell Biol 121:879–886

Oltersdorf T, Fritz LC, Schenk DB, Lieberburg I, Johson-Wood KL, Beattie EC, Ward PJ, Blacher RW, Dovey HF, Sinha S (1989) The secreted form of Alzheimer's amyloid precursor protein with the Kunitz domain is protease nexin-II. Nature 341:144–147

Palmert MR, Podlisny MB, Witker DS, Oltersdorf T, Younkin LH, Selkoe DJ, Younkin SG (1989) The β-amyloid protein precursor of Alzheimer's disease has soluble derivatives found in human brain and cerebrospinal fluid. Proc Natl Acad Sci USA 86:63338–6342

Pike CJ, Burdick D, Walencewicz AJ, Glabe CG, Cotman CW (1993) Neurodegeneration induced by beta-amyloid peptides in vitro: the role of peptide assembly state. J Neurosci 13:1676–1687

Ponte P, Gonzalez-DeWhitt P, Shilling J, Miller J, Hsu D, Greenberg B, Davis K, Wallace W, Lieberburg I, Fuller F (1988) A new A4 amyloid mRNA contains a domain homologous to serine protease inhibitors. Nature 331:525–527

Robakis NK, Ramakrishna N, Wolfe G, Wisniewski HM (1987) Molecular cloning and characterization of a cDNA encoding cerebrovascular and the neuritic plaque amyloid peptides. Proc Natl Acad Sci USA 84:4190–4193

Robakis NK, Altstiel LD, Refolo LM, Anderson JP (1990) Function and metabolism of the protease inhibitor-containing Alzheimer amyloid precursors. In: Miyatake T, Selkoe DJ, Ihara Y (eds) Molecular biology of Alzheimer's disease. Elsevier Science Publishers BV, Amsterdam, pp 179–188

Roch J-M, Shapiro IP, Sundsmo MP, Otero DAC, Refolo LM, Robakis NK, Saitoh T (1992) Bacterial expression, purification, and functional mapping of the amyloid β/A4 protein precursor. J Biol Chem 267:2214–2221

Roch J-M, Masliah E, Roch-Levecq A-C, Otero DAC, Sundsmo MP, Veinbergs I, Saitoh T (1993) Increased synaptic density and memory retention by a biologically active amyloid β/A4 protein precursor peptide. Soc Neurosci Abstr 19:221

Saitoh T, Sundsmo MP, Roch J-M, Kimura N, Cole GM, Schubert D, Oltersdorf T, Schenk DB (1989) Secreted form of amyloid β-protein precursor is involved in the growth regulation of fibroblasts. Cell 58:615–622

Schellenberg GD, Anderson L, O'dahl S, Wisjman EM, Sadovnick AD, Ball MJ, Larson EB, Kuku WA, Martin GM, Roses AD (1991) APP717, APP693, and PRIP gene mutations are rare in Alzheimer disease. Am J Human Genet 49:511–517

Schubert D, Jin L-W, Saitoh T, Cole GM (1989) The regulation of amyloid β protein precursor secretion and its modulatory role in cell adhesion. Neuron 3:689–694

Selkoe DJ, Abraham CR, Podlisny MB, Duffy LK (1986) Isolation of low molecular weight proteins from amyloid plaques in Alzheimer's disease. J Neurochem 146:1820–1834

Smith RP, Higuchi DA, Broze GJ, Jr (1990) Platelet coagulation factor Xla-inhibitor, a form of Alzheimer amyloid precursor protein. Science 248:1126–1128

Strittmatter WJ, Saunders AM, Schmechel D, Pericak-Vance M, Enghild J, Salvesen GS, Roses AD (1993) Apolipoprotein-E-high-avidity binding to β-amyloid and increased frequency of type-4 allele in late-onset familial Alzheimer disease. Proc Natl Acad Sci USA 90:1977–1981

Tanaka S, Nakamura S, Uéda K, Kameyama M, Shiojiri S, Takahashi Y, Kitaguchi N, Ito H (1988) Three types of amyloid precursor mRNA in human brain: their differential expression in Alzheimer's disease. Biochem Biophys Res Commun 157:472–479

Tanzi RE, Gusella JF, Watkins PC, Bruns GAP, St. George-Hyslop P, Van Keuren ML, Patterson D, Pagan S, Kurnit DM, Neve RL (1987) Amyloid β-protein gene: cDNA, mRNA distribution, and genetic linkage near the Alzheimer locus. Science 235:880–884

Tanzi RE, MacClatchey AI, Lamperti ED, Villa-Komaroff LV, Gusella JF, Neve RL (1988) Protease inhibitor domain encoded by an amyloid protein precursor mRNA associated with Alzheimer's disease. Nature 331:528–530

Tanzi RE, Vaula G, Romano DM, Mortilla M, Huang TL, Tupler RG, Wasco W, Hyman BT, Haines JL, Jenkins BJ (1992) Assessment of amyloid beta-protein precursor gene mutations in a large set of familial and sporadic Alzheimer disease cases. Am J Human Genet 51:273–282

Uéda K, Cole G, Sundsmo M, Katzman R, Saitoh T (1989) Decreased adhesiveness of Alzheimer's disease fibroblasts: Is amyloid β-protein precursor involved? Ann Neurol 25:246–251

Van Nostrand WE, Wagner SI, Suzuki M, Choi BH, Farrow JS, Geddes JW, Cotman CW, Cunningham DD (1989) Protease nexin-II, a potent antichymotrypsin, shows identity to amyloid β-protein precursor. Nature 341:546–548

Van Nostrand WE, Schmaier AH, Farrow JS, Cunningham DD (1990) Protease nexin-II (amyloid β-protein precursor): a platelet granule protein. Science 248:745–748

Weidemann A, König G, Bunke D, Fischer P, Salbaum JM, Masters CL, Beyreuther K (1989) Identification, biogenesis, and localization of precursors of Alzheimer's disease A4 amyloid protein. Cell 57:115–126

Yankner BA, Dawes LR, Fisher S, Villa-Komaroff L, Oster-Granite ML, Neve RL (1989) Neurotoxicity of a fragment of the amyloid precursor associated with Alzheimer's disease. Science 245:417–420

Yankner BA, Duffy LK, Kirschner DA (1990a) Neurotrophic and neurotoxic effects of amyloid β-protein: reversal by tachykinin neuropeptides. Science 250:279–282

Yankner BA, Caceres A, Duffy LK (1990b) Nerve growth factor potentiates the neurotoxicity of beta amyloid. proc Natl Acad Sci USA 87:9020–9030

Yoshioka K, Miki T, Katsuya T, Ogihara T, Sakaki Y (1991) The 717Val-lle substitution in amyloid precursor protein is associated with familial Alzheimer's disease regardless of ethnic groups. Biochem Biophys Res Comm 178:1141–1146

Processing of Alzheimer Aβ-Amyloid Precursor Protein: Cell Biology, Regulation, and Role in Alzheimer's Disease

S. Gandy* and P. Greengard

Alzheimer's disease (AD) is characterized by an intracranial amyloidosis that develops in an age-dependent manner and appears to be dependent upon the production of Aβ-amyloid by proteolysis of its integral membrane precursor, the Alzheimer Aβ-amyloid precursor protein (APP). Evidence causally linking APP to AD has been provided by the discovery of mutations within the APP coding sequence that segregate with disease phenotypes in autosomal dominant familial cerebral amyloidoses, including some types of familial AD (FAD). Though FAD is rare (< 10% of all AD), the characteristic clinicopathological features – amyloid plaques, neurofibrillary tangles, synaptic and neuronal loss, neurotransmitter deficits, dementia – are apparently indistinguishable when FAD is compared with typical, common, "non-familial," or sporadic, AD (SAD).

The characterization and regulation of pathways for the cellular processing of APP have been extensively characterized and recent data demonstrate that soluble Aβ-amyloid is released from various cells and tissues in the course of normal cellular metabolism. To date, studies of APP catabolic intermediates and soluble Aβ-amyloid in SAD tissues and fluids have not provided specific SAD-associated changes in APP metabolism. However, studies of some clinically relevant mutant APP molecules from FAD families have yielded evidence that APP mutations can lead to enhanced generation or aggregability of Aβ-amyloid, consistent with a pathogenic role in AD.

In addition, genetic loci for FAD have been discovered which are distinct from the immediate regulatory and coding regions of the APP gene, indicating that defects in molecules other than APP can also specify cerebral amyloidogenesis and FAD. It remains to be elucidated which, if any, of these rare genetic causes of AD is most relevant to our understanding of typical, common SAD.

---

* Department of Neurology and Neuroscience, Cornell University Medical College, 1300 York Avenue, and The Rockefeller University, 1230 York Avenue, New York, NY 10021, USA

C.L. Masters et al. (Eds.)
Amyloid Protein Precursor in Development,
Aging and Alzheimer's Disease
© Springer-Verlag Berlin Heidelberg 1994

Alzheimer's Disease is Associated with an Intracranial Amyloidosis

Amyloid is a generic description applied to a heterogeneous class of tissue protein precipitates which have the common feature of beta-pleated sheet secondary structure, a characteristic which confers affinity for the histochemical dye Congo red (Tomlinson and Corsellis 1984). Amyloids may be deposited in a general manner throughout the body (systemic amyloids) or confined to a particular organ (e.g., cerebral amyloid). AD is characterized by clinical evidence of cognitive failure in association with cerebral amyloidosis, cerebral intraneuronal neurofibrillary pathology, neuronal and synaptic loss, and neurotransmitter deficits (Tomlinson and Corsellis 1984). The cerebral amyloid of AD is deposited around meningeal and cerebral vessels, as well as in gray matter. In gray matter, the deposits coalesce into structures known as plaques. Parenchymal amyloid plaques are distributed in brain in a characteristic fashion, differentially affecting the various cerebral and cerebellar lobes and cortical laminae.

The main constituent of cerebrovascular amyloid was purified and sequenced by Glenner and Wong in 1984. This 40–42 amino acid polypeptide (designated "β protein", Glenner and Wong 1984a,b or, according to Masters et al. 1985, "A4"; now standardized as Aβ by Husby et al. 1993), is derived from a 695–770 amino acid precursor, termed the Aβ-amyloid precursor protein (APP; Fig. 1), which was discovered by molecular cloning (Goldgaber et al. 1987; Tanzi et al. 1987, 1988; Kang et al. 1987; Robakis et al. 1987; Ponte et al. 1988; Kitaguchi et al. 1988).

APP Structure Gives Clues to Some of its Functions

The deduced amino acid sequence of APP predicts a protein with a single transmembrane domain (Goldgaber et al. 1987, Tanzi et al. 1987, 1988; Kang et al. 1987; Robakis et al. 1987; Ponte et al. 1988; Kitaguchi et al. 1988). Isoform diversity is generated by alternative mRNA splicing, and isoforms of 751 and 770 amino acids include a protease inhibitor domain ("Kunitz-type protease inhibitor" domain, or KPI; Ponte et al. 1988; Tanzi et al. 1988; Kitaguchi et al. 1988) in the extracellular region of the APP molecule. The ectodomains of the protease inhibitor-bearing isoforms of APP are identical to molecules which had been identified previously based on their tight association with proteases, and thus were designated "protease nexin II" ("PN-II"; Van Nostrand and Cunningham 1987; Oltersdorf et al. 1989; Van Nostrand et al. 1989). Identical molecules are also present in the platelet alpha-granules, where they were described under the name of "factor XIa inhibitor" (XIaI; Smith et al. 1990; Bush et al. 1990). Upon degranulation of the platelet, factor XIaI/PN-II/APP exerts an antiproteolytic effect on activated factor XIa at late steps of the coagulation cascade.

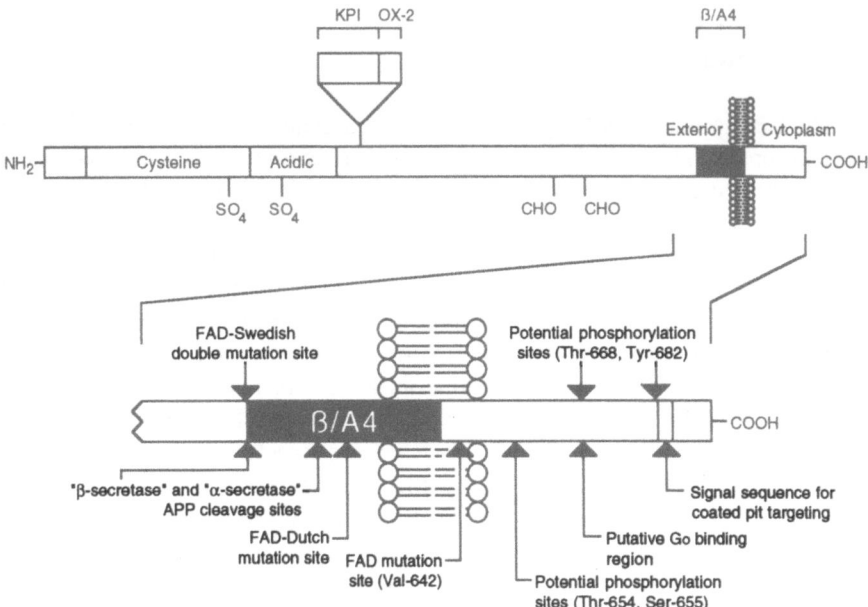

Fig. 1. Structure of the Alzheimer Aβ-amyloid precursor protein (courtesy of Dr. Gregg Caporaso; numbering according to APP$_{695}$, Kang et al 1987. β/A4 domain = Aβ domain; see text or Husby et al. (1993)

Recent evidence suggests that KPI-lacking isoforms may also act as regulators of proteolysis (Miyazaki et al. 1993).

Other physiological role(s) for APP are as yet unknown, although evidence from several independent lines of inquiry suggests that APP may play a role in transmembrane signal transduction (Nishimoto et al. 1993) and/or calcium metabolism (Mattson et al. 1993; Arispe et al. 1993). In addition, potential functional motifs in APP have been recognized by the presence of consensus sequences or by experimental implication. Some of these motifs suggest a role in metal ion binding (Bush et al. 1992), heparin binding (Schubert et al. 1989), cell-cell interaction (Konig et al. 1992), and/or functioning as a receptor for a currently unrecognized ligand (Kang et al. 1987; Chen et al. 1990). In some investigations, Saitoh and colleagues (1989) have accumulated evidence that APP may play a role in regulating cell growth. Recently, novel APP-like proteins (APLPs) have been discovered (Wasco et al. 1992, 1993; Slunt, et al. 1994), suggesting that APP may be a member of a larger family of related molecules. APLPs are highly homologous to APP and to each other, but APLPs lack the Aβ-amyloid domain and therefore cannot serve as precursors to Aβ-amyloid.

APP is Processed via Several Distinct Enzymatic and Subcellular Pathways

APP is initially synthesized and cotranslationally inserted into membranes in the endoplasmic reticulum (ER). Studies of APP metabolism in the presence of either brefeldin A or monensin have, to date, failed to implicate the ER as an important site for discrete proteolytic processing of APP (Caporaso et al. 1992a).

Following its exit from the ER, APP traverses the Golgi apparatus, where it is subjected to N- and O-glycosylation, tyrosyl sulfation, and sialylation (Weidemann et al. 1989; Oltersdorf et al. 1990). APP is also phosphorylated in both the extracellular and cytoplasmic domains and preliminary evidence indicates that some of these events may occur in an early compartment of the central vacuolar pathway (Knops et al., submitted for publication; Suzuki et al., personal communication). In addition, some APP molecules are chondroitin-sulfated in their ectodomains (Shioi et al. 1992).

The proteolytic processing steps for APP have been a subject of intense interest, in part due to early evidence which excluded the possibility that AD was frequently associated with APP gene mutations or with disordered APP transcription (Koo et al. 1990). One attractive possibility, then, was that AD might be a disorder of APP processing. This possibility was strengthened by early evidence for an APP processing pathway which precluded Aβ-amyloid generation (Sisodia et al. 1990; Esch et al. 1990), implying that a defect in this pathway might underlie AD.

Several proteolytic cleavage products of APP processing have now been definitively identified by purification and sequencing. The first to be identified (Weidemann et al. 1989) was a fragment which results primarily from the cleavage which occurs within the Aβ-amyloid domain. A large amino-terminal fragment of the APP extracellular domain ("protease nexin-II" or "PN-II"; Van Nostrand and Cunningham 1987; Oltersdorf et al. 1989; Van Nostrand et al. 1989; or s-APP or APPs, for soluble APP; Citron et al. 1992), is released into the medium of cultured cells and into the cerebrospinal fluid (Weidemann et al. 1989; Palmert et al. 1989; Oltersdorf et al. 1990), leaving a small nonamyloidogenic carboxyl-terminal fragment associated with the cell. This pathway is currently designated the alpha-secretory cleavage/release processing pathway for APP, so-called because the (as-yet undiscovered) enzyme which performs this nonamyloidogenic cleavage/release has been designated "alpha-secretase" (Esch et al. 1990; Seubert et al. 1993). Thus, one important processing event in the biology of APP acts to preclude amyloidogenesis by proteolyzing APP within the Aβ-amyloid domain.

Few details are available concerning the molecular nature of alpha-secretase, although it is very likely to be a member of a class of enzymes which regulates the "shedding" of ectodomains from a wide variety of transmembrane molecules, including growth factor precursors, cell adhesion molecules, receptors, and ectoenzymes (Ehlers and Riordan 1991). Surprisingly, these enzymes appear to act primarily at or near the cell surface and to specify cleavage of substrates at a certain distance from the plasma membrane, largely without regard for the primary sequence surrounding the cleavage site (Sisodia 1992; also Maruyama et al. 1991; Sahasrabudhe et al. 1993). Based on studies of proteolytic processing of the TGF-alpha precursor and the c-kit ligand precursors (which also appear to be cleaved by similar, cell-surface proteinase activities; Pandiella and Massague 1991; Pandiella et al. 1992), it appears that "secretase-like" activities may be heterogeneous at the molecular level (i.e., several individual proteinase species probably exist). This conclusion is based on the observation that, depending upon the substrate assayed, slightly different protease inhibitor sensitivity profiles were obtained in studies of TGF-alpha "secretase" in side-by-side comparison with c-kit ligand family "secretases." Intracellular signal transduction, especially via protein kinase C, is commonly an important regulatory mechanism for processing of molecules via "secretase-like" pathways (see below). The possibility currently exists that the activities of some secretases are regulated by the phosphorylation state of the enzymes themselves; if true, this would provide the first known examples of proteases whose activities are regulated by their states of phosphorylation.

"Alternative" Pathways of APP Metabolism Provide Clues to the Source of Aβ-Amyloid

Due to issues of peptide conformation, peptide aggregation, and antibody reagent insensitivity, the Aβ-amyloid molecule was not initially detected as a normal metabolite of APP, either in brain, cerebrospinal fluid or cell culture systems. In fact, until mid-1992, Aβ-amyloid was generally described as being an "abnormal" metabolite of APP. Instead, early clues into Aβ-amyloidogenesis were provided by the observation of electrophoretic microheterogeneity of carboxyl-terminal fragments of APP. Such microheterogeneity was detected in association with high-level overexpression of human APP using recombinant vaccinia viruses (Wolf et al. 1990), baculoviruses (Gandy et al. 1992a), or stable transfection (Golde et al. 1992), in association with supraphysiological levels of protein phosphorylation (Buxbaum et al. 1990), and in human cerebral vessels (Tamaoka et al. 1992) and cortex (Estus et al. 1992). Antigenic characterization of carboxyl-terminal fragments of APP in cerebral vessels (Tamaoka et al. 1992) and cortex (Estus et al. 1992), in transfected cells (Golde et al. 1992), and in the baculoviral overexpression system (Gandy et al. 1992a) provided the evidence which supported the possibility of "alternative" cleavage of APP molecules, giving rise to carboxyl-terminal fragments containing the complete Aβ-amyloid sequence, which, in turn might give rise to Aβ-amyloid. Protein sequencing of the various putative amyloidogenic carboxyl-terminal species (candidate intermediates in the pathway to Aβ-amyloid deposition) recently provided for their definitive identification (Cheung et al. 1994).

The "alternative" (i.e., non-intra-Aβ) cleavage suggested by this micro-heterogeneity prompted a search for additional intracellular routes for APP trafficking and cleavage. The existence of trafficking routes other than the alpha-secretory cleavage/release processing pathway was also suggested by the estimation that only about 20% of newly synthesized APP molecules are recovered as released molecules (in PC-12 cells; Caporaso et al. 1992b). Since evidence failed to suggest the existence of an important degradative pathway for APP in the ER (Caporaso et al. 1992a), several groups undertook experiments to determine whether acidic (endosomal/lysosomal or trans-Golgi network) compartments of the cell were important in APP metabolism (Cole et al. 1989; Caporaso et al. 1992a; Golde et al. 1992; Haass et al. 1992a; Knops et al. 1992). The possibility of endosomal metabolism of APP was bolstered by the discovery of a clathrin-coated vesicle (CCV) targeting motif in the LDL receptor (Chen et al. 1990). This motif, NPXY, was required for proper internalization of the LDL receptor and was also present in the sequence of the cytoplasmic tail of APP (Fig. 1). The copurification of APP with CCVs was subsequently demonstrated directly (Nordstedt et al. 1993). The fact that APP contains an NPXY motif associates APP with a host of cell-surface receptors and suggests the possibility that APP may be a receptor for an as-yet undiscovered or unrecognized ligand.

In other efforts to dissect the process of Aβ-amyloidogenesis, vesicle-neutralizing agents (such as chloroquine and ammonium chloride) were applied to cultured cells, and these compounds were associated with greatly enhanced recovery of full-length APP and an array of carboxyl-terminal fragments, including nonamyloidogenic and potentially amyloidogenic fragments (Caporaso et al. 1992a; Estus et al. 1992; Golde et al. 1992; Haass et al. 1992a; Knops et al. 1992). A similar array of fragments was recovered from purified lysosomes (Haass et al. 1992a). This led to the formulation that both the potentially amyloidogenic carboxyl-terminal fragments and Aβ-amyloid might be generated primarily in lysosomes. However, no Aβ-amyloid could be recovered from lysosomes (Haass et al. 1993), making this a less likely (but not impossible) scenario. The likelihood that Aβ-amyloid is generated in lysosomes was further diminished by the observation that vesicular neutralization fails to consistently diminish Aβ-amyloid production in certain cell types (Busciglio et al. 1993; see also below), although neutralization-induced stabilization of the standard array of potentially amyloidogenic carboxyl-terminal fragments is consistently apparent.

Aβ-Amyloid is a Normal Constituent of Body Fluids and the Conditioned Medium of Cultured Cells

Until mid-1992, the prevailing notion of Aβ-amyloid was that of an abnormal, potentially toxic species, the production of which was perhaps relatively restricted to the brain in man (and perhaps a few other species), and which occurred primarily in association with aging and AD. This concept became obsolete with the discovery by several groups that a soluble Aβ-amyloid species (presumably a forerunner of the aggregated fibrillar species which is deposited in senile plaque cores) is detectable in body fluids from various species and in the conditioned medium of cultured cells (Haass et al. 1992b; Seubert et al. 1992; Shoji et al. 1992), but is not detectable in the lysates of cultured cells.

This so-called "soluble Aβ-amyloid" is apparently generated in a cellular compartment distal to the ER since brefeldin abolishes its generation and does not result in its accumulation inside cells (Haass et al. 1993). Vesicular neutralization compounds are effective in inhibiting Aβ-amyloid release from some cell types (Shoji et al. 1992), but this is not true for all cell types studied (Busciglio et al. 1993). The precise cellular locus (loci) involved in the amino- and carboxyl-terminal cleavages responsible for Aβ-amyloid generation has not yet been unequivocally established. The consistent inability to recover Aβ-amyloid from cell lysates or from purified vesicles has led to a shift in focus away from the terminal degradative compartments of the cell (i.e., lysosomes) as possible sources for the generation of Aβ-amyloid. One plausible scenario for Aβ-amyloid production is that cleavage at the Aβ-amyloid amino-terminus is catalyzed by β-secretase (see below) in the pre-cell surface limb of the constitutive secretory pathway, perhaps beginning in the trans-Golgi network (TGN). Cell-type-dependent variations in sensitivity of the TGN to neutralizing compounds may explain the observed dissociability of Aβ-amyloid generation from the apparent stabilization by these compounds of potentially amyloidogenic carboxyl-terminal fragments.

Still unexplained is the cellular mechanism by which the carboxyl-terminus of Aβ-amyloid is generated, since this region of the APP molecule resides within an intramembranous domain. A plausible and conventional scenario for this step might involve the trafficking of APP or a potentially amyloidogenic fragment into a multivesicular body where vesiculated APP or an APP fragment may be liberated from the bilayer (Gandy et al. 1992b). This is supported by ultrastructural evidence that multivesicular bodies are immunoreactive for APP epitopes (Caporaso et al. 1994). Once the cleavage which generates the carboxyl-terminus of Aβ-amyloid has occurred, fusion with the plasma membrane of a multivesicular body containing wholly intraluminal Aβ-amyloid could effect release of Aβ-amyloid into the extracellular space.

Evidence Suggests the Existence of an Enzyme, β-Secretase, which Cleaves APP at the Amino Terminus of the Aβ-amyloid Domain

The possibility of heterogeneous cleavage along the constitutive secretory pathway (i.e., cleavage in the pre-cell surface pathway or at the cell surface) was initially discounted (Golde et al. 1992). However, Seubert and colleagues (1993) extended this line of investigation and succeeded in preparing an antibody that was specific for the free methionyl residue which would reside at the predicted carboxyl-terminus of such an alternatively cleaved and released attenuated "PN-II-like" (or "APPs-like") molecule. This species was successfully detected as a component of the PN-II/APPs pool of cleaved and released APP ectodomains. The importance of this activity, designated "β-secretase," was subsequently strengthened by the discovery that a pathogenic FAD mutation in APP results in dramatic increases in Aβ-amyloid generation, which is probably attributable to an increase in β-secretase-type cleavage of the mutant APP (probably because the mutant APP is a better substrate for β-secretase than is wildtype APP; Felsenstein et al. 1994).

APP Mutations in Familial Cerebral Amyloidoses Occur Within or near the Aβ-Amyloid Domain, Segregate with Disease in Affected Kindreds, and Yield APP Molecules which Display Some Pro-Amyloidogenic Properties

Certain mutations associated with familial cerebral amyloidoses have been identified within or near the Aβ-amyloid region of the coding sequence of the APP gene. These mutations segregate with the clinical phenotypes of either hereditary cerebral hemorrhage with amyloidosis, Dutch type (HCHWAD or FAD-Dutch; Fig. 1; van Duinen et al. 1987; Levy et al. 1990; Van Broeckhoven et al. 1990) or more typical FAD (Fig. 1; Goate et al. 1991; Naruse et al. 1991; Murrell et al. 1991; Chartier-Harlin et al. 1991; Mullan et al. 1992a), and provide support for the notion that aberrant APP metabolism is a key feature of AD.

In FAD-Dutch, an uncharged glutamine residue is substituted for a charged glutamate residue at position 693 of APP_{770}. This mutated residue is located in the extracellular region of APP, within the Aβ-amyloid domain, where it apparently exerts its proamyloidogenic effect by generating Aβ-amyloid molecules which bear enhanced aggregation properties (Wisniewski et al. 1991).

Mutations in APP which are apparently pathogenic for more typical FAD have also been discovered. In the first discovered FAD mutation (Goate et al. 1991), an isoleucine residue is substituted for a valine residue at position 717 of APP_{770}, within the transmembrane domain (Fig. 1), at a position just downstream from the carboxyl-terminus of the Aβ-amyloid domain. Although a conservative substitution, the mutation segregates with FAD in pedigrees of American, European and Asian origins, arguing against the possibility that the mutations represent irrelevant polymorphisms. Other pedigrees have been discovered in which affected members have either phenylalanyl (Murrell et al. 1991) or glycyl (Chartier-Harlin et al. 1991) residues at position 717. Neuropathological examination has verified the similarity of these individuals to typical SAD neuropathology (reviewed by Rossor 1992; see also Lantos et al. 1992; Mann et al. 1992; Ghetti et al. 1992; Cairns et al. 1993; Kennedy et al. 1993).

Though the 717 mutant APPs are the most common of the FAD-causing APP mutations, the mechanism by which the 717-mutant APPs exert their effects remains to be clarified. The location of the missense substitution raises the possibility that the mutation may either directly affect proteolytic cleavage (e.g., by leading to the production of extended, perhaps more hydrophobic and thus hyperaggregable Aβ-amyloid molecules; Cai et al. 1993), or that the mutation may otherwise influence the function, trafficking or biology of the APP molecule. Missense mutations in other integral molecules are associated with alternations in their biological activities (e.g., the oncogene neu; Bargmann et al. 1986), their trafficking and proteolysis (e.g., T cell receptor; Bonifacino et al. 1990), or their ability to effect functional physiological changes in response to phosphorylation of their cytoplasmic domains (e.g., CFTR; Schoumacher et al. 1987; Li et al. 1988, 1989; Hwang et al. 1989; Wagner et al. 1991). It has also been hypothesized that the FAD mutation may lead to abnormal APP translation as a result of a disturbance in the secondary structure of APP mRNA (Tanzi and Hyman 1991; Goldgaber, personal communication). Which, if any, of these models accounts for the pathogenesis of APP-717-mutant FAD remains a mystery.

Another FAD pedigree has been discovered and has proven to be substantially more informative in elucidating the cell biological consequences of the pathogenic mutation. In a large Swedish kindred, tandem missense mutations occur at the amino terminus of the Aβ-amyloid domain (Mullan et al. 1992a). Transfection of cultured cells with APP molecules containing the "Swedish" missense mutations results in the production of six- to eight-fold excess soluble Aβ-amyloid above that generated from wildtype APP (Citron et al. 1992; Cai et al. 1993). This is the first (and, to date, only) example of AD apparently caused by excessive Aβ-amyloid production. Based upon the models of FAD-Dutch and FAD-Swedish, an important issue for clarification in SAD will be to establish whether hyperaggregation or hyperproduction of Aβ-amyloid (or neither) is an important predisposing factor(s) to this much more commonly encountered clinical entity.

Signal Transduction via Protein Phosphorylation Regulates the Relative Utilization of APP Processing Pathways

As noted, the protease which cleaves APP within the Aβ-amyloid domain, as part of the nonamyloidogenic cleavage/release pathway ("alpha-secretase"), and the proteases which cleave APP at other sites within the molecule to generate Aβ-amyloid ("β-secretase" and perhaps others) have not yet been identified. Nevertheless, some progress has been made toward understanding the regulation of APP cleavage. For example, the relative utilization of the various alternative APP processing pathways appears to be at least partially cell-type determined, with transfected AtT20 cells secreting virtually all APP molecules (Overly et al. 1991), whereas glia release little or none (Haass et al. 1991). In neuronal-like cells, the state of differentiation also plays a role in determining the relative utilization of the pathways (Baskin et al. 1992; Hung et al. 1992), with the differentiated neuronal phenotype being associated with relatively diminished basal utilization of the nonamyloidogenic alpha-secretase cleavage/ release pathway (Hung et al. 1992).

Certain signal transduction systems that involve protein phosphorylation are potent regulators of APP cleavage, acting in some cases, perhaps, by altering the relative activity of nonamyloidogenic cleavage by alpha-secretase. The role of protein kinase C (PKC) in this process has received the most attention. In many types of cultured cells, activation of PKC by phorbol esters dramatically stimulates APP proteolysis (Buxbaum et al. 1990) and cleavage/release (Caporaso et al. 1992b; Gillespie et al. 1992; Sinha and Lieberburg 1992) via the alpha-secretase pathway. PKC-stimulated alpha-secretory cleavage of APP may also be induced by the application of neurotransmitters and other first messenger compounds whose receptors are linked to PKC (Nitsch et al. 1992; Buxbaum et al. 1992; Lahiri et al. 1992). Okadaic acid, an inhibitor of protein phosphatases 1 and 2A (Cohen et al. 1990), also increases APP proteolysis and release via the alpha-secretase pathway (Buxbaum et al. 1990; Caporaso et al. 1992b). Thus, either stimulation of PKC or inhibition of protein phosphatases 1 and 2A is sufficient to produce a dramatic acceleration of nonamyloidogenic APP degradation. Furthermore, this PKC-activated processing can be demonstrated to occur at the expense of amyloidogenic APP degradation, resulting in diminished generation of Aβ-amyloid (Sinha, personal communication; Buxbaum et al. 1993; Hung et al. 1993).

These results suggest that defects in signal-dependent regulation of APP cleavage may contribute to the pathogenesis of AD, a possibility supported by evidence that deficits in cholinergic neurotransmission (Davies and Maloney 1976) and in protein kinase C activity (Cole et al. 1988; Van Huynh et al. 1989; Masliah et al. 1991) accompany AD. By extension, then, the possibility exists that pharmacological modulation of APP metabolism via signal transduction might be therapeutically beneficial in individuals with AD (Gandy et al. 1991, 1992b; Gandy and Greengard 1992). Complicating these notions, however, is the observation that PKC is also a potent regulator of APP expression (Goldgaber et al. 1989), although these pleiotropic effects of PKC may be dissociable at the level of PKC isoenzyme involved (Hata et al. 1993). In addition to the attention to regulation of the nonamyloidogenic alpha-secretase pathway as a source of candidate etiologic defects and therapeutic opportunities, it may also be fruitful to study the potentially amyloidogenic β-secretase pathway in an analogous fashion. Further work will be required to elucidate the importance of signal transduction systems as important candidate defects or therapeutic targets in AD. The enormous pharmacological experience with compounds that affect signal transduction makes such an approach particularly attractive for targeting therapy. The probable causal relationship between aberrant protein phosphorylation and neurofibrillary tangle formation (another component of Alzheimer structural pathology) adds to the attractiveness of protein phosphorylation pathways as potential therapeutic targets in AD.

The mechanism by which stimulation or inhibition of intracellular protein phosphorylation regulates the processing of APP (including evaluation of the effect of changing the phosphorylation state of APP *per se*) remains to be fully elucidated. Protein kinase C rapidly phosphorylates a seryl residue in the cytoplasmic domain of APP (Fig. 1), using either a synthetic peptide (Gandy et al. 1988; Suzuki et al. 1992) or APP holoprotein (Suzuki et al. 1992) as substrate. Moreover, APP species are phosphorylated on this and other seryl and threonyl residues in intact cells and in brain (Suzuki et al., manuscript in preparation; Oishi et al., personal communication). Characterization of the various APP residues phosphorylated in intact cells is underway to determine which sites of phosphorylation are utilized and to determine the possible existence of novel APP phosphorylation sites and APP kinases (Knops et al. 1993; Hung and Selkoe 1994; Suzuki et al. 1994; Oishi et al., personal communication). Once the sites for APP phosphorylation in intact cells are established, analysis of the processing of phosphorylation-site mutant APP molecules can be used to elucidate the role of direct phosphorylation of APP.

This approach has already been applied to certain cytoplasmic phosphorylation sites in APP (da Cruz e Silva et al. 1993; Hung and Selkoe 1994; Vitek et al., personal communication). These experiments have demonstrated that changes in the phosphorylation state of the APP cytoplasmic domain are not necessary in order for the phenomenon of phosphorylation-regulated alpha-secretory cleavage of APP to occur. These observations have led to the proposal that proteins of the processing/cleavage/release pathway may be phosphoprotein mediators of "regulated" or "activated processing" (da Cruz e Silva et al. 1993; Hung and Selkoe 1994).

Activation of proteolysis by phosphorylation has been demonstrated for a number of integral membrane proteins, including the polyimmunoglobulin receptor (pIgR; Casanova et al. 1990), the transforming growth factor-alpha (TGF-alpha) precursor (Pandiella and Massague 1991), and the receptor for colony-stimulating factor-1 (CSF1R; Downing et al. 1989). Direct phosphorylation of pIgR appears to be crucial to the activation of its trafficking and processing; phosphorylation of the TGF-alpha precursor has not been demonstrated; CSF1R is known to be a phosphoprotein, but the relationship between its phosphorylation and its proteolysis is not yet established.

In general terms, the possible mechanisms for activated processing of integral molecules can be conceptualized as involving either activation or redistribution of either the substrate (i.e., APP) or the enzyme (i.e., secretase). Based on the APP cytoplasmic tail mutational analyses described above (da Cruz e Silva et al. 1993; Hung and Selkoe 1994; Vitek et al., personal communication), the "substrate activation" model (Gandy et al. 1988, 1991, 1992b) is inadequate to completely explain activated processing of APP.

Furthermore, in recent immunofluorescent studies of APP in cultured cells which were incubated in the absence or presence of PKC- activating phorbol esters (Caporaso et al. 1994), no obvious phorbol-dependent redistribution of APP immunoreactivity was apparent at steady-state. A more detailed analysis of APP distribution following PKC activation is underway, as suggested by the model of Luini and De Matteis (1993).

Along a related line of investigation, Bosenberg and colleagues (1993) have succeeded in demonstrating apparently faithful activated processing of TGF-alpha precursor in porated cells in the virtual absence of cytosol, and in the presence of N-ethylmaleimide or 2.5 M NaCl. The preservation of activated processing under such conditions suggests that extensive vesicular trafficking is probably not required for activated processing of TGF-alpha, and is consistent with a model of enzyme activation by direct phosphorylation. Studies are underway to determine whether activated APP processing has similar features.

Beyond Aβ-Amyloid: Other Molecular Factors in Amyloidogenesis, and Factors Differentiating Aging-Related Cerebral Amyloidosis from AD

Since APP can be metabolized along several nonamyloidogenic or potentially amyloidogenic pathways. AD might be a clinicopathological phenotype that is due to a metabolic imbalance of the relative utilization of nonamyloido-genic pathway(s) versus potentially amyloidogenic pathway(s). To examine a possible correlation between APP metabolic pathway utilization and AD, some investigators have sought to identify AD-related changes in APP metabolism. Diminished levels of the large amino-terminal fragment of APP have been reported in the cerebrospinal fluid from patients with AD and from patients with the cerebrovascular Aβ-amyloidosis HCHWAD or FAD-Dutch (van Nostrand et al. 1992a,b). According to these reports, decreased levels of the released APP amino-terminal fragment were characteristic of the CSF from AD and FAD-Dutch patients, but not that from age-matched controls, although there was some overlap between AD patients and patients with non-Alzheimer-type dementia. To date, however, AD-specific changes in the levels of potentially amyloidogenic carboxyl-terminal fragments have not been observed in AD cortex (Nordstedt et al. 1991; Estus et al. 1992). Further, as noted in a preceding section, the metabolism of some mutant APP molecules and their carboxyl-terminal fragments in transfected cells appears to proceed in standard fashion (Cai et al. 1993; Felsenstein and Lewis-Higgins 1993; including apparently "normal" secretory cleavage), unperturbed by the presence of either the $APP^{717\text{-Ile}}$ FAD mutation or the $APP^{693\text{-Gln}}$ FAD-Dutch mutation (numbering according to APP_{770} isoform).

CSF levels of soluble Aβ-amyloid in normal aging and AD have been investigated to determine whether a correlation exists between CSF soluble Aβ-amyloid levels and the predisposition to AD. An initial study failed to detect an obvious relationship (Shoji et al. 1992), and that observation has been recently confirmed (Wisniewski et al. 1993). Thus, there appear to be other important factors – perhaps downstream events in the metabolism of APP fragments or soluble Aβ-amyloid – that play key roles in Aβ-fibrillogenesis. In support of this latter possibility is the evidence that an important effect of the FAD-Dutch mutation is to accelerate Aβ-amyloid fibril formation (Wisniewski et al. 1991). Factors contributing to Aβ-amyloid deposition and fibril formation may include the processing of soluble Aβ-amyloid into an aggregated form (Burdick et al. 1992; Dyrks et al. 1992) and/or the association of Aβ-amyloid with other molecules, such as alpha-1-ACT (Abraham et al. 1988), heparan sulfate proteoglycan (Snow et al. 1992), apolipoprotein E (Wisniewski and Frangione 1992; Strittmatter et al. 1993), and P component (Wisniewski and Frangione 1992). In addition, deposited Aβ-amyloid plaques may serve as nucleation foci and act to recruit additional Aβ-amyloid deposition (Maggio et al. 1992).

Events beyond Aβ-amyloid deposition may also be crucial in determining the eventual toxicity of Aβ-amyloid plaques. While aggregation of Aβ-amyloid is important for *in vitro* models of neurotoxicity (Mattson and Rydel 1992; Pike et al. 1993), the relevance of these phenomena for the pathogenesis of AD is unclear, since Aβ-amyloid deposits may occur in normal aging, in the absence of any evident proximate neuronal injury (Crystal et al. 1988; Masliah et al. 1990; Berg et al. 1993; Delaere et al. 1993). This finding suggests that other events must distinguish "simple" cerebral amyloidosis from "full-blown" AD. One intriguing possible contributing factor is the association of complement components with Aβ-amyloid (Rogers et al. 1992). In cerebellum, where Aβ-amyloid deposits appear to cause no injury, plaques are apparently free of associated complement, while in the forebrain, complement associates with plaques, perhaps becoming activated and injuring the surrounding cells (Lue and Rogers 1992). Other, as-yet undiscovered, plaque-associated molecules may also play important roles.

It is also possible that Alzheimer neuropathology may be a final end product which can develop through a host of independent initiating molecular abnormalities, analogous to the manner in which either disorders of oxygen radical metabolism (Rosen et al. 1993) or of cytoskeletal protein expression (Brady 1993; Cote et al. 1993; Xu et al. 1993) can lead to a clinicopathological picture of motor neuron disease. Similarly, in the case of AD, it is unknown whether, for example, in some situations cytoskeletal phosphorylation abnormalities could be initiating events, and Aβ-amyloid deposits could occur secondarily. In support of this possibility is the recent demonstration that toxin- or lesion-induced nerve terminal degeneration can be associated with altered, potentially amyloidogenic APP metabolism (Iverfeldt et al. 1993). Further, Aβ-amyloid deposition may "decorate" the periphery of amyloid plaques primarily composed of prion protein (Ikeda et al. 1993).

The most promising leads for furthering our understanding of the molecular pathology of AD beyond APP metabolism lie in elucidating the role of apolipoprotein E allelic variation in determining predisposition to SAD (Saunders et al. 1993 and in the eventual discovery of the gene which causes the most common form of FAD, a form caused by a gene which resides on chromosome 14 (Schellenberg et al. 1992; St George-Hyslop pet al. 1992; Van Broeckhoven et al. 1992; Mullan et al 1992b). The identity of this gene is entirely unknown: it may represent a molecule which regulates APP expression or degradation, analogous to the lysozyme protease enzyme defect which was recently discovered to underlie hereditary systemic amyloidosis (Pepys et al. 1993). Alternatively, the chromosome 14 mutant molecule may implicate neurofibrillary components or may point in an entirely unexpected direction. In any event, discovery of the chromosome 14 FAD gene may prove to be an important step toward the eventual unravelling of the molecular basis of typical, common SAD, and it is this information which offers the most promise for ultimately providing us with a full understanding of AD and making possible its rational treatment.

Acknowledgements. This work was supported USPHS grants AG-11508 (to S.G.), and AG-09464 and AG-10491 (to P.G.).

S.G. is the recipient of a Cornell Scholar Award in the Biomedical Sciences. The authors thank Drs. S. Sisodia and D. Selkoe for critical review of the manuscript.

References

Abraham CR, Selkoe DJ, Potter H (1988) Immunochemical identification of the serine protease inhibitor α_1-antichymotrypsin in the brain amyloid deposits of Alzheimer's disease. Cell 52:487–501

Arispe N, Rojas E, Pollard HB (1993) Alzheimer disease amyloid β protein forms calcium channels in bilayer membranes: Blockade by tromethamine and aluminum. Proc Natl Acad Sci USA 90:567–571

Bargmann C, Hung M, Weinberg R (1986) Multiple independent activations of the *neu* oncogene by a point mutation altering the transmembrane domain of p185. Cell 45:649–657

Baskin F, Rosenberg R, Davis RM (1992) Morphological differentiation and proteoglycan synthesis regulate Alzheimer amyloid precursor protein processing in PC-12 and human astrocyte cultures. J Neurosci Res 32:274–279

Berg L, McKeel DW, Miller JP, Baty J, Morris JC (1993) Neuropathological indexes of Alzheimer's disease in demented and nondemented persons aged 80 years and older. Arch Neurol 50:349–358

Bonifacino J, Cosson P, Klausner R (1990) Colocalized transmembrane determinants for ER degradation and subunit assembly explain the intracellular fate of TCR chains. Cell 63:503–513

Bosenberg MW, Pandiella A, Massague J (1993) Activated release of membrane-anchored TGF-α in the absence of cytosol. J Cell Biol 122:95–101

Brady ST (1993) Motor neurons and neurofilaments in sickness and in health. Cell 73:1–3

Burdick D, Soreghan B, Kwon M, Kosmoski J, Knauer M, Henschen A, Yates J, Cotman C, Glabe C (1992) Assembly and aggregation properties of synthetic Alzheimer's A4/β amyloid peptide analogs. J Biol Chem 267:546–554

Busciglio J, Gabuzda DH, Matsudaira P, Yankner B (1993) Generation of β-amyloid in the secretory pathway in neuronal and nonneuronal cells. Proc Natl Acad Sci USA 90:2092–2096

Bush AI, Martins RN, Rumble B, Moir R, Fuller S, Milward E, Currie J, Ames D, Weidemann A, Fischer P, Multhaup G, Beyreuther K, Masters CL (1990) The amyloid precursor protein of Alzheimer's disease is released by human platelets. J Biol Chem 265:15977–15983

Bush AI, White S, Thomas LD, Williamson TG, Van Tiggelen CJ, Currie J, Small DH, Moir RD, Li Q-X, Rumble B, Monning U, Beyreuther K, Masters C (1992) An abnormality of plasma amyloid protein precursor in Alzheimer's disease. Ann Neurol 32:57–65

Buxbaum JD, Gandy SE, Cicchetti P, Ehrlich ME, Czernik AJ, Fracasso RP, Ramabhadran TV, Unterbeck AJ, Greengard P (1990) Processing of Alzheimer β/A4 amyloid precursor protein: Modulation by agents that regulate protein phosphorylation. Proc Natl Acad Sci USA 87:6003–6006

Buxbaum JD, Oishi M, Chen HI, Pinkas-Kramarski R, Jaffe EA, Gandy SE, Greengard P (1992) Cholinergic agonists and interleukin 1 regulate processing and secretion of the Alzheimer β/A4 amyloid protein precursor. Proc Natl Acad Sci USA 89:10075–10078

Buxbaum JD, Koo EH, Greengard P (1993) Protein phosphorylation inhibits production of Alzheimer amyloid β/A4 peptide. Proc Natl Acad Sci USA 90:9195–9198

Cai X-D, Golde TE, Younkin SG (1993) Release of excess amyloid β protein from a mutant amyloid β protein precursor. Science 259:514–516

Cairns NJ, Chadwick A, Lantos PL, Levy R, Rossor MN (1993) βA4 protein deposition in familial Alzheimer's disease with the mutation in codon 717 of the βA4 amyloid precursor protein gene and sporadic Alzheimer's disease. Neurosci Lett 149:137–140

Caporaso GL, Gandy SE, Buxbaum JD, Greengard P (1992a) Chloroquine inhibits intracelluar degradation but not secretion of Alzheimer β/A4 amyloid precursor protein. Proc Natl Acad Sci USA 89:2252–2256

Caporaso GL, Gandy SE, Buxbaum JD, Ramabhadran TV, Greengard P (1992b) Protein phosphorylation regulates secretion of Alzheimer β/A4 amyloid precursor protein. Proc Natl Acad Sci USA 89:3055–3059

Caporaso G, Takei K, Gandy S, Matteoli M, Mundigl O, Greengard P, de Camilli P (1994) Morphologic and biochemical analysis of the intracellular trafficking of the Alzheimer β/A4 amyloid precursor protein. J Neurosci, in press

Casanova JE, Breitfeld PP, Ross SA, Mostov KE (1990) Phosphorylation of the polymeric immunoglobulin receptor required for its efficient transcytosis. Science 248:742–745

Chartier-Harlin M-C, Crawford F, Houlden H, Warren A, Hughes D, Fidani L, Goate A, Rossor M, Roques P, Hardy J, Mullan M (1991) Early-onset Alzheimer's disease caused by mutations at codon 717 of the β-amyloid precursor protein gene. Nature 353:844–846

Chen W-J, Goldstein JL, Brown MS (1990) NPXY, a sequence often found in cytoplasmic tails, is required for coated pit-mediated internalization of the low density lipoprotein receptor. J Biol Chem 265:3116–3123

Cheung TT, Ghiso J, Shoji M, Cai X-D, Golde T, Gandy S, Frangione B, Younkin S. (1994) Characterization by radiosequencing of the carboxyl-terminal derivatives produced from normal and mutant amyloid β protein precursors. Amyloid, in press

Citron M, Oltersdorf T, Haass C, McConlogue L, Hung AY, Seubert P, Vigo-Pelfrey C, Lieberburg I, Selkoe DJ (1992) Mutation of the β-amyloid precursor protein in familial Alzheimer's disease increases β-protein production. Nature 360:672–674

Cohen P, Holmes CFB, Tsukitani Y (1990) Okadaic acid: A new probe for the study of cellular regulation. Trends Biochem Sci 15:98–102

Cole G, Dobkins KR, Hansen LA, Terry RD, Saitoh T (1988) Decreased levels of protein kinase C in Alzheimer brain. Brain Res 452:165–174

Cole GM, Huynh TV, Saitoh T (1989) Evidence for lysosomal processing of amyloid β-protein precursor in cultured cells. Neurochem Res 14:933–939

Cote F, Collard J-F, Julien J-P (1993) Progressive neuronopathy in transgenic mice expressing the human neurofilament heavy gene: A mouse model of amyotrophic lateral sclerosis. Cell 73:35–46

Crystal H, Dickson D, Fuld P, Masur D, Scott R, Mehler M, Masdeu J, Kawas C, Aronson M, Wolfson L (1988) Clinico-pathologic studies in dementia: Nondemented subjects with pathologically confirmed Alzheimer's disease. Neurology 38:1682–1687

da Cruz e Silva O, Iverfeldt K, Oltersdorf T, Sinha S, Lieberburg I, Ramabhadran T, Suzuki T, Sisodia S, Gandy S, Greengard P (1993) Regulated cleavage of Alzheimer β-amyloid precursor protein in the absence of the cytoplasmic tail. Neuroscience 57:873–877

Davies P, Maloney AJF (1976) Selective loss of central cholinergic neurons in Alzheimer's disease. Lancet II, 1403

Delaere P, He Y, Fayet G, Duyckaerts C, Hauw JJ (1993) βA4 deposits are constant in the brain of the oldest old: An immunocytochemical study of 20 French centenarians. Neurobiol Aging 14:191–194

Downing JR, Roussel MF, Sherr CJ (1989) Ligand and protein kinase C downmodulate the colony-stimulating factor 1 receptor by independent mechanisms. Mol Cell Biol 9:2890–2896

Dyrks T, Dyrks E, Hartmann T, Masters C, Beyreuther K (1992) Amyloidogenicity of βA4 and βA4-bearing fragments by metal catalyzed oxidation. J Biol Chem 267:18210–18217

Ehlers MRW, Riordan JF (1991) Membrane proteins with soluble counterparts: Role of proteolysis in the release of transmembrane proteins. Biochemistry 30:10065–10074

Esch FS, Keim PS, Beattie EC, Blacher RW, Culwell AR, Oltersdorf T, McClure D, Ward PJ, (1990) Cleavage of amyloid β peptide during constitutive processing of its precursor. Science 248:1122–1124

Estus S, Golde T, Kunishita T, Blades D, Lowery D, Eisen M, Usiak M, Qu X, Tabira T, Greenberg B, Younkin S (1992) Potentially amyloidogenic, carboxyl-terminal deriviatives of the amyloid protein precursor. Science 255:726–728

Felsenstein K, Lewis-Higgins L (1993) Processing of the β-amyloid precursor protein carrying the familial, Dutch-type, and a novel recombinant C-terminal mutation. Neurosci Lett 152:185–189

Felsenstein KM, Hunihan LW, Roberts SB (1994) Altered cleavage and secretion of a recombinant β-APP bearing the Swedish familial Alzheimer's disease mutation. Nature Genetics 6:251–256

Gandy S, Greengard P (1992) Amyloidogenesis in Alzheimer's disease: Some possible therapeutic opportunities. Trends Pharmacol Sci 13:108–113

Gandy SE, Bhasin R, Ramabhadran TV, Koo EL, Price DL, Goldgaber D, Greengard P (1992a) Alzheimer β/A4-amyloid precursor protein: Evidence for putative amyloidogenic fragment. J Neurochem 58:383–386

Gandy SE, Buxbaum JD, Greengard P (1991) Signal transduction and the pathobiology of Alzheimer's disease. In: Iqbal K, Crapper McLachlan DR, Winblad B, Wisniewski HM (eds) Alzheimer's disease, basic mechanisms, diagnosis and therapeutic strategies. John Wiley & Sons Ltd., New York, pp 155–172

Gandy SE, Buxbaum JD, Greengard P (1992b) A cell biological approach to the therapy of Alzheimer-type cerebral βA4-amyloidosis. In: Khachaturian ZS, Blass JP (eds) Alzheimer's disease, new treatment strategies. Marcel Dekker, Inc., New York, pp 175–192

Gandy S, Czernik AJ, Greengard P (1988) Phosphorylation of Alzheimer disease amyloid precursor peptide by protein kinase C and Ca^{2+}/calmodulin-dependent protein kinase II. Proc Natl Acad Sci USA 85:6218–6221

Ghetti B, Murrell J, Benson MD, Farlow MR (1992) Spectrum of amyloid β-protein immunoreactivity in hereditary Alzheimer disease with a guanine to thymine missense change at position 1924 of the APP gene. Neurosci Lett 571:133–139

Gillespie SL, Golde TE, Younkin SG (1992) Secretory processing of the Alzheimer amyloid β/A4 protein precursor is increased by protein phosphorylation. Biochem Biophys Res Commun 187:1285–1290

Glenner GG, Wong CW (1984a) Alzheimer's disease: Initial report of the purification and characterization of a novel cerebrovascular amyloid protein. Biochem Biophys Res Commun. 120:885–890

Glenner GG, Wong CW (1984b) Alzheimer's disease and Down's syndrome: Sharing of a unique cerebrovascular amyloid fibril protein. Biochem Biophys Res Commun 122:1131–1135

Goate A, Chartier-Harlin, M-C, Mullan M, Brown J, Crawford F, Fidani L, Giuffra L, Haynes A, Irving N, James L, Mant R, Newton P, Rooke K, Roques P, Talbot C, Pericak-Vance M, Roses A, Williamson R, Rossor M, Owen M, Hardy J (1991) Segregation of a missense mutation in the amyloid precursor protein gene with familial Alzheimer's disease. Nature 349:704–706

Golde TE, Estus S, Younkin LH, Selkoe DJ, Younkin SG (1992) Processing of the amyloid protein precursor to potentially amyloidogenic derivatives. Science 255:728–730

Goldgaber D, Lerman MI, McBride OW, Saffiotti U, Gajdusek DC (1987) Characterization and chromosomal localization of a cDNA encoding brain amyloid of Alzheimer's disease. Science 235:877–880

Goldgaber D, Harris HW, Hla T, Maciag T, Donnelly RJ, Jacobsen JS, Vitek MP, Gajdusek DC (1989) Interleukin 1 regulates synthesis of amyloid β-protein precursor mRNA in human endothelial cells. Proc Natl Acad Sci USA 86:7606–7610

Haass C, Hung AY, Selkoe DJ (1991) Processing of β-amyloid precursor protein in microglia and astrocytes favors an internal localization over constitutive secretion. J Neurosci 11:3783–3793

Haass C, Koo, EH, Mellon A, Hung AY, Selkoe DJ (1992a) Targeting of cell-surface β-amyloid precursor protein in lysosomes: Alternative processing into amyloid-bearing fragments. Nature 357:500–503

Haass C, Schlossmacher MG, Hung AY, Vigo-Pelfrey C, Mellon A, Ostaszewski BL, Lieberburg I, Koo EH, Schenk D, Teplow DB, Selkoe DJ (1992b) Amyloid β-peptide is produced by cultured cells during normal metabolism. Nature 359:322–325

Haass C, Hung AY, Schlossmacher MG, Teplow DB, Selkoe DJ (1993) β-amyloid peptide and a 3-kDa fragment are derived by distinct cellular mechanisms. J Biol Chem 268:3021–3024

Hata A, Akita Y, Suzuki K, Ohno S (1993) Functional divergence of protein kinase C family members. J Biol Chem 268:9122–9129

Hung AY, Koo EH, Haass C, Selkoe DJ (1992) Increased expression of β-amyloid precursor protein during neuronal differentiation is not accompanied by secretory cleavage. Proc Natl Acad Sci USA 89:9439–9443

Hung AY, Haass C, Nitsch RM, Qiu WQ, Citron M, Wurtman RJ, Growdon JH, Selkoe DJ (1993) Activation of protein kinase C inhibits cellular production of the amyloid β-protein. J Biol Chem 268:22959–22962

Hung AY, Selkoe DJ (1994) Selective ectodomain phosphorylation and regulated cleavage of β-amyloid precursor protein. EMBO J 13:534–542

Husby G, Araki S, Benditt EP, Glenner GG, Natvig JB, Westermark P (1993) Nomenclature of amyloid and amyloidosis. Bull WHO 71:105–108

Hwang T-C, Lu L, Gruenet DC, Huganir R, Guggino WB (1989) Cl⁻ channels in CF: Lack of activation by protein kinase C and cAMP-dependent protein kinase. Science 244:1351–1353

Ikeda S, Yanagisawa N, Glenner G, Allsop D (1993) Gerstmann-Straussler-Scheinker disease showing β-protein amyloid deposits in the peripheral regions of PrP-immunoreactive amyloid plaques. Neurodegeneration 1:281–288

Iverfeldt K, Walaas SI, Greengard P (1993) Altered processing of Alzheimer amyloid precursor protein in response to neuronal degeneration. Proc Natl Acad Sci USA 90:4146–4150

Kang J, Lemaire H-G, Unterbeck A, Salbaum JM, Masters CL, Grzeschik K-H, Multhaup G, Beyreuther K, Müller-Hill B (1987) The precursor of Alzheimer's disease amyloid A4 protein resembles a cell-surface receptor. Nature 325:733–736

Kennedy AM, Newman S, McCaddon A, Ball J, Roques P, Mullan M, Hardy J, Chartier-Harlin M-C, Frackowiak RSJ, Warrington EK, Rossor MN (1993) Familial Alzheimer's disease: A pedigree with a missense mutation in the amyloid precursor protein gene (amyloid precursor protein 717 valine to glycine). Brain 116:309–324

Kitaguchi N, Takahashi Y, Tokushima Y, Shiojiri S, Ito H (1988) Novel precursor of Alzheimer's disease amyloid protein shows protease inhibitory activity. Nature 331:530–532

Knops J, Lieberburg I, Sinha S (1992) Evidence for a nonsecretory, acidic degradation pathway for amyloid precursor protein in 293 cells. J Biol Chem 267:16022–16024

Knops J, Gandy S, Greengard P, Lieberburg I, Sinha S (1993) Serine phosphorylation of the secreted extracellular domain of APP. Biochem Biophys Res Commun 197:380–385

Konig G, Monning U, Czeck C, Prior R, Baniti R, Schreiter-Gasser U, Bauer J, Masters CL, Beyreuther K (1992) Identification and expression of a novel alternative splice form of the βA4 amyloid precursor protein. (APP) mRNA in leucocytes and brain microglial cells. J Biol Chem 267:10804–10809

Koo E, Sisodia S, Cork L, Unterbeck A, Bayney R, Price D (1990) Differential expression of amyloid precursor protein mRNAs in cases of Alzheimer's disease and in aged nonhuman primates. Neuron 2:97–104

Lahiri DK, Nall C, Farlow M (1992) The cholinergic agonist carbachol reduces intracellular β-amyloid precursor protein in PC 12 and C6 cells. Biochem Int 28:853–860

Lantos PL, Luthert PJ, Hanger D, Anderton BH, Mullan M, Rossor M (1992) Familial Alzheimer's disease with the amyloid precursor protein position 717 mutation and sporadic Alzheimer's disease have the same cytoskeletal pathology. Neurosci Lett 137:221–224

Levy E, Carmen MD, Fernandez-Madrid IJ, Power MD, Lieberburg I, van Duinen SG, Bots GThAM, Luyendijk W, Frangione B (1990) Mutation of the Alzheimer's disease amyloid gene in hereditary cerebral hemorrhage, Dutch type. Science 248:1124–1126

Li M, McCann J, Liedtke C, Nairn A, Greengard P, Welsh M (1988) Cyclic AMP-dependent protein kinase opens chloride channels in normal but not cystic fibrosis airway epithelium. Nature 331:358–360

Li M, McCann JD, Anderson MP, Clancy JP, Liedtke CM, Nairn AC, Greengard P, Welsh MJ (1989) Regulation of chloride channels by protein kinase C in normal and cystic fibrosis airway epithelia. Science 244:1353–1356

Lue L-F, Rogers J (1992) Full complement activation fails in diffuse plaques of the Alzheimer's disease cerebellum. Dementia 3:308–313

Luini A, De Matteis MA (1993) Receptor-mediated regulation of constitutive secretion. Trends in Cell Biol 3:290–292

Maggio JE, Stimson ER, Ghilard JR, Allen CJ, Dahl CE, Whitcomb DC, Vigna SR, Vinters HV, Labenski ME, Mantyh PW (1992) Reversible in vitro growth of Alzheimer disease β-amyloid plaques by deposition of labeled amyloid peptide. Proc Natl Acad Sci USA 89:5462–5466

Mann DMA, Jones D, Snowden JS, Neary D, Hardy J (1992) Pathological changes in the brain of a patient with familial Alzheimer's disease having a missense mutation at codon 717 in the amyloid precursor protein gene. Neurosci Lett 137:225–228

Maruyama K, Kametani F, Usami M, Yamao-Harigaya W, Tanaka K (1991) "Secretase", Alzheimer amyloid protein precursor secreting enzyme is not sequence specific. Biochem Biophys Res Commun 179:1670–1676

Masliah E, Terry RD, Mallory M, Alford M, Hansen LA (1990) Diffuse plaques do not accentuate synapse loss in Alzheimer's disease. Am J Pathol 137:1293–1297

Masliah E, Cole GM, Hansen LA, Mallory M, Albright T, Terry RD, Saitoh T (1991) Protein kinase C alteration is an early biochemical marker in Alzheimer's disease. J Neurosci 11:2759–2767

Masters CL, Simms G, Weinman NA, Multhaup G, McDonald BL, Beyreuther K (1985) Amyloid plaque core protein in Alzheimer disease and Down syndrome. Proc Natl Acad Sci USA 82:4245–4249

Mattson MP, Cheng B, Culwell AR, Esch FS, Lieberburg I, Rydel RE (1993) Evidence for excitoprotective and intraneuronal calcium-regulating roles for secreted forms of the β-amyloid precursor protein. Neuron 10:243–254

Mattson MP, Rydel R (1992) β-amyloid precursor protein and Alzheimer's disease: The peptide plot thickens. Neurobiol Aging 13:617–621

Miyazaki K, Hasegawa M, Funahashi K, Umeda M (1993) A metalloproteinase inhibitor domain in Alzheimer amyloid protein precursor. Nature 362:839–841

Mullan MF, Crawford K, Axelman H, Houlden L, Lilius B, Winblad L, Lannfelt (1992a) A pathogenic mutation for probable Alzheimer's disease in the APP gene at the N-terminus of β-amyloid. Nature Genet 1:345–347

Mullan M, Houlden H, Windelspecht M, Fidani L, Lombardi C, Diaz P, Rossor M, Crook R, Hardy J, Duff K, Crawford F (1992b) A locus for familial early-onset Alzheimer's disease on the long arm of chromosome 14, proximal to the α_1-antichymotrypsin gene. Nature Genet 2:340–342

Murrell J, Farlow M, Ghetti B, Benson MD (1991) A mutation in the amyloid precursor protein associated with hereditary Alzheimer disease. Science 254:97–99

Naruse S, Igarashi S, Kobayashi H, Aoki K, Inuzuka T, Kaneko K, Shimizu T, Iihara K, Kojima T, Miyatake T, Tsuji S (1991) Missense mutation Val-Ile in exon 17 of amyloid precursor protein gene in Japanese familial Alzheimer's disease. Lancet 337:978–979

Nishimoto I, Okamoto T, Matsuura Y, Takahashi S, Okamoto T, Murayama Y, Ogata E (1993) Alzheimer amyloid protein precursor complexes with brain GTP-binding protein G_0. Nature 362:75–79

Nitsch RM, Slack BE, Wurtman RJ, Growdon JH (1992) Release of Alzheimer amyloid precursor derivatives stimulated by activation of muscarinic acetylcholine receptors. Science 258:304–307

Nordstedt C, Gandy SE, Alafuzoff I, Caporaso G, Iverfeldt K, Grebb JA, Winblad B, Greengard P (1991) Alzheimer β/A4 amyloid precursor protein in human brain: Aging-associated increases in holoprotein and in a proteolytic fragment. Proc Natl Acad Sci USA 88:8910–8914

Nordstedt C, Caporaso GL, Thyberg J, Gandy SE, Greengard P (1993) Identification of the Alzheimer β/A4 amyloid precursor protein in clathrin-coated vesicles purified from PC12 cells. J Biol Chem 268:608–612

Oltersdorf T, Fritz LC, Schenk DB, Lieberburg I, Johnson-Wood KL, Beattie EC, Ward PJ, Blacher RW, Dovey HF, Sinha S (1989) The secreted form of the Alzheimer's amyloid precursor protein with the Kunitz domain is protease nexin-II. Nature 341:144–147

Oltersdorf T, Ward PJ, Henriksson T, Beattie EC, Neve R, Lieberburg I, Fritz LC (1990) The Alzheimer amyloid precursor protein: Identification of a stable intermediate in the biosynthetic/degradative pathway. J Biol Chem 265:4492–4497

Overly CC, Fritz LC, Lieberburg I, McConlogue L (1991) The β-amyloid precursor protein is not processed by the regulated secretory pathway. Biochem Biophys Res Comm 181:513–519

Palmert MR, Berman-Podlisny M, Witker DS, Oltersdorf T, Younkin LH, Selkoe DJ, Younkin SG (1989) The β-amyloid protein precursor of Alzheimer disease has soluble derivatives found in human brain and cerebrospinal fluid. Proc Natl Acad Sci USA 86:6338–6342

Palmert MR, Podlisny MB, Witker DS, Oltersdorf T, Younkin LH, Selkoe DJ, Younkin SG (1989) The β-amyloid protein precursor of Alzheimer disease has soluble derivatives found in human brain and cerebrospinal fluid. Proc Natl Acad Sci USA 86:6338–6342

Pandiella A, Massagué J (1991) Cleavage of the membrane precursor for transforming growth factor α is a regulated process. Proc Natl Acad Sci USA 88:1726–1730

Pandiella A, Bosenberg MW, Huang EJ, Besmer P, Massagué J (1992) Cleavage of membrane-anchored growth factors involves distinct protease activities regulated through common mechanisms. J Biol Chem 267:24028–24033

Pepys MB, Hawkins PN, Booth DR, Vigushin DM, Tennent GA, Soutar AK, Totty N, Nguyen O, Blake CCF, Terry CJ, Feest TG, Zalin AM, Hsuan (1993) Human lysozyme gene mutations cause hereditary systemic amyloidosis. Nature 362:553–557

Pike CJ, Burdick D, Walencewicz AJ, Glabe CG, Cotman CW (1993) Neurodegeneration induced by β-amyloid peptides in vitro: The role of peptide assembly state. J Neurosci 13:1676–1687

Ponte P, Gonzalez-DeWhitt P, Schilling J, Miller J, Hsu D, Greenberg B, Davis K, Wallace W, Lieberburg I, Fuller F, Cordell B (1988) A new A4 amyloid mRNA contains a domain homologous to serine proteinase inhibitors. Nature 331:525–527

Robakis NK, Ramakrishna N, Wolfe G, Wisniewski HM (1987) Molecular cloning and characterization of a cDNA encoding the cerebrovascular and neuritic plaque amyloid peptides. Proc Natl Acad Sci USA 84:4190–4194

Rogers J, Cooper NR, Webster S, Schultz J, McGeer PL, Styren SD, Civin WH, Brachova L, Bradt B, Ward P, Lieberburg I (1992) Complement activation by β-amyloid in Alzheimer disease. Proc Natl Acad USA 89:10016–10020

Rosen DR, Siddique T, Patterson D, Figlewicz DA, Sapp P, Hentati A, Donaldson D, Goto J, O'Regan JP, Deng H-X, Rahmani Z, Krizus A, McKenna-Yasek D, Cayabyab A, Gaston SM, Berger R, Tanzi RE, Halperin JJ, Herzfeldt B, Van den Bergth R, Hung W-Y, Bird T, Deng G, Mulder DW, Smyth C, Laing NG, Soriano E, Pericak-Vance MA, Haines J, Rouleau GA, Gusella JS, Horvitz HR, Brown RH (1993) Mutations in Cu/Zn superoxide dismutase gene are associated with familial amyotrophic lateral sclerosis. Nature 362:59–62

Rossor M (1992) Familial Alzheimer's disease. In: Rossor M (ed) Bailliere's clinical neurology: unusual dementias. Baillere Tindall, Philadelphia, 517–534

Sahasrabudhe SR, Spruyt MA, Muenkel HA, Blume AJ, Vitek MP, Jacobsen JS (1992) Release of amino-terminal fragments from amyloid precursor protein reporter and mutated derivatives in cultured cells. J Biol Chem 267:25062–25608

Saitoh T, Sundsmo M, Roch J-M, Kimura N, Cole G, Schubert D, Oltersdorf T, Schenk DB (1989) secreted form of amyloid β protein precursor is involved in the growth regulation of fibroblasts. Cell 58:615–622

Saunders AM, Strittmatter WJ, Schmechel D, St George-Hyslop PH, Pericak-Vance MA, Joos SH, Rosi BL, Gusella JF, Crapper-MacLachlan DR, Alberts MJ, Hulette C, Crain B, Goldgaber D, Roses AD (1993) Association of apolipoprotein E allele ε4 with late-onset familial and sporadic Alzheimer's disease. Neurology 43:1467–1472

Schellenberg GD, Bird TD, Wijsman EM, Orr HT, Anderson L, Nemens E, White JA, Bonnycastle

L, Weber JL, Alonso ME, Potter H, Heston LL, Martin GM (1992) Genetic evidence for a familial Alzheimer's disease locus on chromosome 14. Science 258:668–671

Schoumacher RA, Shoemaker RL, Halm DR, Tallant EA, Wallace RW, Frizzel RA (1987) Phoshorylation fails to activate chloride channels from cystic fibrosis airway cells. Nature 330:752–754

Schubert D, LaCorbiere M, Saitoh T, Cole G (1989) Characterization of an amyloid β precursor protein that binds heparin and contains tyrosine sulfate. Proc Natl Acad Sci USA 86:2066–2069

Seubert P, Vigo-Plefrey C, Esch F, Lee M, Dovey H, Davis D, Sinha S, Schlossmacher M, Whaley J, Swindlehurst C, McCormack R, Wolfert T, Selkoe D, Lieberburg I, Schenk D (1992) Isolation and quantification of soluble Alzheimer's β-peptide from biological fluids. Nature 359:325–327

Seubert P, Oltersdorf T, Lee MG, Barbour R, Blomquist C, Davis DL, Bryant K, Fritz LC, Galasko D, Thal LJ, Lieberburg I, Schenk DB (1993) Secretion of β-amyloid precursor protein cleaved at the amino terminus of the β-amyloid peptide. Nature 361:260–263

Shackelford DA, Trowbridge IS (1986) Identification of lymphocyte integral membrane proteins as substrates for protein kinase C. J Biol Chem 261:8334–8341

Shioi J, Anderson JP, Ripellino JA, Robakis NK (1992) Chondroitin sulfate proteoglycan form of the Alzheimer's β-amyloid precursor. J Biol Chem 267:13819–13822

Shoji M, Golde TE, Ghiso J, Cheung TT, Estus S, Shaffer LM, Cai X-D, McKay DM, Tintner R, Frangione B, Younkin SG (1992) Production of the Alzheimer amyloid β protein by normal proteolytic processing. Science 258:126–129

Sinha S, Lieberburg I (1992) Normal metabolism of the amyloid precursor protein (APP). Neurodegeneration 1:169–175

Sisodia SS (1992) β-amyloid precursor protein cleavage by a membrane-bound protease. Proc Natl Acad Sci USA 89:6075–6079

Sisodia SS, Koo EH, Beyreuther K, Unterbeck A, Price DL (1990) Evidence that β-amyloid protein in Alzheimer's disease is not derived by normal processing. Science 248:492–495

Slunt HH, Thinakaran G, Von Koch C, Lo ACY, Tanzi RE, Sisodia SS (1994) Expression of a ubiquitous cross-reactive homologue of the mouse β-amyloid precursor protein (APP) J Biol Chem 269:2637–2644

Smith RP, Higuchi DA, Broze GJ, Jr (1990) Platelet coagulation factor XIₐ-inhibitor, a form of Alzheimer amyloid precursor protein. Science 248:1126–1128

Snow AD, Sekiguchi R, Nochlin D, Kimata K, Schreier WA, Morgan DG (1992) A rat model to study the effects of βAP-containing amyloid in brain. Soc Neurosci Abstr 18:1465

St George-Hyslop P, Haines I, Rogaev E, Mortilla M, Vaula G, Pericak-Vance M, Foncin J-F, Montesi M, Bruni A, Sorbi S, Rainero I, Pinessi L, Pollen D, Polinsky R, Nee L, Kennedy J, Macciardi F, Rogaeva E, Liang Y, Alexandrova N, Lukiw W, Schlumpf K, Tanzi R, Tsuda T, Farrer L, Cantu J-M, Duara R, Amaducci L, Bergamini L, Gusella J, Roses A, Crapper-McLachlan D (1992) Genetic evidence for a novel familial Alzheimer's disease locus on chromosome 14. Nature Genet 2:330–334

Strittmatter WJ, Saunders AM, Schmechel D, Pericak-Vance M, Enghild J, Salvesen GS, Roses AD (1993) Apolipoprotein E: High-avidity binding to β-amyloid and increased frequency of type 4 allele in late-onset familial Alzheimer disease. Proc Natl Acad Sci USA 90:1977–1981

Suzuki T, Nairn AC, Gandy SE, Greengard P (1992) Phosphorylation of Alzheimer amyloid precursor protein by protein kinase C. Neuroscience 48:755–761

Suzuki T, Oishi M, Marshak DR, Czernik AJ, Nairn AC, Greengard P (1994) Cell cycle-dependent regulation of the phosphorylation and metabolism of the Alzheimer amyloid precursor protein. EMBO J., in press

Tamaoka A, Kalaria RN, Lieberburg I, Selkoe D (1992) Identification of a stable fragment of the Alzheimer amyloid precursor containing the β-protein in brain microvessels. Proc Natl Acad Sci USA 89:1345–1349

Tanzi RE, Gusella JF, Watkins PC, Bruns GAP, St George-Hyslop P, Van Keuren ML, Patterson D, Pagan S, Kurnit DM, Neve RL (1987) Amyloid β protein gene: cDNA, mRNA distribution, and genetic linkage near the Alzheimer locus. Science 235:880–884

Tanzi RE, McClatchey AI, Lamperti ED, Villa-Komaroff L, Gusella JF, Neve RL (1988) Protease inhibitor domain encoded by an amyloid protein precursor mRNA associated with Alzheimer's disease. Nature 31:528–530

Tanzi R, Hyman B (1991) Alzheimer's mutation. Nature 350:564

Tomlinson BE, Corsellis JAN (1984) Ageing and the dementias *In*: Adams JH, Corsellis JAN, Duchen LW, (eds) Greenfield's neuropathology. Fourth edition. John Wiley & Sons, Inc., New York, pp 951–1025

Van Broeckhoven C, Haan J, Bakker E, Hardy JA, Van Hul W, Wehnert A, Vegter-Van der Vlis M, Roos RAC (1990) Amyloid β protein precursor gene and hereditary cerebral hemorrhage with amyloidosis (Dutch). Science 248 : 1120–1122

Van Broeckhoven C, Backhovens H, Crusts M, De Winter G, Bruyland M, Cras P, Martin J-J (1992) Mapping of a gene predisposing to early-onset Alzheimer's disease to chromosome 14q24.3. Nature Genet 2 : 335–339

van Duinen SG, Castaño EM, Prelli F, Bots GThAM, Luyendijk W, Frangione B (1987) Hereditary cerebral hemorrhage with amyloidosis in patients of Dutch origin is related to Alzheimer disease. Proc Natl Acad Sci USA 84 : 5991–5994

Van Huynh T, Cole G, Katzman R, Huang K-P, Saitoh T (1989) Reduced protein kinase C immunore- activity and altered protein phosphorylation in Alzheimer's disease fibroblasts. Arch Neurol 46 : 1195–1199

Van Nostrand WE, Cunningham DD (1987) Purification of protease nexin II from human fibroblasts. J Biol Chem 262 : 8508–8514

Van Nostrand WE, Wagner SL, Suzuki M, Choi BH, Farrow JS, Geddes JW, Cotman CW, Cunning- ham DD (1989) Protease nexin II, a potent antichymotrypsin, shows identity to amyloid β-protein precursor. Nature 341 : 546–549

Van Nostrand W, Wagner S, Shankle WR, Farrow JS, Dick M, Rozemuller JM, Kuiper MA, Wolters EC, Zimmerman J, Cotman CW, Cunningham DD (1992a) Decreased levels of soluble amyloid β-protein precursor in cerebrospinal fluid of live Alzheimer disease patients. Proc Natl Acad Sci USA 89 : 2551–2555

Van Nostrand WE, Wagner SL, Haan J, Bakker E, Roos RA (1992b) Alzheimer's disease and hereditary cerebral hemorrhage with amyloidosis-Dutch type share a decrease in cerebrospinal fluid levels of amyloid β-protein precursor. Ann Neurol 32 : 215–218

Wagner J, Cozens A, Schulman H, Gruenert D, Stryer L, Gardner P (1991) Activation of chloride channels in normal and cystic fibrosis airway epithelial cells by multifunctional calcium/calmodulin- dependent protein kinase. Nature 349 : 793–796

Wasco W, Bupp K, Magendantz M, Gusella JF, Tanzi RE, Solomon F (1992) Identification of a mouse brain cDNA that encodes a protein related to the Alzheimer disease-associated amyloid β protein precursor. Proc Natl Acad Sci USA 89 : 10758–10762

Wasco W, Gurubhagavatula S, Paradis Md, Romano DM, Sisodia SS, Hyman BT, Neve RL, Tanzi RE (1993) Isolation and characterization of APLP2 encoding a homologue of the Alzheimer's associated amyloid β protein precursor. Proc Natl Acad Sci USA 5 : 95–100

Weidemann A, König G, Bunke D, Fischer P, Salbaum JM, Masters CL, Beyreuther K (1989) Identification, biogenesis, and localization of precursors of Alzheimer's disease A4 amyloid protein. Cell 57 : 115–126

Wisniewski T, Frangione B (1992) Apolipoprotein E : A pathological chaperone in patients with cerebral and systemic amyloid. Neurosci Lett 135 : 235–238

Wisniewski T, Ghiso J, Frangione B (1991) Peptides homologous to the amyloid protein of Alzheimer's disease containing a glutamine for glutamic acid substitution have accelerated amyloid fibril formation. Biochem Biophys Res Commun 179 : 1247–1254

Wisniewski T, Wegiel J, Wisniewski HM, Frangione B (1993) Alzheimer's amyloid β subunit is present in preamyloid deposits and in CSF. Neurology 43 : A422

Wolf D, Quon D, Wang Y, Cordell B (1990) Identification and characterization of C-terminal fragments of the β-amyloid precursor produced in cell culture. EMBO J 9 : 2079–2084

Xu Z, Cork LC, Griffin JW, Cleveland DW (1993) Increased expression of neurofilament subunit NF-L produces morphological alterations that resemble the pathology of human motor neuron disease. Cell 73 : 23–33

Studies of APP Biology: Analysis of APP Secretion and Characterization of an APP Homologue, APLP2

S. S. Sisodia*, H. H. Slunt, C. Van Koch, A. C. Y. Lo, and G. Thinakaran

Abstract

β-Amyloid precursor proteins (APP) are integral membrane glycoproteins encoded by alternatively spliced transcripts derived from a single gene on chromosome 21 (Müller-Hill and Beyreuther 1989; Selkoe 1989). Biochemical studies have demonstrated that APP mature through the constitutive secretory pathway and that a fraction of molecules are secreted into the conditioned medium following endoproteolytic cleavage within the Aβ sequence. In this report, we define the cellular site of APP cleavage as the plasma membrane. We also provide strong evidence for the role of APP cytoplasmic sequences on intracellular trafficking and endocytosis of newly synthesized APP. Additional studies are presented that describe the identification and characterization of a novel APP homologue, APLP2. APLP2 mRNA are expressed ubiquitously and at high levels relative to APP in rodent tissue; the neuronal expression of APLP2 has been demonstrated by *in situ* hybridization. *In vitro* studies indicate that APLP2 matures through the constitutive secretory pathway and that soluble APLP2 derivatives are secreted. Importantly, several antibodies elicited against APP epitopes cannot discriminate between APP and APLP2, suggesting that numerous reports purported to follow APP may have followed APLP2 as well.

Introduction

Alzheimer's disease is a neurodegenerative disorder characterized by the presence of numerous senile plaques and neurofibrillary tangles in the cerebral cortex and hippocampus of affected individuals (Wisniewski and Terry 1973; Kemper 1984; Goedert et al. 1991). The principal protein in plaques is Aβ (Glenner and Wong 1984; Masters et al. 1985), an ~ 4-kD amyloidogenic peptide, derived from larger APP (Kang et al. 1987). APP are ubiquitously expressed integral membrane glycoproteins of 695, 714, 751, and 770 amino

---

* Neuropathology Laboratory, The Johns Hopkins University School of Medicine, 558 Ross Research Building, 720 Rutland Avenue, Baltimore, MD 21205-2196, USA

C.L. Masters et al. (Eds.)
Amyloid Protein Precursor in Development,
Aging and Alzheimer's Disease
© Springer-Verlag Berlin Heidelberg 1994

acids (Kang et al. 1987; Kitaguchi et al. 1988; Ponte et al. 1988; Tanzi et al. 1988; Golde et al. 1990) encoded by alternatively spliced mRNA. The two largest forms contain a domain structurally and functionally homologous to the Kunitz family of protease inhibitors (KPI; Kitaguchi et al. 1988; Ponte et al. 1988; Tanzi et al. 1988). In cultured cells, APP mature through the constitutive secretory pathway and are modified by the addition of N- and O-linked oligosaccharides and tyrosine sulfation (Weidemann et al. 1989). Full-length APP appear on the plasma membrane with the nearly concomitant appearance of C-terminal truncated derivatives in the conditioned medium. Some plasma membrane-bound molecules are internalized and degraded by endosomal/lysosomal pathways (Golde et al. 1992; Haass et al. 1992a). Although biochemical mechanism(s) involved in the generation of $A\beta$ are presently unknown, soluble $A\beta$ is normally secreted from cultured cells and is present in human cerebrospinal fluid (Haass et al. 1992b; Seubert et al. 1992; Shoji et al. 1992). The first set of experiments focus on the cellular site of APP cleavage and discuss the role of sequences in the APP cytoplasmic domain on APP trafficking and internalization.

Despite advances in our understanding of APP structure and metabolism (Selkoe 1991; Goedert et al. 1991; Hardy and Mullan 1992), little is known regarding the physiological functions of APP. Although evidence favors a role for the soluble form of APP-751, or protease nexin II, in wound healing (Oltersdorf et al. 1989; Smith et al. 1990; Van Nostrand et al. 1990), the function(s) of APP in the brain and other tissues remains uncertain, but roles for APP in the maintenance of synaptic interactions (Schubert 1989), cell-to-cell contact (Shivers et al. 1988), organization of the extracellular matrix (Narindrasorasak et al. 1992), mitogenesis (Saitoh et al. 1989), and as a receptor coupled to the trimeric G protein, G_0 (Nishimoto et al. 1993), have been suggested. However, the identification of human cDNA that encodes an APP-related molecule, termed APLP1 (Wasco et al. 1992), is consistent with the view that APP are a member of a larger gene family. In the second set of studies, we will present experiments that examine the expression of a second APP-related protein, APLP2, and provide evidence that APP-specific antibodies are unable to discriminate APP from APLP2.

Results

APP Cleavage Occurs on the Plasma Membrane

We and others have used molecular biological and biochemical approaches to confirm that the APP ectodomain is secreted following endoproteolytic cleavage between residues 16 (lysine) and 17 (leucine) of the $A\beta$ sequence (Esch et al. 1990; Sisodia et al. 1990; Anderson et al. 1991; Wang et al. 1991). Below, we extend those observations to examine the cellular site of APP cleavage.

Weidemann and colleagues (1989) demonstrated the presence of full-length precursors on the cell surface. To address whether plasma membrane precursors

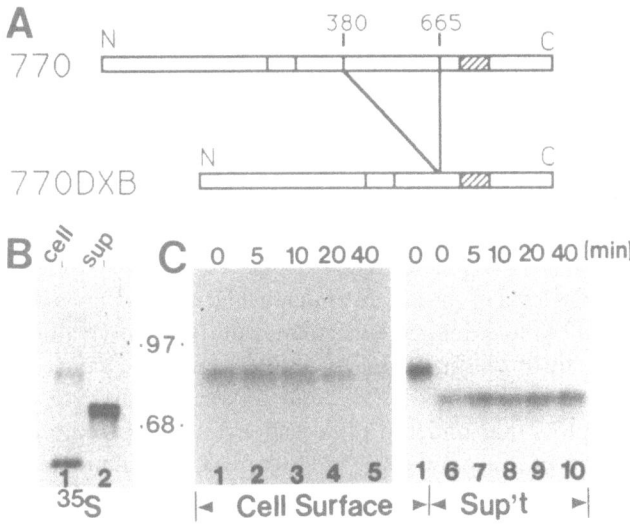

Fig. 1. APP cleavage occurs on the plasma membrane. **A** Structure of wild-type APP-770 and truncated analogue 770DXB. Hatched box, APP transmembrane domain. **B** 770DXB is cleaved and secreted. Lanes 1 and 2, [^{35}S] methionine-labeled immunoprecipitates from cell lysate or supernatant (sup), respectively, derived from a stable cell line (C7DXB) that constitutively expresses 770DXB polypeptides. Immunoprecipitation utilized APP-specific polyclonal antibody RGP-3 elicited against a synthetic peptide corresponding to residues 45–62 of APP (a kind gift from Dr. George Perry, Case Western Reserve University, Cleveland). **C** 770DXB is cleaved at the plasma membrane. CD7DXB cells were surface radioiodinated at 4 °C and then placed in prewarmed growth medium. 770DXB-related polypeptides were immunoprecipitated from cell pellets (lanes 1–5) or conditioned medium (lanes 6–10) at 0 min (1 and 6), 5 min (2 and 7), 10 min (3 and 8), 20 min (4 and 9), or 40 min (5 and 10). Sup't, supernatant

are substrates for cleavage, we analyzed a Chinese hamster ovary (CHO) cell line (C7DXB) that overexpresses an APP-770 minigene (770DXB) that encodes APP-770 deleted of 285 residues of the APP extracellular domain but retains the entire cytoplasmic and transmembrane regions and 35 residues of the adjacent extracellular domain (Fig. 1A). Following [^{35}S]methionine labeling and immunoprecipitation, 770 DXB molecules appear as immature 55-kiloDalton (kD) and mature $\sim$ 85-kD species in cell lysates (Fig. 1B), lane 1) and as $\sim$ 70-kD molecules in conditioned media (Fig. 1B, lane 2). C7DXB cells were surface labeled with [^{125}I] at 4 °C, resulting in the labeling of $\sim$ 85-kD mature 770DXB polypeptides (Fig. 1C, lane 1). Upon returning cells to prewarmed culture media, 770DXB polypeptides in cell lysates and conditioned media were assayed over a 45-min period. In Figure 1C, we demonstrate that the full-length forms have a half-life of 5-10 min and, more importantly, that a truncated $\sim$ 70-kD 770DXB-related species is detected in culture media at the earliest ($\sim$ 30 sec) time point and accumulates during the next 10 minutes. The rapid kinetics of this process is inconsistent with a model whereby membrane-bound

APP are recycled, cleaved intracellularly, and then secreted. Thus, these data are consistent with APP cleavage that occur in the plasma membrane.

Sequences on the APP Cytoplasmic Tail are Required for Trafficking and Endocytosis

Early pulse-chase experiments indicated that only a fraction of newly synthesized APP is secreted (Weidemann et al. 1989). Indeed, we demonstrated that APP deleted of the last 16 amino acids of the APP cytoplasmic tail were secreted at a 2–3-fold higher level than wild-type polypeptides (Sisodia et al. 1990). Contained within these 16 residues is the sequence YENPTY that, in part, resembles the motif, NPXY, that is present in the cytoplasmic tail of a number of receptors that undergo rapid endocytosis (e.g., receptors for epidermal growth factor (EGF), low-density lipoprotein (LDL), mannose-6-phosphate), mutations of the tyrosine residue severely compromise the efficiency of internalization of parent molecules (Collawn et al. 1991). To define more clearly the requirement of

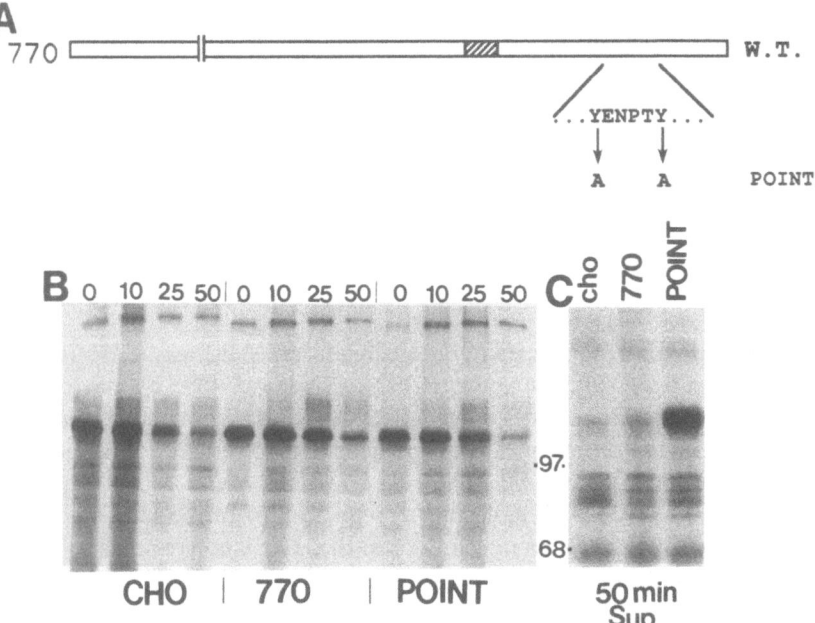

Fig. 2. APP harboring mutations within the endocytic targeting signal are efficiently secreted. **A** Structure of wild-type (W.T.) APP-770 and APP-770 containing tyrosine-alamine substitutions in the endocytic targeting signal (POINT). **B** Pulse-chase analysis. CHO cells or CHO cells stably transfected with APP-770 or "POINT" were pulse labeled with [^{35}S] methionine for 10 min and then chased for 10, 25, or 50 min. Cell lysates were prepared at each time point and immunoprecipitated with APP-specific antibodies. **C** Secretion of APP-related derivatives. An aliquot of supernatant (Sup) at the 50-min chase time point was fractionated by SDS-PAGE

the YENPTY sequence on internalization, we analyzed mutant APP molecules in which the tyrosine residues in the YENPTY sequence were replaced by alanine. Stable CHO cell lines expressing wild-type or mutant APP (POINT; Fig. 2A) were assayed by pulse-chase analysis (Fig. 2B), and the secretion of soluble APP-770 derivatives was analyzed (Fig. 2C). Although the synthetic rates and maturation of APP-770 and POINT were identical (Fig. 2B, lane 0), the secretion of soluble APP derived from POINT molecules was ≥ 3-fold higher than derivatives generated from APP-770 (Fig. 2C). We argue that the increased retention of internalization-defective precursors on the plasma membrane increases the probability of endoproteolytic cleavage and results in elevated levels of soluble APP forms.

To confirm that cell-surface cleavage was responsible for the increased secretion of APP-derivatives from cells that express APP with altered cytoplasmic sequences, we compared the extent of secretion of newly synthesized, cell surface forms of wild-type APP to APP deleted of the YENPTY motif (ΔYY) from cell lines that express these molecules (Fig. 3). We established that the synthetic rates of the wild-type and mutant APP were identical (Fig. 3A). In short pulse-chase and immunoprecipitation analysis, both molecules mature with identical kinetics and exhibit similar levels of glycosylated species (Fig. 3B). Biotinylation of live cells at 4 °C at the end of the pulse-chase paradigm and precipitation of cell-surface forms with streptavidin revealed that ∼ 4-fold higher levels of mutated APP molecules appeared on the cell surface (Fig. 3C). This result indirectly suggests that the YENPTY signal may have a regulatory role in the delivery of APP to the plasma membrane. In any event, upon warming to 37 °C, cells that express mutant APP release a large fraction of surface-bound molecules (Fig. 3D), whereas cells expressing

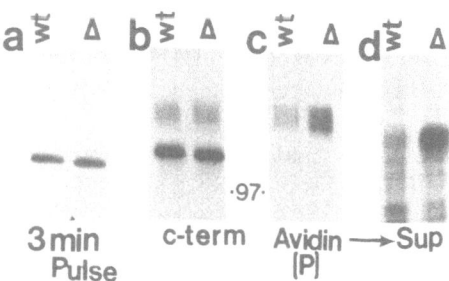

Fig. 3. Sequence in the APP cytoplasmic domain involved in intracellular trafficking and endocytosis. **a** CHO cell lines that overexpress APP-770 (wt) or APP deleted of the YENPTY sequence in the cytoplasmic tail (Δ) were pulse labeled for 3 min with [^{35}S] methionine and APP was immunoprecipitated from cell lysates. **b–c** WT or Δ cell lines were pulse labeled for 10 min and then chased for 25 min. Cells were cooled to 4 °C and then reacted with NHS S-S biotin. Cells were lysed and immunoprecipitated with APP-specific C-terminal (C-term) antibodies. One-fifth of the immunoprecipitate is shown in **b**. Four-fifths of the immunoprecipitate was reprecipitated with streptavidin and fractionated. **d** A parallel set of cultured cells was labeled with [^{35}S] methionine for 10 min, chased for 25 min, and subsequently reacted with NHS S-S biotin at 4 °C. Cells were placed at 37 °C for 10 min, and the conditioned medium was precipitated with streptavidin. Sup, supernatant

wild-type molecules secrete considerably lower levels of APP derivatives. Notably, because the ratio of secreted molecules derived from wild-type APP and mutant APP is ~ 1:10 and the ratio of respective cell-surface forms is ~ 1:4, we argue that, in addition to its role in regulating plasma membrane delivery, the YENPTY sequence also serves as an internalization signal. More importantly, these studies reinforce the idea that plasma membrane cleavage is the preponderant pathway for the generation of soluble APP derivatives in cultured cells.

Identification of a cDNA-Encoding APLP2

We screened a mouse embryo cDNA library with a probe that encodes the last 104 residues of APP at low stringency. Two classes of cDNA were identified: strongly hybridizing cDNA derived from the mouse APP gene and a set of cDNA encoded by a related but nonidentical gene. The longest cDNA in the latter class (clone D2) contained a 3628-base pair (bp) sequence encoding a 751 amino acid polypeptide that, over most of its length, is highly homologous to mouse APP-751 (Fig. 4). Following an unusually long hydrophobic sequence at the N-terminus that resembles a signal peptide, the homologue is ~ 72% identical with the cysteine-rich domain of APP, including alignment of the 12 cysteine residues. The region is followed by a highly acidic domain both in the homologue and in APP. Downstream of this region, amino acids 309–365 of the homologue contains a domain with 68% identity to the protease inhibitor insert of APP-751. This domain retains the invariant cysteine residues and the P1-reactive site (cysteine-arginine-alanine; amino acids 319–321) contained within all Kunitz protease inhibitors. This region is followed by a stretch of 202 residues (amino acids 364–565) with 64% identity to amino acids 346–548 of APP-751. Surprisingly, the next 113 amino acids of the APP homologue have no homology to the corresponding region of APP. Despite the conspicuous absence of the extracellular 28-residue segment of Aβ within this region in the homologue, the homology between the homologue and APP resumes precisely at the NH$_2$ terminus of the respective transmembrane

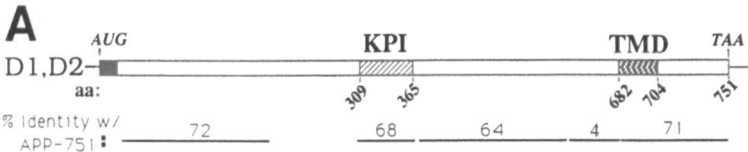

Fig. 4. Structure of APLP2 cDNA and comparison to APP-751. The structure of the full-length (cDNA) encoding APLP2 was isolated from whole mouse 8.5-day embryo libraries. The positions of the signal peptide (dark box), KPI, and transmembrane domain (TMD) are indicated as well as the percent identity between subregions of APLP2 with APP-751. AUG and TAA denote the translation, initiation, and termination codons of APLP2

domains and continues through to the termination condon (at the 71% identity level).

Neuronal Expression of APLP2

We confirmed the cellular expression of APLP2 in mouse brain by *in situ* hybridization analysis. To generate a probe specific for APLP2, sequences that encode the region highly divergent from APP (residues 568 to 681 of mouse APLP2) were subcloned, and [^{35}S]-labeled riboprobes were synthesized in the sense and antisense orientations. Radioactive probes of identical specific activities were hybridized to consecutive 12-μm coronal sections of mouse brain. In Figure 5A, we document specific hybridization to antisense probe to neuronal populations in neocortex, hippocampus, and thalamus, with virtually undetectable hybridization with the sense probe (Fig. 5B).

Expression of mRNA Encoding APLP2 and APP in Peripheral Tissue

We examined the relative levels of steady-state mRNA that encode APP and APLP2 in selected adult mouse tissue, using a quantitative reverse transcriptase-polymerase chain reaction (RT-PCR) method (Fig. 6 A, B). A schematic of the strategy is presented in Figure 6A. Total RNA, reverse transcribed with random hexamer primers, was subjected to PCR amplification, using a set of degenerate primers that hybridized with highly conserved, identically positioned sequences within APLP2 or APP cDNA. Thus, PCR generates 444-bp products in a mixture that contains APP and APLP2 cDNA templates; subsequent digestion with Xho I only cleaves the APP-derived product to 260 bp and 184 bp. Because the sense primer is [^{32}P] end labeled, only the 444-bp (APLP2) and 260-bp (APP) fragments are detected by autoradiography. Relative to APP mRNA, APLP2 transcripts are expressed at 1.2-, 0.6-, 0.4-, 1.2-, and 2.2-fold levels in heart, brain, kidney, lung, and testes, respectively (Fig. 6B), and at 2.8- and 10.4-fold levels in thymus and liver, respectively (Fig. 6B, lanes 1, 4, respectively).

APLP2 Matures Through the Secretory Pathway

The conservation of structural motifs between APLP2 and APP suggested that the polypeptides might undergo similar maturation pathways. Initially, we examined the insertion of APLP2 into microsomal membranes by programming a rabbit reticulocyte translation system that contained canine pancreatic microsomal membranes with 5′m^{7}G-capped transcripts encoding APLP2. This reaction resulted in the synthesis of a polypeptide with an apparent molecular mass of $\sim$ 115 kD (Fig. 7A, lane 1). The digestion of a parallel reaction with

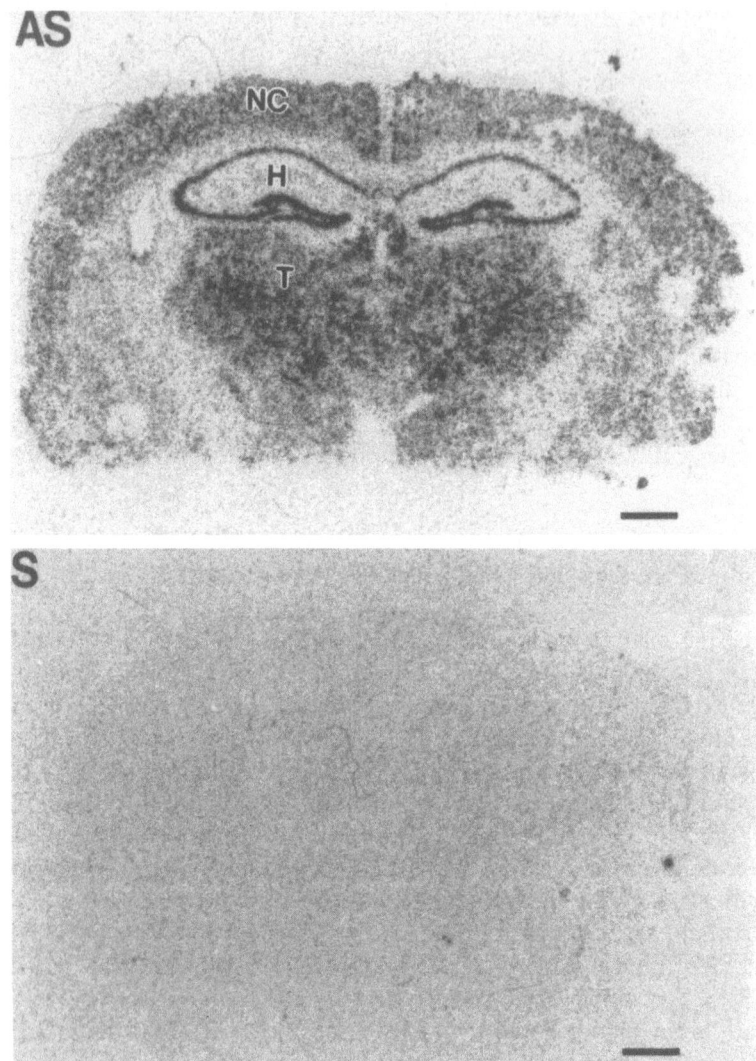

Fig. 5. *In situ* hybridization. Antisense (AS) and sense (S) APLP2 probe hybridization to adult mouse brain. NC, H, and T represent neocortex, hippocampus, and thalamus, respectively

proteinase K resulted in conversion of APLP2 into a slightly shortened protease-resistant polypeptide (Fig. 7A, lane 2); complete digestion of the latter form is only observed after disruption of membrane integrity by detergent (Fig. 7A, lane 3). Thus, the protease-dependent truncation of APLP2 by $\sim$ 5 kD (Fig. 7A, lane 3) is consistent with the digestion of a short cytoplasmic domain of APLP2. We conclude that APLP2 adopts a topology typical of type-I integral membrane proteins.

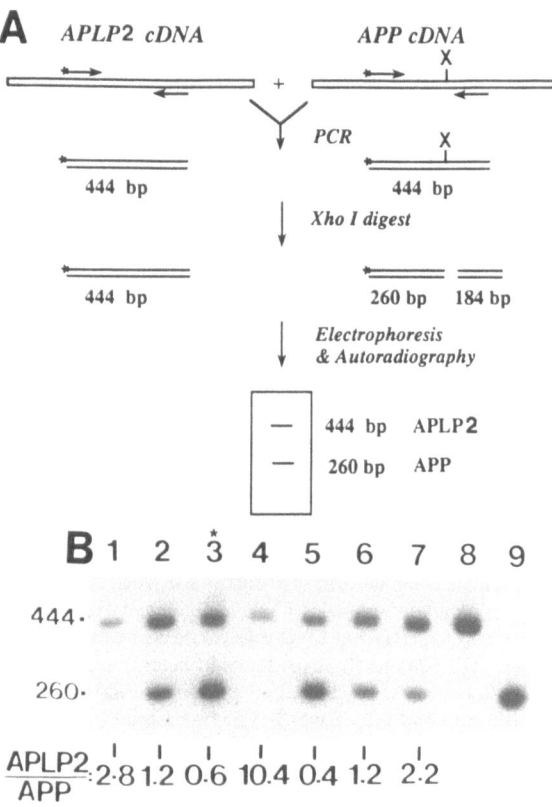

Fig. 6. Quantitative PCR analysis of APLP2 and APP mRNA in adult mouse brain and systemic tissue. See text for details of the strategy for PCR quantification. Autoradiogram of PT-PCR analysis. Positions of 444-bp (APLP2) and 260-bp (APP) fragments are indicated, as are the ratios of APLP2 to APP PCR products. Note that the PCR product generated from the mouse APP cDNA template is digested to completion (lane 8), indicating that the residual 444-bp product in lanes 1–7 represents a *bona fide* APLP2-encoding fragment

To compare the maturation of APLP2 with APP in cultured cells, we transiently transfected cDNA that encode either APLP2 or APP-770 (Sisodia et al. 1990) into CHO cells, African green monkey kidney (COS-1) cells, or mouse neuroblastoma cells (N_2A). Figures 7B, C depict the analysis in transfected CHO cells. A polyclonal antisera raised against APP-695 residues 645–694 (Ab369; Buxbaum et al. 1990; Nordstedt et al. 1991) immunoprecipitated a closely migrating doublet of ~ 115 kD from detergent extracts prepared from untransfected CHO cells labeled with [^{35}S] methionine (Fig. 7B, lane 1). CHO cells transfected with a cDNA-encoding human APP-770 (Sisodia et al. 1990) expressed increased amounts of APP-770 that comigrate with the lower band of the doublet and higher molecular weight Golgi-modified forms of APP-770 (Fig. 7B, lane 2). On the other hand, CHO cells transfected with a

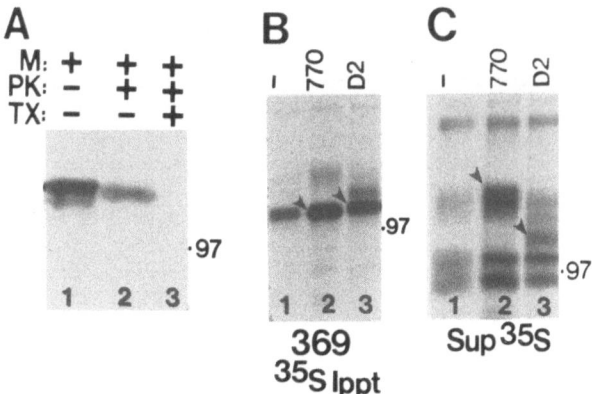

Fig. 7. Biogenesis and maturation of APLP2. **A** *In vitro* translation of APLP2 mRNA in the presence of canine pancreatic membranes. Full-length 5' capped transcripts encoding APLP2 mRNA were incubated in a rabbit reticulocyte lysate in the presence of microsomal membranes at 37 °C for 60 min (lane 1). Parallel reactions were subsequently digested for 15 min at 4 °C with 0.1 mg/ml proteinase K (PK) (lane 2) alone or with PK and 0.1% Triton X-100 (TX) (lane 3). **B** Synthesis of human APP-770 and mouse APLP2 in transfected CHO cells. Lanes 1–3 represent Ab369 immunoprecipitable, [^{35}S] methionine-labeled polypeptides synthesized in untransfected CHO cells (lane 1) or in CHO cells transfected with cDNA encoding human APP-770 (lane 2) or mouse APLP2 (lane 3). Arrowheads in lanes 2 and 3 indicate immature forms of APP-770 and APLP2, respectively. **C** Secretion of soluble APP-770 and mouse APLP2-related derivatives from transfected CHO cells. Lanes 1–3 represent total [^{35}S] methionine-labeled polypeptides in conditioned media from untransfected CHO cells (lane 1) or CHO cells that express human APP-770 (lane 2) or mouse APLP2 (lane 3). Arrowheads in lanes 2 and 3 indicate soluble APP-770- or APLP2-related derivatives, respectively. Sup, supernatant

cDNA-encoding mouse APLP2 synthesized a polypeptide that migrated with the upper band of the doublet and an additional form of ~ 125 kD that likely represents APLP2 forms containing additional oligosaccharide modifications (Fig. 7B, lane 3). Parallel analysis of conditioned media revealed the secretion of soluble derivatives of ~ 125 kD (Fig. 7C, lane 2) or ~ 105 kD (Fig. 7C, lane 3) from cells that express APP-770 or APLP2, respectively. Although the soluble APLP2 derivatives lack the cytoplasmic domain (data not shown), the cellular site for cleavage and the sequence flanking the scissile bond in APLP2 remain to be established.

APP Antibodies Cross React with APLP2

The observation that antibody 369 recognizes APLP2 led us to examine the cross reactivity of other antibodies generated against independent APP epitopes. As expected, Ab369 recognized APP or APLP2 equally in immunoblotting studies of cell lysates prepared from COS-1 cells transfected with cDNA-encoding APP-770 (Fig. 8A, lane 2) or APLP2 (Fig. 8A, lane 3), respectively. Antibody 22C11, raised against bacterially synthesized human APP-695,

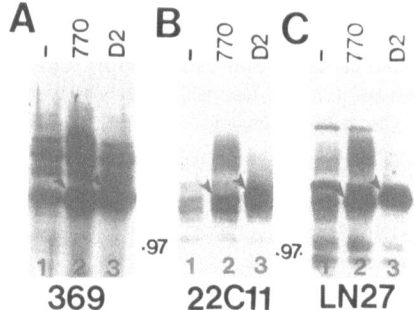

Fig. 8. APP and APLP2 cannot be discriminated by APP antibodies. Panels A–C represent immunoblots of COS-1 cell extracts probed with Ab369, 22C11, or LN27, respectively. Lanes 1–3 represent extracts prepared from untransfected COS-1 cells or COS-1 cells transfected with cDNA that express human APP-770 cDNA or mouse APLP2, respectively. Arrowheads in lanes 2 and 3 indicate immature forms of APP-770 and APLP2, respectively. The molecular weight marker is shown in kD

was also unable to distinguish between APP-770 and APLP2 in extracts prepared from COS-1 cells transfected with cDNA encoding APP-770 (Fig. 8B, lane 2) or APLP2 (Fig. 8B, lane 3). Extensive serial dilutions of 22C11 and 369 antibodies revealed that these reagents have equivalent avidities for APP and APLP2 (data not shown). Finally, we examined the reactivity of monoclonal antibody LN21 generated against soluble APP-751 forms produced by *Spodoptera frugiperda* ovarian cells infected with a human APP-751-encoding baculovirus vector. LN21 was unable to discriminate between APP-770 and APLP2 in COS-1 cells that express these polypeptides (Fig. 8C, 2, 3). Thus, we have documented that a wide array of "anti-APP" antibodies fails to discriminate APP from APLP2.

Acknowledgments. The authors thank Drs. Donald L. Price (The Johns Hopkins School of Medicine) and Ian Trowbridge (Salk Institute) for invaluable discussions. This work was supported by grants from the U.S. Public Health Service (NIH AG 05146, NS 20471) and American Health Assistance Foundation.

References

Anderson JP, Esch FS, Keim PS, Sambamurti K, Lieberburg I, Robakis NK (1991) Exact cleavage site of Alzheimer amyloid precursor in neuronal PC-12 cells. Neurosci Lett 128:126–128

Buxbaum JD, Gandy SE, Cicchetti P, Ehrlich ME, Czernik AJ, Fracasso RP, Ramabhadran TV, Unterbeck AJ, Greengard P (1990) Processing of Alzheimer β/A4 amyloid precursor protein: modulation by agents that regulate protein phosphorylation. Proc Natl Acad Sci USA 87:6003–6006

Collawn JF, Kuhn LA, Liu L-FS, Tainer JA, Trowbridge IS (1991) Transplanted LDL and mannose-6-phosphate receptor internalization signals promote high-efficiency endocytosis of the transferrin receptor. EMBO J 10: 3247–3253

Esch FS, Keim PS, Beattie EC, Blacher RW, Culwell AR, Oltersdorf T, McClure D, Ward PJ (1990) Cleavage of amyloid β peptide during constitutive processing of its precursor. Science 248: 1122–1124

Glenner GG, Wong CW (1984) Alzheimer's disease: initial report of the purification and characterization of a novel cerebrovascular amyloid protein. Biochem Biophys Res Commun 120: 885–890

Goedert M, Sisodia SS, Price DL (1991) Neurofibrillary tangles and β-amyloid deposits in Alzheimer's disease. Curr Opin Neurobiol 1: 441–447

Golde TE, Estus S, Usiak M, Younkin LH, Younkin SG (1990) Expression of β amyloid protein precursor mRNAs: recognition of a novel alternatively spliced form and quantitation in Alzheimer's disease using PCR. Neuron 4: 253–267

Golde TE, Estus S, Younkin LH, Selkoe DJ, Younkin SG (1992) Processing of the amyloid protein precursor to potentially amyloidogenic derivatives. Science 255: 728–730

Haass C, Koo EH, Mellon A, Hung AY, Selkoe DJ (1992a) Targeting of cell-surface β-amyloid precursor protein to lysosomes: alternative processing into amyloid-bearing fragments. Nature 357: 500–503

Haass C, Schlossmacher MG, Hung AY, Vigo-Pelfrey C, Mellon A, Ostaszewski BL, Lieberburg I, Koo EH, Schenk D, Teplow DB, Selkoe DJ (1992b) Amyloid β-peptide is produced by cultured cells during normal metabolism. Nature 359: 322–325

Hardy J, Mullan M (1992) Alzheimer's disease: In search of the soluble. Nature 359: 268–269

Kang J, Lemaire H-G, Unterbeck A, Salbaum JM, Masters CL, Grzeschik K-H, Multhaup G, Beyreuther K, Müller-Hill B (1987) The precursor of Alzheimer's disease amyloid A4 protein resembles a cell-surface receptor. Nature 325: 733–736

Kemper T (1984) Neuroanatomical and neuropathological changes in normal aging and in dementia. In: Albert ML (ed) Clinical neurology of aging. Oxford University Press, New York, pp 9–52

Kitaguchi N, Takahashi Y, Tokushima Y, Shiojiri S, Ito H (1988) Novel precursor of Alzheimer's disease amyloid protein shows protease inhibitory activity. Nature 331: 530–532

Masters CL, Simms G, Weinman NA, Multhaup G, McDonald BL, Beyreuther K (1985) Amyloid plaque core protein in Alzheimer disease and Down syndrome. Proc Natl Acad Sci USA 82: 4245–4249

Müller-Hill B, Beyreuther K (1989) Molecular biology of Alzheimer's disease. Annu Rev Biochem 58: 287–307

Narindrasorasak S, Lowery DE, Altman RA, Gonzalez-DeWhitt PA, Greenberg BD, Kisilevsky R (1992) Characterization of high affinity binding between laminin and Alzheimer's disease amyloid precursor proteins. Lab Invest 67: 643–652

Nishimoto I, Okamoto T, Matsuura Y, Takahashi S, Okamoto T, Murayama S and Ogata E (1993) Alzheimer amyloid protein precursor complexes with brain GTP-binding protein G_0. Nature 362: 75–79

Nordstedt C, Gandy SE, Alafuzoff I, Caporaso GL, Iverfeldt K, Grebb JA, Winblad B, Greengard P (1991) Alzheimer β/A4-amyloid precursor protein in human brain: aging-associated increases in holoprotein and in a proteolytic fragment. Proc Natl Acad Sci USA 88: 8910–8914

Oltersdorf T, Fritz LC, Schenk DB, Lieberburg I, Johnson-Wood KL, Beattie EC, Ward PJ, Blacher RW, Dovey HF, Sinha S (1989) The secreted form of the Alzheimer's amyloid precursor protein with the Kunitz domain is protease nexin-II. Nature 341: 144–147

Ponte P, Gonzalez-DeWhitt P, Schilling J, Miller J, Hsu D, Greenberg B, Davis K, Wallace W, Lieberburg I, Fuller F, Cordell B (1988) A new A4 amyloid mRNA contains a domain homologous to serine proteinase inhibitors. Nature 331: 525–532

Saitoh T, Sundsmo M, Roch J-M, Kimura T, Cole G, Schubert D, Oltersdorf T, Schenk DB (1989) Secreted form of amyloid β protein precursor is involved in the growth regulation of fibroblasts. Cell 58: 615–622

Schubert D (1989) The biological roles of heparan sulfate proteoglycans in the nervous system. Neurobiol Aging 10:504–506

Selkoe DJ (1989) Biochemistry of altered brain proteins in Alzheimer's disease. Annu Rev Neurosci 12:463–490

Selkoe DJ (1991) The molecular pathology of Alzheimer's disease. Neuron 6:487–498

Seubert P, Vigo-Pelfrey C, Esch F, Lee M, Dovey H, Davis D, Sinha S, Schlossmacher M, Whaley J, Swindlehurst C, McCormack R, Wolfert R, Selkoe D, Lieberburg I, Schenk D (1992) Isolation and quantification of soluble Alzheimer's β-peptide from biological fluids. Nature 359:325–327

Shivers BD, Hilbich C, Multhaup G, Salbaum M, Beyreuther K, Seeburg PH (1988) Alzheimer's disease amyloidogenic glycoprotein: expression pattern in rat brain suggests a role in cell contact. EMBO J 7:1365–1370

Shoji M, Golde TE, Ghiso J, Cheung TT, Estus S, Shaffer LM, Cai X-D, McKay DM, Tintner R, Frangione B, Younkin S (1992) Production of the Alzheimer amyloid β protein by normal proteolytic processing. Science 258:126–129

Sisodia SS, Koo EH, Beyreuther K, Unterbeck A, Price DL (1990) Evidence that β-amyloid protein in Alzheimer's disease is not derived by normal processing. Science 248:492–495

Smith RP, Higuchi DA, Broze GJ Jr (1990) Platelet coagulation factor XI_a-inhibitor, a form of Alzheimer amyloid precursor protein. Science 248:1126–1128

Tanzi RE, McClatchey AI, Lampert ED, Villa-Komaroff L, Gusella JF, Neve RL (1988) Protease inhibitor domain encoded by an amyloid protein precursor mRNA associated with Alzheimer's disease. Nature 331:528–530

Van Nostrand WE, Schmaier AH, Farrow JS, Cunningham DD (1990) Protease nexin-II (amyloid β-protein precursor): a platelet α-granule protein. Science 248:745–748

Wang R, Meschia JF, Cotter RJ, Sisodia SS (1991) Secretion of the β/A4 amyloid precursor protein. Identification of a cleavage site in cultured mammalian cells. J Biol Chem 266:16960–16964

Wasco W, Bupp K, Magendantz M, Gusella JF, Tanzi RE, Solomon F (1992) Identification of a mouse brain cDNA that encodes a protein related to the Alzheimer disease-associated amyloid-beta-protein precursor. Proc Natl Acad Sci USA 89: 10758–10762

Weidemann A, König G, Bunke D, Fischer P, Salbaum JM, Masters CL, Beyreuther K (1989) Identification, biogenesis, and localization of precursors of Alzheimer's disease A4 amyloid protein. Cell 57:115–126

Wisniewski HM, Terry RD (1973) Reexamination of the pathogenesis of the senile plaque. In: Zimmerman HM (ed) Progress in neuropathology, Vol. II. Grune & Stratton, New York, pp 1–26

Transmembrane APP is Distributed into Two Pools and Associated with Polymerized Cytoskeleton

B. Allinquant*, K. L. Moya, C. Bouillot, and A. Prochiantz

Introduction

βA4 peptide is the major component of extracellular amyloid deposits present in the brain of patients with Alzheimer's disease. The sequence of βA4 indicates that it is cleaved from the larger amyloid precursor protein (APP). APP is encoded by a single gene which yields, by alternative splicing, three major isoforms designated APP770, APP751, APP695. Sequence analysis suggests that APP is a transmembrane protein having a long N-terminal extracellular domain, a transmembrane region and a short cytoplasmic tail (Kang et al. 1987).

APP is thought to be primarily processed by two major cellular pathways. In one pathway, the precursor is cleaved within the βA4 region, releasing a long N-terminal fragment into extracellular fluids (Palmert et al. 1989; Esch et al. 1990). The second major pathway involves other cleavage steps yielding βA4-containing C-terminal fragments. These fragments then appear to be re-endocytosed and degraded within lysosomes (Estus et al. 1992; Golde et al. 1992).

Recently, the production and release of βA4 into conditioned medium have been observed in cultures of human mixed brain cells and the βA4 peptide has been detected in human cerebrospinal fluids (Haass et al. 1992; Seubert et al. 1992). The cellular pathway leading to the formation of βA4 and to its extracellular deposit is still speculative, and the cellular sources of the peptide also remain to be established. The high amount of APP immunoreactivity in neuronal structures in the vicinity of amyloid plaques (Martin et al. 1991) suggests that neurons are a good candidate source for βA4 extracellular deposits. Thus it is of particular interest to elucidate the mechanisms of APP processing and secretion by neurons.

Cortical Embryonic Neurons *in vitro* Express Only Full-length Transmembrane APP Isoforms

Pure cortical embryonic rat neurons (E15, E16) in primary culture under conditions precluding synaptogenesis (Lafont et al. 1992) express a major

---

* CNRS, URA 1414, ENS, 46 rue d'Ulm, Paris, France

C.L. Masters et al. (Eds.)
Amyloid Protein Precursor in Development,
Aging and Alzheimer's Disease
© Springer-Verlag Berlin Heidelberg 1994

transmembrane isoform at 105 kd which probably corresponds to APP 695 predominantly expressed in neurons. Minor quantities of other transmembrane proteins which could correspond to post-translationally modified forms of APP 695 are also present. In our *in vitro* conditions, neuronal differentiation is clearly visible after two to three days in vitro (DIV) and we observed that APP expression increases with neuronal differentiation, as also reported for hippocampal cells in culture (Hung et al. 1992). However, this APP remains associated with the membrane-enriched fraction, suggesting that APP is associated with the plasma membrane or membranous organelles. In addition, no secreted APP can be observed in the conditioned medium during differentiation; this is similar to the absence of secreted forms in primary cultures of rat astrocytes and microglia (Haass et al. 1991) and is in contrast to the presence of cleaved and secreted forms of all major APP isoforms in human mixed brain cell cultures (Haass et al. 1992; Seubert et al. 1993).

Transmembrane APP Isoforms in Polarized Neurons are Distributed into Two Pools

In immunocytochemical studies, we never detected APP at the surface of non-fixed live cells in culture, a finding consistent with an absence of cleavage and secretion thought to occur at the plasma membrane (Sisodia 1992). Fixation of the cells with 4% paraformaldehyde results in the visualization of APP in 40% of the neurons with specific staining of axonal segments and/or cell bodies (Fig. 1a). Triton-X100 permeabilization after fixation results in 100% of the cells

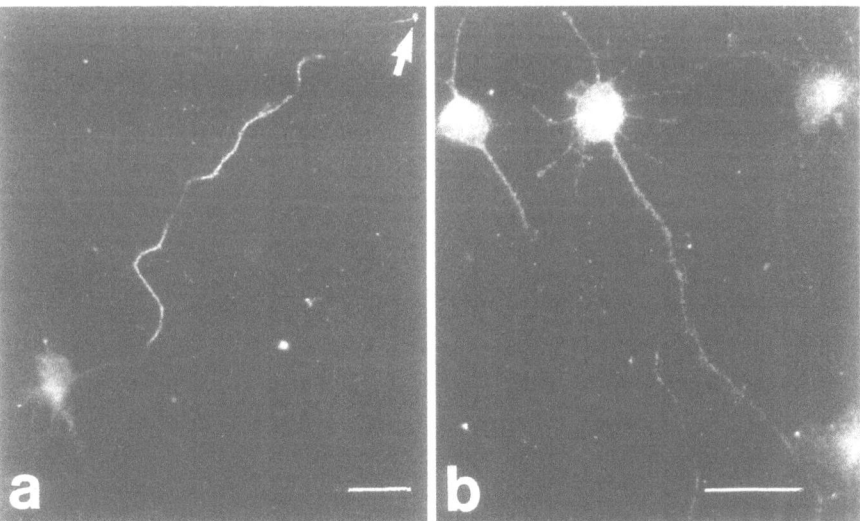

Fig. 1. APP immunoreactivity in fixed cells without (a) or with (b) triton X100 permeabilization. Note the presence of APP detected at the growth cone in fixed cells in the absence of detergent (arrow). Scale bar: 10 μm

being immunoreactive for APP and extends the staining to all compartments, including dendrites (Fig. 1b). In the presence of Triton-X100, no difference in the intensity of labeling between axons and dendrites can be observed, and APP immunoreactivity is highest in the cell bodies.

These differences in the distribution and intensity of APP immuno-reactivity under different permeabilization conditions suggest the presence of two pools of APP. One pool is restricted to axons and cell bodies and appears to be closest to the cell surface. The second pool is more widespread in the neuron and is only accessible after detergent permeabilization, suggesting that it is more interior within the cell and may thus be associated with the cytoskeleton.

In experiments designed to mimic calcium-mediated secretion, we found that, upon ionophore-triggered calcium entry (ionomycin or A23187), APP closest to the surface of axons and cell bodies is highly augmented and is observed in the entire neuronal population. However, APP remains mem-brane-associated, uncleaved and devoid of any further post-translational modification.

Transmembrane APP of Polarized Neurons is Associated with the Cytoskeleton

APP has already been reported to be associated with the detergent-insoluble cytoskeleton in C6 and PC12 cell lines and also in adult rat brains (Refolo et al. 1991). Similarly, we observed the presence of APP in the detergent-insoluble cytoskeleton fraction of cortical embryonic neurons at five DIV. To investigate if this association involves the C-terminal region of APP, we extracted microtubules from adult rat brain and repolymerized them in the presence of either secreted APP isoforms lacking the C-terminus or full-length transmembrane APP. We found that full-length APP associates with the polymerized cytoskeleton, while APP lacking the C-terminal does not (Table 1).

Table 1. Transmembrane and secreted APP in rat cortical embryonic neurons and rat adult brain extracts

	Transmembrane APP	Secreted APP
Neurons in culture	yes	no
Adult brain	yes	yes
APP associated with cytoskeleton	yes	no

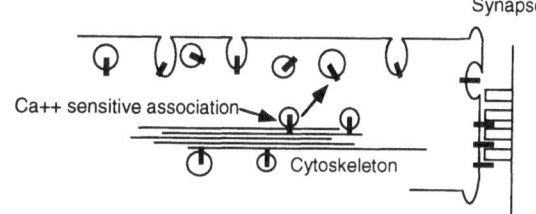

Fig. 2. Hypothetical model of the effects of calcium entry on transmembrane APP in differentiated rat embryonic neurons

Conclusions

Neurons differentiating *in vitro* only contain transmembrane forms of APP which can associate with polymerized cytoskeleton, probably through their C-terminus. This APP is not detectable at the surface of live cells and is distributed into two pools, as depicted in Figure 2. One pool is localized at or near the surface of axons and cell bodies whereas the other is spread throughout all compartments (cell bodies, axons, dendrites) and is more interior, thus requiring detergent permeabilization to be immunodetected.

Upon calcium entry, APP-containing vesicles associated with the cytoskeleton are freed and accumulate under the plasma membrane of axons and cell bodies (Fig. 2). Such APP may be sequestered within invaginations of the membrane and thus inaccessible to antibodies in non-fixed live cells. Another possibility is that APP has an extremely short half-life at the neuronal surface, cycling very rapidly with the plasma membrane, a possibility consistent with the presence of APP in clathrin-coated vesicles (Nordstedt et al. 1993).

In cultures of differentiating cortical neurons, APP is not stabilized at the cell surface and cannot be cleaved and secreted. Stabilization of the precursor may require a target element such as might be present during the establishment of synaptic contacts. It is noteworthy that in another series of experiments we observed an increased synthesis and rapid axonal transport of some APP isoforms at the time of target contact and synaptogenesis (Moya et al. 1994). In addition, a relative abundance of APP has been reported at synaptic sites (Schubert et al. 1991) and there is some evidence that APP may mediate cell-cell interactions, perhaps through its association with target-derived cell or substrate adhesion molecules (Breen et al. 1991; Schubert et al. 1989; Klier et al. 1989; Schubert 1991).

Taken together, converging evidence suggests that APP is involved in cell-cell interactions and may participate in synaptic plasticity. It will therefore be of considerable interest to more directly examine the factors that may stabilize APP at the neuronal surface and catalyze its subsequent processing. This will be achieved by the *in vitro* reconstitution of conditions favorable to the establishment of synaptic functions.

References

Breen KC, Bruce M, Anderton BH (1991) Beta amyloid precursor protein mediates neuronal cell-cell and cell-surface adhesion. J Neurosci Res 28:90–100

Esch FS, Keim EC, Blacher RW, Culwell AR, Oltersdorf T, McClure D, Ward PJ (1990) Cleavage of amyloid β peptide during constitutive processing of its precursor. Science 248:1122–1124

Estus S, Golde TE, Kunishita T, Blades D, Lowery D, Eisen M, Usiak M, Qu X, Tabira T, Greenberg BD, Younkin SG (1992) Potentially amyloidogenic, carboxyl-terminal derivatives of the amyloid protein precursor. Science 255:726–728

Golde TE, Estus S, Younkin LH, Selkoe DJ, Younkin SG (1992) Processing of the amyloid protein precursor to potentially amyloidogenic derivatives. Science 255:728–730

Haass C, Hung AY, Selkoe DJ (1991) Processing of β-amyloid precursor protein in microglia and astrocytes favors an internal localization over constitutive secretion. J Neurosci 11:3783–3793

Haass C, Schlossmacher MG, Hung AY, Vigo-Pelfrey C, Mellon A, Ostaszewski BL, Lieberburg I, Koo EH, Schenk D, Teplow DB, Selkoe DJ (1992) Amyloid β-peptide is produced by cultured cells during normal metabolism. Nature 359:322–325

Hung AY, Koo EH, Haass C, Selkoe DJ (1992) Increased expression of β-amyloid precursor protein during neuronal differentiation is not accompanied by secretory cleavage. Proc Natl Acad Sci USA 89:9439–9443

Kang J, Lemaire HG, Unterbeck A, Salbaum JM, Masters CL, Grzeschik KH, Multhaup G, Beyreuther K, Müller-Hill B (1987) The precursor of Alzheimer's disease amyloid A4 protein resembles a cell-surface receptor. Nature 325:733–736

Klier FG, Cole G, Stallcup W, Schubert D (1992) Amyloid β-protein precursor is associated with extracellular matrix. Brain Res. 515:336–342

Lafont F, Rouget M, Triller A, Prochiantz A, Rousselet A (1992) In vitro control of neuronal polarity by glycosaminoglycans. Development 114:17–29

Martin LJ, Sisodia SS, Koo EH, Cork LC, Dellovade TL, Weidemann, A, Beyreuther K, Masters C, Price DL (1991) Amyloid precursor protein in aged nonhuman primates. Proc Natl Acad Sci USA 88:1461–1465

Moya KL, Benowitz LI, Schneider GE, Allinquant B (1994) The amyloid precursor protein is developmentally regulated and correlated with synaptogenesis. Dev Biology 161:597–603

Nordstedt C, Caporaso GL, Thyberg J, Gandy SE, Greengard P (1993) Identification of the Alzheimer β/A4 amyloid precursor protein in clathrin-coated vesicles purified from PC12 cells. J Biol Chem 268:608–612

Palmert MR, Podlisny MB, Witker DS, Olderstorf T, Younkin LH, Selkoe DJ, Younkin SG (1989) The β-amyloid protein precursor of alzheimer disease has soluble derivatives found in human brain and cerebrospinal fluid. Proc Natl Acad Sci USA 86:6338–6342

Refolo LM, Wittenberg IS, Friedrich Jr VL, Robakis NK (1991) The Alzheimer amyloid precursor is associated with the detergent-insoluble cytoskeleton. J Neurosci 11:3888–3897

Schubert D (1991) The possible role of adhesion in synaptic modification. Trends Neurosci 15:127–130

Schubert D, Jin LW, Saitoh T, Cole G (1989) The regulation of amyloid β protein precursor secretion and its modulatory role in cell adhesion. Neuron 3:689–694

Shubert W, Prior R, Weidemann A, Dircksen H, Multhaup G, Masters CL, Beyreuther K (1991) Localization of Alzheimer βA4 amyloid precursor protein at central and peripheral synaptic sites. Brain Res 563:184–194

Seubert P, Vigo-Pelfrey C, Esch F, Lee M, Dovey H, Davis D, Sinha S, Schlossmacher M, Whaley J, Swindlehurst C, McCormack R, Wolfert R, Selkoe D, Lieberburg I, Schenk D (1992) Isolation and quantification of soluble Alzheimer's β-peptide from biological fluids. Nature 359:325–327

Seubert P, Oltersdorf T, Lee MG, Barbour R, Blomquist C, Davis DL, Bryant, K, Fritz LC, Galasko D, Thal LJ, Lieberburg I, Schenk DB (1993) Secretion of β-amyloid precursor protein cleaved at the amino terminus of the β-amyloid peptide Nature 361:260–263

Sisodia SS (1992) β-Amyloid precursor protein cleavage by a membrane-bound protease. Proc Natl Acad Sci USA 89:6075–6079

Isolation and Characterisation of Novel Metalloproteases from Embryonic Mouse Hippocampus

A. Thorpe*, V. Samtani, A. Gittner, W. Mills, and S.-J. Richards

Introduction

Alzheimer's disease (AD) is a debilitating neurodegenerative condition which is currently being investigated via a wide range of clinical and molecular approaches. β-amyloid forms part of the amyloid precursor protein (APP) and its deposition in dense extracellular plaques is one of the hallmarks of AD (Glenner and Wong 1984; Masters et al. 1985). The processing of APP leading to the production of β-amyloid is being extensively studied both *in vivo* and *in vitro*. Since β-amyloid is produced by the proteolytic cleavage of APP (Kang et al. 1987), there is evidence for as yet uncharacterized protease activity at the earliest stages of AD neuropathology (Sisodia et al. 1990; Seubert et al. 1993). The β-amyloid domain is embedded in the plasma membrane and it was initially assumed that membrane damage must precede proteolytic action in order for the full length peptide to be released. Since it was shown that β-amyloid is present within intracellular lysosomal organelles (Benowitz et al. 1989), much work has concentrated on the routes of APP processing, with evidence for the targetting of up to half of the APP produced directly into the lysosomal pathway (Caporaso et al. 1992a,b). However, the cellular location of β-amyloid production and the enzymes which cleave APP in either the "normal" pathway, which results in secreted proteins with C terminal β amyloid fragments, or an alternative processing pathway, resulting in the complete β-amyloid peptide, have still to be identified.

Metalloproteases in Alzheimer's Disease

The presence of a 57 amino acid Kunitz protease inhibitor region in two isoforms of APP (APP_{751} and APP_{770}; Tanzi et al. 1988; Ponte et al. 1988; Kitaguchi et al. 1988) has implicated serine proteases in the proteolytic processing of APP. More recently, a metalloprotease inhibitor domain has been

---

* Developmental Neurobiology Group, Department of Medicine, University of Cambridge, Addenbrooke's Hospital, Hills Road, Cambridge CB2 QQ, UK

C.L. Masters et al. (Eds.)
Amyloid Protein Precursor in Development,
Aging and Alzheimer's Disease
© Springer-Verlag Berlin Heidelberg 1994

a

Endopeptidase 24·11 (human, rat, rabbit)
Fibroblast collagenase (human)
Stromelysin (human)
Gelatinase (human)
Stromelysin, transin 1 and 2 (rat)
Endopeptidase 24.15 (rat)
Aminopeptidase N (human)
Digestive protease (crayfish)
Surface protease (*Leishmania* sp.)
Neutral protease (*B. subtilis*)
Neutral protease (*Serratia* sp.)
Peptidase N (*E. coli*)
Thermolysin (*B. stearothermophilus*)

```
Endopeptidase 24·11 (human, rat, rabbit)   V I G H E I T H G F D
Fibroblast collagenase (human)             V A A H E L G H S L G
Stromelysin (human)                        V A A H E I G H S L G
Gelatinase (human)                         V A A H E F G H A M G
Stromelysin, transin 1 and 2 (rat)         V A A H E L G H S L G
Endopeptidase 24.15 (rat)                  T Y F H E F G H V M H
Aminopeptidase N (human)                   V I A H E L A H Q W F
Digestive protease (crayfish)              T I I H E L M H A I G
Surface protease (Leishmania sp.)          V V T H E M T H A L G
Neutral protease (B. subtilis)             V T A H E M T H G V T
Neutral protease (Serratia sp.)            T F T H E I G H A L G
Peptidase N (E. coli)                      V I G H E Y F H N W T
Thermolysin (B. stearothermophilus)        V V G H E L T H A V T
```

b

```
5' CAT GAA TTT TTT CAT  3'
    C   G C C ACC    C
        A G GGA
        G     G
```

Fig. 1. a Conserved amino acid sequence in a number of zinc-dependent metalloproteases (Jongeneel et al. 1989; Pierotti et al. 1990). b Degenerate oligonucleotide probe synthesised to the consensus sequence of metalloproteases. The complexity of this probe was reduced from 3456 to 216 by inserting inosine at sites of quadruple degeneracy

identified in the C-terminal glycosylated region of secreted forms of APP (Miyazaki et al. 1993), implicating the matrix metalloprotease gelatinase A in the neurodegenerative cascade.

The family of zinc-dependent metalloproteases has a unique consensus sequence (see Fig. 1) which comprises three neutral amino acids, the sequence HEXXH (single letter amino acid code) and then two hydrophobic residues (Jongeneel et al. 1989). The consensus sequence in the matrix-degrading metalloproteinases (MMPs) has an additional conserved residue (HEXGH). The MMPs are a group of related enzymes which show highly regulated expression and coordinated modes of action in the extracellular matrix (see Matrisian 1992 for review). Three such enzymes which are Ca^{2+} dependent were isolated from human post mortem hippocampus and, furthermore, were shown to have significantly higher levels of activity in AD tissues compared to controls (Backstrom et al. 1992). Proteases and their inhibitors are in a dynamic equilibrium controlling physiological processes within many tissues (Travis and Salveson, 1983), and there is evidence that serine proteases often act as activators for the metalloproteases (Murphy et al. 1980; Okada et al. 1988). It may be that such a system is operating within APP processing, with a complex balance of the proteolytic enzymes and Ca^{2+} controlling different pathways and ultimately resulting in a variety of enzymatic products.

It is clear that, in order to understand the problems arising in APP processing within AD which result in such abnormally high levels of β-amyloid, the normal processing pathways of APP must first be elucidated and the responsible proteolytic enzymes identified. Therefore, we aim to isolate and characterise novel members of the metalloprotease family as candidate proteases for the processing of APP and the production of neurotoxic β-amyloid.

Isolation of Novel Metalloproteases

A 15-base degenerate oligonucleotide probe was synthesised to the consensus sequence of the zinc-dependent metalloproteases (Fig. 1). This probe was end-labelled with $[\gamma^{32}P]$ ATP using polynucleotide kinase (NBL) and was then used to screen an embryonic day 16 (E16) mouse hippocampal cDNA library. After three rounds of screening, several positive recombinants were identified. The presence of the metalloprotease degenerate probe sequence was confirmed in two of these clones by PCR analysis using the probe and a λgt10 primer. Double stranded DNA sequencing (Sequenase) of parts of both clones has shown, after comparison with gene sequences stored in the EMBL database, that both clones are novel.

Northern blotting revealed that two of the recombinants, clones 7 and 8, are expressed in both adult and embryonic mouse brain, while Southern blots of several unrelated human DNA samples which were probed with clone 7 confirmed the presence of the sequence in the human genome. Interestingly, one of the human samples displayed a possible polymorphism, indicating that a recombination event may have taken place at some stage. Expression was more specifically localised using in situ hybridisation. Frozen adult mouse brain sections were cut coronally at 10 μm on a microtome, fixed in 4% paraformaldehyde and dehydrated through ascending ethanol concentrations. Radioactivity labelled clone 7 was hybrisidised overnight at 42 °C (Chirgwin et al. 1979). Sections were emulsion treated and visualised on X-ray film. High levels of expression were observed in the cell bodies of layers CA1-4 of the hippocampus and pyramidal, granular, stellate and Bergman glia cells of the cerebellum, with low background expression throughout the brain (Fig. 2).

Conclusions

The isolation of novel proteases found in high abundance in the hippocampus and neocortex is an exciting discovery in view of the potential role of aberrant proteolytic cleavage within AD amyloid plaque deposition. The metalloprotease family has previously been demonstrated to play an active role in protein secretion within the CNS and has been implicated in the pathological process by an elevated presence in AD brain tissues investigated at postmortem.

The data presented here on the two novel proteases isolated from a hippocampal cDNA library are preliminary and further characterisation is in progress. Any role of these proteases in the aetiology of AD is currently under investigation.

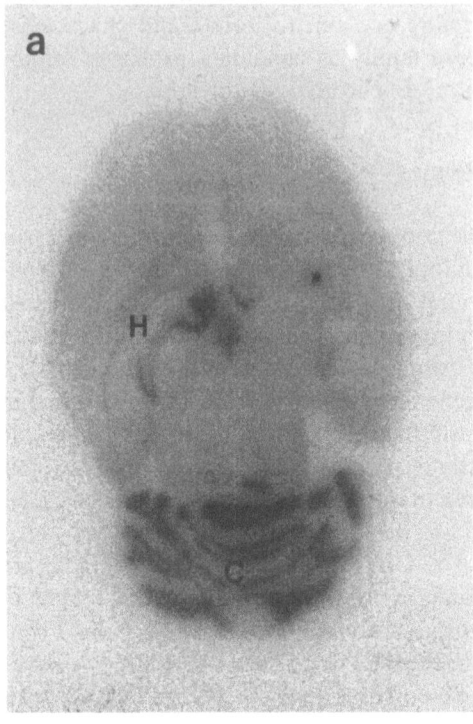

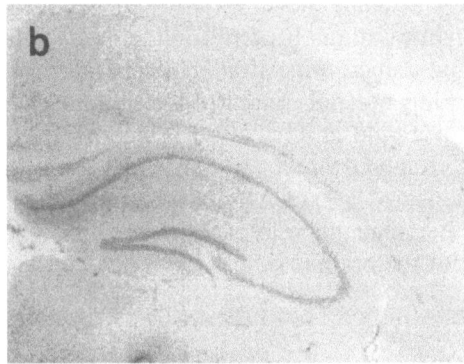

Fig. 2. *In situ* hybridisation of adult mouse brain with clone 7. **a** 10 μm horizontal section of the brain showing high expression in the hippocampus (H) and cerebellum (C). **b** Expression is more specifically located in layers CA1-4 of the hippocampus

References

Backstrom JR, Miller CA, Tökés ZA (1992) Characterization of neutral proteinases from Alzheimer-affected and control brain specimens: Identification of calcium-dependent metalloproteinases from the hippocampus. J Neurochem 58:983–992

Benowitz LI, Rodriguez W, Paskevich P, Mufson EJ, Schenk D, Neve RL (1989) The amyloid precursor protein is concentrated in neuronal lysosomes in normal and Alzheimer disease subjects. Expl Neurology 106:237–250

Caporaso GL, Gandy SE, Buxbaum JD, Greengard P (1992a) Chloroquine inhibits intracellular degradation but not secretion of Alzheimer β/A4 amyloid precursor protein: Modulation by agents that regulate protein phosphorylation. Proc Natl Acad Sci USA 89:2252–2256

Caporaso GL, Gandy SE, Buxbaum JD, Ramabhadran TV, Greengard P (1992b) Protein phosphorylation regulates secretion of Alzheimer β/A4 amyloid precursor protein. Proc Natl Acad Sci USA 89:3055–3059

Chirgwin JM, Przybyla AE, MacDonald RJ, Rutter WJ (1979) Isolation of biologically active ribonucleic acid from sources enriched in ribonuclease. Biochemistry 18:5294–5299

Glenner GG, Wong CW (1984) Alzheimer's disease: initial report of the purification and characterisation of a novel cerebrovascular amyloid protein. Biochem Biophys Res Commun 120:885–890

Jongeneel CV, Bouvier J, Bairoch A (1989) A unique signature identifies a family of zinc-dependent metallopeptidases. FEBS Lett 242:211–214

Kang J, Lemaire H-G, Unterbeck A, Salbaum JM, Masters CL, Grzeschik K-H, Multhaup G, Beyreuther K, Müller-Hill B (1987) The precursor of Alzheimer's disease amyloid A4 protein resembles a cell-surface receptor. Nature 197:192–193

Kitaguchi N, Takahashi Y, Tokushima Y, Shiojiri S, Ito H (1988) Novel precursor of Alzheimer's disease amyloid protein shows protease inhibitory activity. Nature 331:530–532

Masters CL, Simms G, Weinman NA, Multhaup G, McDonald BL, Beyreuther K (1985) Amyloid plaque core protein in Alzheimer disease and Down syndrome. Proc Natl Acad Sci USA 82:4245–4249

Matrisian LM (1992) The matrix-degrading metalloproteinases. BioEssays 14:455–463

Miyazaki K, Hasegawa M, Funahashi K, Umeda M (1993) A metalloproteinase inhibitor domain in Alzheimer amyloid protein precursor. Nature 362:839–841

Murphy G, Bretz U, Baggiolini M, Reynolds JJ (1980) The latent collagenase and gelatinase of human polymorphonuclear neutrophil leucocytes. Biochem J 192:517–525

Okada Y, Harris ED, Nagase H (1988) The precursor of a metalloendopeptidase from human rheumatoid synovial fibroblasts. Purification and mechanisms of activation by endopeptidases and 4-aminophenylmercuric acetate. Biochem J 254:731–741

Pierotti A, Dong K-W, Glucksman MJ, Orlowski M, Roberts JL (1990) Molecular cloning and primary structure of rat testes metalloendopeptidase EC 3.4.24.15. Biochemistry 29:10323–10329

Ponte P, Gonzalez-DeWhitt P, Schilling J, Miller J, Hsu D, Greenberg B, Davis K, Wallace W, Lieberburg I, Fuller F, Cordell B (1988) A new A4 amyloid mRNA contains a domain homologous to serine protease inhibitors. Nature 331:525–527

Seubert P, Oltersdorf T, Lee MG, Barbour R, Blomquist C, Davis DL, Bryant K, Fritz LC, Galasko D, Thal LJ, Lieberburg I, Schenk DB (1993) Secretion of β-amyloid precursor protein cleaved at the amino terminus of the β-amyloid peptide. Nature 361:260–263

Sisodia SS, Koo EH, Beyreuther K, Unterbeck A, Price DL (1990) Evidence that β-amyloid protein in Alzheimer's disease is not derived by normal processing. Science 248:492–495

Tanzi RE, McClatchey AI, Lamperti ED, Villa-Komaroff L, Gusella JF, Neve RL (1988) Protease inhibitor domain encoded by an amyloid precursor protein mRNA associated with Alzheimer's Disease. Nature 331:528–530

Travis J, Salveson GS (1983) Human plasma proteinase inhibitors. Ann Rev Biochem 52:655–709

A Transgenic Mouse Model of Alzheimer's Disease

*B. Cordell** and *L. Higgins*

Summary

Transgenic technology can be successfully applied to develop a small animal model of Alzheimer's disease. We describe a transgenic mouse which has been genetically programmed for neuronal overexpression of the 751 amino acid isoform of the human amyloid precursor protein and which displays histological features of Alzheimer's disease. These features include extracellular deposits of human amyloid derived from the transgene and aberrancies in the neuronal cytoskeleton. Both of these structures increase in frequency with the age of the animal, paralleling the human condition. While the typical transgenic mouse presents with an early Alzheimer's disease-like phenotype, occasionally some mice show advanced histopathology. Characteristics of more mature Alzheimer's disease-like pathology include large amyloid deposits associated with gliosis and dystrophic neurites. These results indicate the murine brain is capable of reproducing features of Alzheimer's disease, providing validity to the transgenic approach in obtaining a small animal model for study and therapeutic development.

Introduction

Amyloid plaque formation is the major histopathological hallmark of Alzheimer's disease. While the amyloid plaque is unique to Alzheimer's disease, its role in the development of this pathogenic state is unclear. It has been argued that amyloid plaque formation is a major etiological factor leading to the Alzheimer's disease phenotype. Conversely, the plaque has been viewed as an epiphenomenon with little contribution to the pathological condition. Recent evidence, however, suggests that amyloid deposition may not only be a pathological marker but may also play a direct role in the pathogenesis of Alzheimer's disease (Goate et al. 1991; Murrell et al. 1991).

One of the problems in determining the role of amyloid plaque formation in Alzheimer's disease has been the lack of easily studied small animal models

* Scios Nova Inc., 2450 Bayshore Parkway, Mountain View, CA 94043, USA

C.L. Masters et al. (Eds.)
Amyloid Protein Precursor in Development,
Aging and Alzheimer's Disease
© Springer-Verlag Berlin Heidelberg 1994

which spontaneously develop amyloid deposits. Other than in humans, naturally occurring amyloid deposits have been observed only in aged monkeys, bears, and certain strains of dogs (Wisniewski et al. 1970; Selkoe et al. 1987; Giaccone et al. 1990). These animals present significant challenges and limitations to defining the pathological contribution of amyloid deposition, as well as to study the mechanisms leading to amyloid plaque formation. Transgenic technology offers the opportunity to address these issues experimentally. Transgenesis also provides the potential of a small animal model of Alzheimer's disease which would be valuable for therapeutic development.

Several groups, including this laboratory, have reported production of transgenic mice displaying deposits of amyloid in their brains (Quon et al. 1991; Wirek et al. 1991; Kawabata et al. 1991). Unfortunately, two of these reports have been retracted, leaving the field skeptical about the application of transgenic technology to Alzheimer's disease research. The transgenic mouse model which we developed remains the only successful model to date (Quon et al. 1991). Since our initial report describing this transgenic mouse model of amyloid deposition, these animals have been more fully characterized for similarities to the human disease. Here we describe that this transgenic mouse model has a number of histopathological features which parallel those seen in Alzheimer's disease. In addition, our results indicate that the murine brain is inherently capable of producing advanced Alzheimer's disease-like pathology, validating transgenesis as an approach to study this disease.

Experimental Strategy
for Transgenic Mouse Model Development

The amyloid constituent of cerebrovascular, diffuse and neuritic plaques in the Alzheimer's disease brain is a 39–43 amino acid peptide referred to as β-amyloid. β-amyloid is derived from the β-amyloid precursor protein (β-APP; Kang et al. 1987). Several isoforms of β-APP exist which are generated by alternative splicing of a single primary RNA transcript (Ponte et al. 1988; Tanzi et al. 1988; Kitaguchi et al. 1988). The predominant β-APP isoform in brain is a 695 amino acid precursor protein, β-APP695, which is expressed almost exclusively in neurons (Ponte et al. 1988; Neve et al. 1988). The second major isoform in brain of 751 amino acids, β-APP751, contains a Kunitz serine protease inhibitor (KPI) domain and, in contrast to β-APP695, is expressed ubiquitously (Ponte et al. 1988; Neve et al. 1988). Alterations in the expression levels of β-APP695 and β-APP751 have been observed in Alzheimer's disease brain. In general the data indicate that isoforms harboring the KPI domain are selectively elevated in Alzheimer's disease brain (Johnson et al. 1988, 1990; Golde et al. 1990). In fact, with collaborators, we conducted a study which demonstrated that increased levels of β-APP751 mRNA in hippocampal and entorhinal cortical neurons could be directly correlated with amyloid plaque density (Johnson et al. 1990).

We elected to apply this disease-specific alteration of β-APP isoform expression in our experimental strategy to produce a transgenic mouse model of Alzheimer's disease. Therefore, we genetically programmed mice to recreate this imbalance of neuronal β-APP isoforms. To do so, transgenic mice were generated in which elevated β-APP751 isoform expression occurred in a neuron-specific manner. This was achieved by linking the human cDNA encoding β-APP751 to the rat neuron-specific enolase promoter (NSE:β-APP751). Six founder mice were identified to be carrying the transgene. These founders were bred to homozygous pedigrees and each was shown to stably transmit the NSE:β-APP751 transgene to all progeny. Furthermore, each pedigree was characterized and shown to express the transgene at both the RNA and protein levels (Quon et al. 1991). While each NSE:β-APP751 pedigree had widely different increases in RNA levels of the transgene varying from several to 50-fold over endogenous murine β-APP RNA, only a two- to three-fold increase in β-APP protein levels was observed in each line. These data suggest that β-APP expression is under tight translational control. This result has implications for pathogenic mechanisms possibly occurring in Alzheimer's disease. Lack of β-APP translational control may represent yet another mechanism to promote the disease state. Mice from these six NSE:β-APP751 pedigrees, in addition to wild type mice of the parental strain, constituted the set of animals used to characterize the histopathological consequences of neuronal over-expression of human β-APP751.

Transgenic Mice Have β-Amyloid Deposits in Their Brains

The NSE:β-APP751 and wild type mice were surveyed for production of β-amyloid immunoreactive deposits in their brains, employing standard immunohistochemical methodology. Tissue sections were prepared and stained with a number of β-amyloid-specific antibodies, including a monoclonal antibody, 4.1 mAb, produced in our laboratory, as well as several polyclonal antisera used by others in the field. All antibodies were raised against human β-amyloid synthetic peptides and have been used in specific staining of plaques in Alzheimer's disease brain tissue. As a result of staining with each antibody, extracellular immunoreactive deposits were revealed in brain sections from NSE:β-APP751 mice which were not seen in sections from wild type mice, identically stained (Fig. 1), which we have previously reported (Quon et al. 1991).

Fig. 1. Immunohistochemical staining of β-amyloid deposits in NSE:β-APP751 transgenic mouse brain using 4.1 mAb. A CA-1 hippocampal field. B, C parietal cortex. D thalamus. Magnification, 350×

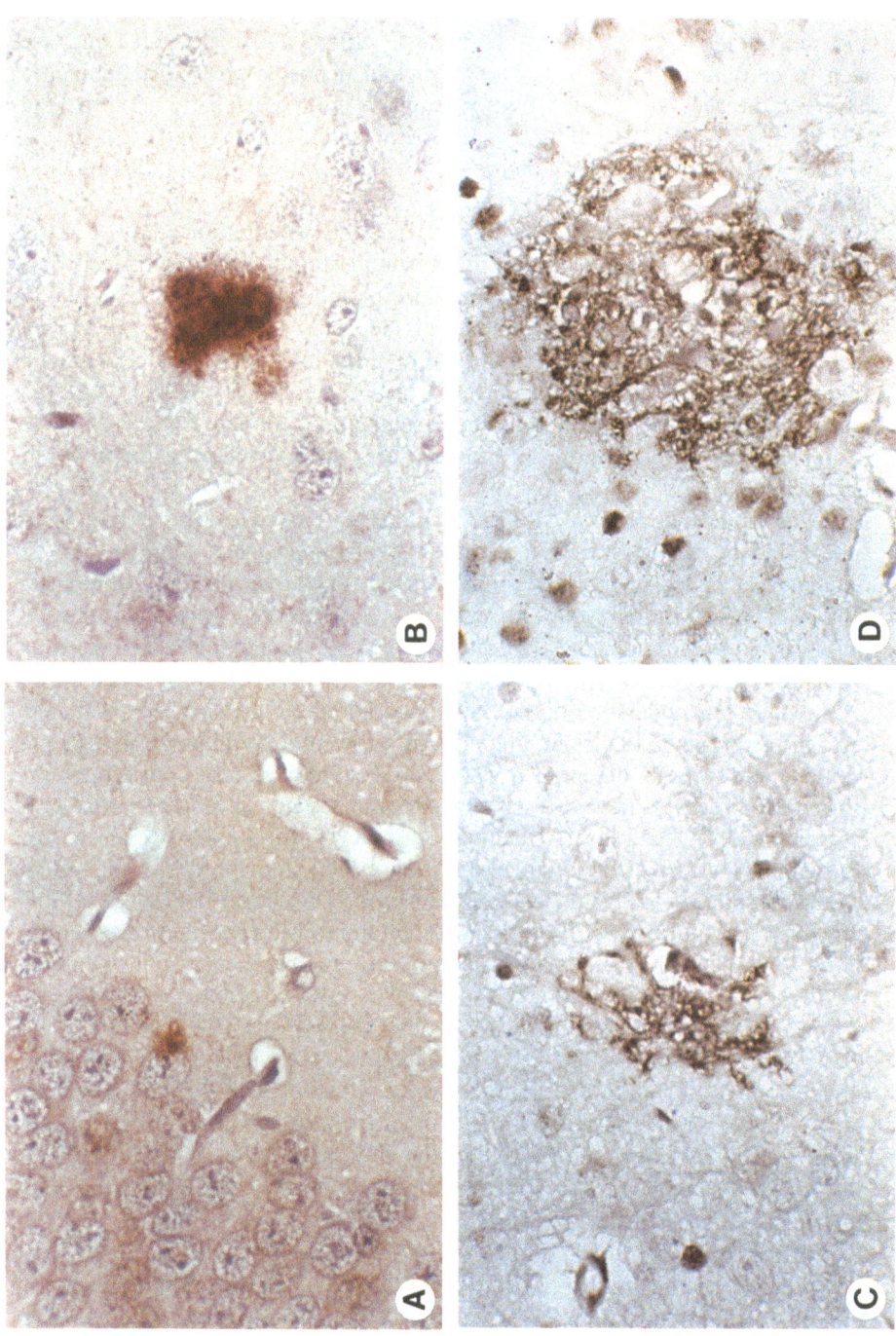

The immunoreactive deposits present in the transgenic brains vary in size and morphology. The deposits are typically 10–50 µm in diameter and are seen to be diffuse or compact. The β-amyloid deposits were most frequently observed in the cortex and hippocampus, were occasionally seen in the thalamus, and were never found in the cerebellum. Immunoreactive staining of these structures could be competed by the synthetic peptide β-amyloid immunogen.

The monoclonal 4.1 mAb was most extensively used in our analysis of the transgenic mice because of its low background staining and high sensitivity. In a survey of a large number of animals spanning the six NSE:β-APP751 pedigrees, 4.1 mAb detected β-amyloid deposits in 27% of the brain sections from NSE:β-APP751 animals (three sections per animal examined). Immunoreactive deposits were detected in 67% of the 33 NSE:β-APP751 animals used in the study, including members of all six NSE:β-APP751 pedigrees. Presumably if more sections had been surveyed more animals would have scored positive.

Data from the NSE:β-APP751 animals employed in this study were subdivided by sex and transgene hemi- or homozygosity. Comparing the frequency of deposits in male and female mice revealed no difference. However, animals homozygous for the transgene displayed twice the frequency of β-amyloid immunoreactive deposits in their brains compared to hemizygous animals.

To place our understanding of the β-amyloid immunoreactive deposits that form in the brains of the transgenic mice into the context of human pathology, we compared these deposits to β-amyloid immunoreactive structures in Alzheimer's disease and Down's syndrome brain tissue. Since individuals with Down's syndrome develop Alzheimer's disease by the fourth decade of life (Burger and Vogel 1973; Wisniewski et al. 1985), the Down's brain offers a temporal glimpse of events in the progression of Alzheimer's disease pathology. In young adult Down's brain, 4.1 mAb immunohistochemistry reveals only diffuse β-amyloid deposits; mature plaques are not yet seen at this age. This observation is in agreement with published reports describing immature Alzheimer's disease pathology in Down's brain (Allsop et al. 1989; Giaccone et al. 1989; Mann and Esiri 1989). The 4.1 mAb immunoreactivity in NSE:β-APP751 mouse brain is morphologically similar to the diffuse deposits seen in the young adult Down's brain. As with young Down's syndrome brain tissue, classic mature plaques were not observed in the transgenic mouse brain. Thus, β-amyloid deposits in NSE:β-APP751 brain most closely resemble the amyloid deposits in early Alzheimer's disease-like pathology.

Further evidence that NSE:β-APP751 transgenic mice display early Alzheimer's disease pathology with predominantly diffuse, pre-amyloid deposits was obtained using a number of classic histological reagents. The staining revealed that deposits in the transgenic mouse can be stained with methenamine silver, which stains both diffuse deposits and plaques in Alzheimer's disease brain. Only in rare cases do the transgenic murine brains stain with modified

Bielschowsky silver method, which stains only mature neuritic plaques in Alzheimer's disease brain. Thioflavin S, which stains plaques and occasionally preplaques in the human tissue, was found to stain deposits infrequently in the transgenic mouse brain. Congo red interacts only with β-amyloid in a highly β-pleated sheet conformation such as is found in mature plaques. Congo red staining of the NSE:β-APP751 mouse brain tissue failed to produce the typical birefringence of amyloid when viewed under polarized light (Table 1). Taken together, these data describe a profile of the deposits in the transgenic mouse brain that closely resembles that seen in early Alzheimer's disease pathology such as in the young adult Down's brain (Allsop et al. 1989; Giaccone et al. 1989).

Based on results of several assays, the monoclonal antibody, 4.1 mAb, appears to recognize an epitope in the first 17 amino acids of human β-amyloid. Since rodent β-amyloid differs from the human sequence at three residues within this epitope – positions 5, 10, and 13 of the peptide sequence (Yamada et al. 1987) – we evaluated 4.1 mAb for its species specificity. In an ELISA format against mouse and human β-amyloid synthetic peptides encompassing residues 1–17 and 1–28, the antibody recognized all human peptides but did not react with murine counterparts, even when high concentrations of peptide or antibody were assayed. In addition, murine β-amyloid peptide did not compete 4.1 mAb immunoreactivity in the staining of plaques in human Alzheimer's disease brain sections whereas identical concentrations of the human β-amyloid homologue abolished 4.1 mAb immunoreactivity. Therefore, the deposits present in NSE:β-APP751 transgenic mouse brain appear to be derived from the transgene which is expressing human β-APP751. It is possible the human β-amyloid sequence is important to deposition and plaque formation. β-amyloid deposition has not been observed in wild type rodent brain, yet is frequently seen in animals with the same primary β-amyloid sequence as humans, such as non-human primates, bears, and dogs (Johnstone et al. 1991; Podlisny et al. 1991).

Table 1. Staining characteristics of deposits in NSE:β-APP751 mouse brain and early Down's syndrome are similar

Stain	NSE:β-APP751	Early DS[a]	Late DS/AD
β-amyloid antibodies	+	+	+
Methenamine silver	+	+	+
Bielschowsky silver	±	±	+
Thioflavin S	±	±	+
Congo red	−	−	+

[a] Abbreviations: DS, Down's syndrome; AD, Alzheimer's disease.
Histology was performed on transgenic mice using standard protocols for each stain. Results are compared with the human staining profile (Allsop et al. 1989; Giaccone et al. 1989; Mann and Esiri 1989)

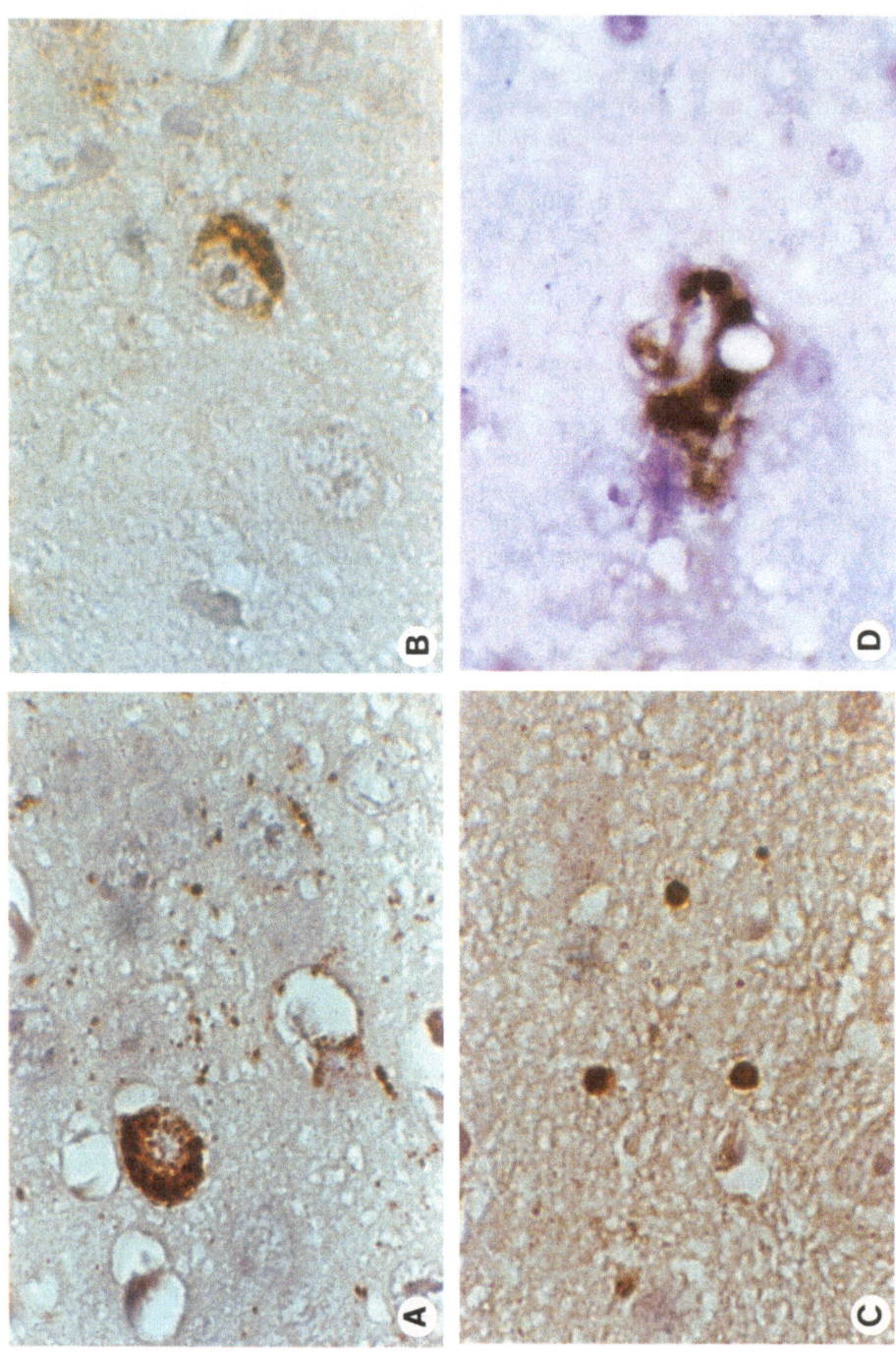

Transgenic Mice Have Other Histopathological Features

A second major histological feature of Alzheimer's disease brain is neurofibrillary tangles composed, in part, of an abnormally phosphorylated form of the microtubule associated protein tau. An extensively documented antibody that histologically stains only abnormal tau in neurofibrillary tangles is Alz50 (Wolozin et al. 1986). NSE: β-APP751 brain sections were stained with Alz50 to assay for aberrancies in tau. The staining revealed immunoreactive neurons and processes as well as fields of puncta in the neuropil (Fig. 2). The aberrant subcellular localization of tau to the neuronal soma seen in the transgenic mice stained with Alz50 is identical to the abnormal subcellular distribution of tau observed in Alzheimer's disease. Stained neuronal soma in the NSE: β-APP751 mice were exclusively localized to the cerebral cortex (both deep and superficial layers), thalamus, and amygdala. Immunoreactive processes were frequently noted in these same brain regions and occasionally in the hippocampus. This Alz50 staining profile was unique to the transgenic mice and was not found in sections from wild type mice. As in the case of β-amyloid immunoreactivity, Alz50 staining of NSE: β-APP751 mouse brains is most similar to the pathology present in young adult Down's brain and not in the late-stage Alzheimer's disease brain (Mann and Esiri 1989; Mann et al. 1989). The transgenic mice demonstrate that β-APP751 overexpression and/or β-amyloid deposition can lead to cytoskeletal pathology as defined by Alz50 immunoreactivity. This finding is illustrated, in part, in a simple hypothetical cascade of pathological events that we propose is occurring in Alzheimer's disease (Fig. 3). That preamyloid promotes abnormalities in tau is consistent with observations of Down's pathology in which preamyloid formation is seen to precede neurofibrillary tangle formation (Wisniewski et al. 1985). We propose that neurofibrillary tangles ultimately promote neuronal loss which, in turn, culminates in the behavioral manifestations of dementia.

Frequency of β-Amyloid and Alz50 Immunoreactivities in Transgenic Mice Increases with Age

As described, the transgenic mice display a number of histopathologic characteristics of early Alzheimer's disease. The mice further parallel the human condition in that the number of β-amyloid deposits and abnormal Alz50-immunoreactive structures seen in NSE: β-APP751 transgenic brains increases with age of the animal. We selected a single NSE: β-APP751 pedigree for which

---

Fig. 2. Aberrant Alz50 immunoreactive structures in NSE: β-APP751 transgenic mouse brain. **A, B** Stained cortical neuronal soma and puncta. **C, D** Stained thalamic swollen dystrophic neurites. Magnification, 860 ×

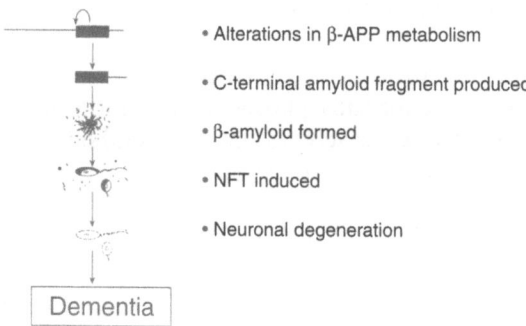

- Alterations in β-APP metabolism
- C-terminal amyloid fragment produced
- β-amyloid formed
- NFT induced
- Neuronal degeneration

Dementia

Fig. 3. Proposed pathogenic cascade in Alzheimer's disease. β-APP and NFT denote β-amyloid precursor protein and neurofibrillary tangles, respectively. The black box represents the β-amyloid domain within the precursor

Table 2. Age-related increase of β-amyloid and Alz50 immunoreactive structures in NSE: β-APP751 mouse brains

Age (months)	% sections positive for β-amyloid immunoreactive deposits	% sections with abnormal Alz50 immunoreactive structure
2–3	29 (n = 35)	33 (n = 36)
22	49 (n = 35)	69 (n = 36)

Twelve mice in each age group from a single NSE: β-APP751 pedigree, all homozygous for the transgene, were employed for this study. Three midline coronal sections were stained with 4.1 mAb for β-amyloid immunoreactivity and three for Alz50 immunoreactivity, then scored blind by two investigators. Values for old and young groups are statistically different ($p < 0.05$, one tailed).

we had a large number of young (2–3 months) and old (22 months) homozygous mice to examine. The study, conducted blind by the investigators scoring the brain sections, revealed that the frequency of β-amyloid immunoreactive deposits increased with age; nearly twice the frequency in the old set of animals compared with that in the young set was observed (Table 2). Similarly, Alz50-immunoreactive structures occurred at twice the frequency in the older population of NSE: β-APP751 mice (Table 2). It will be of interest to further characterize the transgenic mice with respect to possible changes in neurotransmitters, synaptic quality, and memory/learning capabilities for other alterations which may reflect events occurring in the pathogenic process.

Advanced Histopathology can be Achieved in the Transgenic Mouse

A concern in attempts to develop a transgenic model of Alzheimer's disease is the possibility that the murine brain is inherently incapable of producing mature

Alzheimer's disease-like histopathology. From our characterization, the NSE: β-APP751 transgenic mice most frequently produce diffuse extracellular β-amyloid deposits and modest intraneuronal abnormal tau immunoreactive structures. These results demonstrate that the murine brain is capable of reproducing at least two early events in Alzheimer's disease-like pathology. However, we have observed, albeit rarely, NSE: β-APP751 transgenic mice with a much more mature appearing pathology. The 4.1 mAb immunoreactivity of brain sections from several NSE: β-APP751 mice revealed large deposits of 100–250 μm with extensive β-amyloid immunoreactivity. These large deposits are infrequent in that they have only been observed in 4% of the transgenic mice thus far examined, but appear to be specific in that such structures have never been seen in wild type control mice or in mice transgenic for other human β-APP constructs.

These rare mice displayed several very large regions of β-amyloid immunoreactivity, often in the thalamus (Fig. 1D). The deposits were interspersed with vacuolated regions and were associated with elongated, abnormal appearing neurons. Other areas of the brain, including those near the large deposits, appeared normal. An antibody to glial fibrillary acidic protein highlighted extensive gliosis in affiliation with the large β-amyloid immunoreactive deposits. All of these features – vacuolization, gliosis, dense extracellular β-amyloid, and morphologically abnormal cells – are characteristic of Alzheimer's disease plaques. Alz50 immunohistochemistry of sections from this type of transgenic mouse produced globular staining associated with the large β-amyloid deposits (Fig. 2C, D) that is reminiscent of dystrophic neurites or swollen boutons typically found associated with mature plaques in Alzheimer's disease tissue stained with Alz50. As expected, these same mice revealed neuritic abnormalities typically associated with human plaques when stained with modified Bielschowsky silver salts. Given the very limited murine life span (24 months for this strain) compared to the period of time spanning many decades for the progression of Alzheimer's disease pathology, the occurrence of even a small subset of transgenic mice with extensive histopathology is remarkable. The next challenge in improving this small animal model of Alzheimer's disease will be to produce advanced state pathology consistently.

Although the occurrence of advanced histopathology in the transgenic mouse is infrequent, this finding demonstrates that the murine brain is capable of producing a mature Alzheimer's disease-like histopathology.

Conclusions

The results we have obtained with these transgenic mice should provide renewed confidence in the application of transgenic methods to the development of a small animal model of Alzheimer's disease. Only a single alteration was made in these animals, yet a number of pathological events were seen to develop. This has permitted us to begin to define the causal interrelationship among the histological features of the disease. The transgenic approach also allows other purported molecular mechanisms of pathogenesis to be tested.

This current transgenic mouse model typically exhibits features resembling an early stage of Alzheimer's disease. The immature Alzheimer's disease-like phenotype in these transgenic mice allows evaluation of putative environmental risk factors of the disease, as well as additional genes that may also be implicated in Alzheimer's disease, any of which may promote more frequent late stage pathology in the mice. Some mice, however, proceed to develop mature Alzheimer's disease-like histopathology. This is an important observation since it indicates that the murine brain is capable of recapitulating many of the advanced characteristics of Alzheimer's disease.

Last, this existing model and future transgenic mouse models of Alzheimer's disease will prove valuable in assessing potential therapeutics for this disease, including, but not exclusively, those designed to prevent amyloid deposition.

Acknowledgments. We thank our colleagues at Scios Nova, who contributed to the research described, and Marion Merrell Dow, Inc., who sponsors this research.

References

Allsop D, Haga S-I, Haga C, Ikeda S-I, Mann DMA, Ishii T (1989) Early senile plaques in Down's syndrome brains show a close relationship with cell bodies of neurons. Neuropath Applied Neurobiol 15:531–542

Burger PC, Vogel FC (1973) The development of the pathological changes of Alzheimer's disease and senile dementia in patients with Down's syndrome. Am J Pathol 73:457–476

Giaccone G, Tagliavini F, Linoli G, Bouras C, Frigerio L, Frangione B, Bugiani O (1989) Down syndrome patients: Extracellular preamyloid deposits precede neuritic degeneration and senile plaques. Neurosci Lett 97:232–238

Giaccone G, Verga L, Finazzi M, Pollo B, Tagliavini F, Frangione B, Bugiani O (1990) Cerebral preamyloid deposits and congophilic angiopathy in aged dogs. Neurosci Lett 114:178–183

Goate A, Chartier-Harlin M-C, Mullan M, Brown J, Crawford F, Fidani L, Giuffra L, Haynes A, Irving N, James L, Mant R, Newton P, Rooke K, Roques P, Talbot C, Pericak-Vance M, Roses A, Williamson R, Rossor M, Owen M, Hardy J (1991) Segregation of a missense mutation in the amyloid precursor protein with familial Alzheimer's disease. Nature 349:704–706

Golde TE, Estus T, Usiak M, Younkin L, Younkin S (1990) Expression of β-amyloid protein precursor mRNAs: recognition of a novel alternatively spliced form and quantitation in Alzheimer's disease using PCR. Neuron 4:253–267

Johnson SA, Pasinetti GM, May PC, Cordell B, Finch CE (1988) Selective reduction of mRNA for the β-amyloid precursor protein that lacks the Kunitz-type protease inhibitor motif in cortex of Alzheimer's disease. Exp Neurol 102:264–268

Johnson SA, McNeill T, Cordell B, Finch CE (1990) Relation of neuronal APP-751/APP-695 mRNA ratio and neuritic plaque density in Alzheimer's disease. Science 248:854–857

Johnstone EM, Chaney MO, Norris FH, Pascual R, Little SP (1991) Conservation of the sequence of the Alzheimer's disease amyloid peptide in dog, polar bear and five other mammals by cross-species polymerase chain reactions. Mol Brain Res 10:299–305

Kang J, Lemaire H-G, Unterbeck A, Salbaum JM, Masters CL, Grzeshik K-H, Multhaup G, Beyreuther K, Müller-Hill B (1987) The precursor of Alzheimer's disease amyloid A4 protein resembles a cell-surface receptor. Nature 325:733–736

Kawabata S, Higgins GA, Gordon JW (1991) Amyloid plaques, neurofibrillary tangles and neuronal loss in brains of transgenic mice overexpressing a C-terminal fragment of human amyloid precursor protein. Nature 354:476–478

Kitaguchi N, Takahashi Y, Tokushima Y, Shiojiri S, Ito H (1988) Novel precursor of Alzheimer's disease amyloid protein shows protease inhibitory activity. Nature 331:530–532

Mann DNA, Esiri MM (1989) The pattern of acquisition of plaques and tangles in the brains of patients under 50 years of age with Down's syndrome. J Neurol Sci 89:169–179

Mann DMA, Prinja D, Davies CA, Ihara Y, Delacourte A, Défossez A, Mayer RJ, Landon M (1989) Immunocytochemical profile of neurofibrillary tangles in Down's syndrome patients of different ages. J Neurol Sci 92:247–260

Murrell J, Farlow M, Ghetti B, Benson MD (1991) A mutation in the amyloid precursor protein associated with hereditary Alzheimer's disease. Science 254:97–99

Neve RL, Finch EA, Dawes LP (1988) Expression of the Alzheimer amyloid protein gene transcript in the human brain. Neuron 1:669–677

Podlisny MB, Tolan D, Selkoe DJ (1991) Homology of the amyloid β-protein precursor in monkey and human supports a primate model for β-amyloidosis in Alzheimer's disease. Am J Pathol 138:1423–1425

Ponte P, Gonzalez-DeWhitt P, Schilling J, Miller J, Hsu D, Greenberg B, Davies K, Wallace W, Leiberburg I, Fuller F, Cordell B (1988) A new A4 amyloid contains a domain homologous to serine protease inhibitors. Nature 331:525–527

Quon D, Wang Y, Catalano R, Scardina JM, Murakami K, Cordell B (1991) Formation of β-amyloid protein deposits in brains of transgenic mice. Nature 352:239–241

Selkoe DJ, Bell DS, Podlisny MB, Price DL, Cork LC (1987) Conservation of brain amyloid proteins in aged mammals and humans with Alzheimer's disease. Science 235:873–877

Tanzi RE, McCleatchey AI, Lamperti ED, Villa-Kamaroff L, Gusella JF, Neve RL (1988) Protease inhibitor domain encoded by an amyloid protein precursor mRNA associated with Alzheimer's disease. Nature 331:528–530

Wirek DO, Bayney R, Ramabhadran TV, Fracasso RP, Hart JH, Hauer PE, Hsiau P, Pekar SK, Scangos GA, Trapp BD, Unterbeck AJ (1991) Deposits of amyloid β protein in the central nervous system of transgenic mice. Science 253:323–325

Wisniewski H, Johnson AB, Raine CS, Kay WJ, Terry RD (1970) Senile plaques and cerebral amyloidosis in aged dogs: a histochemical study. Lab Invest 1970; 23:287–296

Wisniewski KE, Wisniewski HM, Wen GY (1985) Occurrence of neuropathological changes and dementia of Alzheimer's Diseases in Down's syndrome. Ann Neurol 17:278–282

Wolozin BL, Pruchnicke A, Dickson DW, Davies P (1986) A neuronal antigen in the brains of Alzheimer patients. Science 232:647–650

Yamada T, Hiroyuki S, Furuya H, Miyata T, Goto I, Sakaki Y (1987) Complementary DNA for the mouse homolog of the human amyloid beta protein precursor. Biochem Biophys Research Comm 149:665–671

Amyloid in Alzheimer's Disease and Animal Models

D. L. Price*, B. T. Lamb, J. D. Gearhart, L. J. Martin, L. C. Walker, E. H. Koo, D. R. Borchelt, and S. S. Sisodia

Summary

Animal models provide unique opportunities to analyze mechanisms of β-amyloid protein (Aβ) amyloidogenesis. One set of studies in control animals was designed to identify the neural cells that express the amyloid precursor protein (APP) and to characterize the transport and processing of APP *in vivo*. APP is synthesized by neurons and transported by fast axonal transport to terminals, where it may play a role in cell-cell and synaptic interactions. A second group of investigations focused on amyloidogenesis in aged nonhuman primates. In late middle life, monkeys develop age-associated impairments in performance on cognitive/memory tasks and begin to show brain abnormalities, including deposits of Aβ and formation of neurites. Amyloid is readily demonstrable in proximity to APP-enriched swollen axonal terminals and dendrites, suggesting that neurons may be one source of Aβ. However, in ways not yet clear, astrocytes, microglia, and vascular cells may also contribute to the formation of Aβ. In the neuropil of brain, alterations in the normal biology of APP may lead not only to the formation of amyloid fibrils but may also impair synaptic interactions, resulting in synaptic disjunction and disconnection. More recently, in a third set of experiments, we have begun to examine transgenic mice, generated by the yeast artificial chromosome (YAC)-embryonic stem (ES) cell technique. These animals express the entire human APP gene and transgene expression that approximates levels of endogenous APP. These mice, trisomic for APP, may develop Alzheimer's disease (AD)-type pathology, as occurs in individuals with Down's syndrome (trisomy 21). Finally, recent research is designed to produce transgenic mice with AD-linked APP mutations; these studies are essential for determining some of the genetic/molecular/biochemical mechanisms that cause AD-type brain lesions in familial AD (FAD). The strategies that have proved valuable in aged monkeys will be very helpful in studies of these mice. Both nonhuman primate and transgenic models will permit the testing of therapeutic approaches designed to ameliorate some of the abnormalities that occur in humans with AD. In conclusion, this review

* Neuropathology Laboratory, The Johns Hopkins University School of Medicine, 558 Ross Research Building, 720 Rutland Avenue, Baltimore, MD 21205-2196, USA

C.L. Masters et al. (Eds.)
Amyloid Protein Precursor in Development,
Aging and Alzheimer's Disease
© Springer-Verlag Berlin Heidelberg 1994

summarizes briefly the features of AD relevant to these studies and outlines some of our research focusing on the biology of APP in neural tissues and animal models, including aged nonhuman primates and transgenic mice.

Alzheimer's Disease

AD, the most common disease associated with cognitive impairment in the elderly (McKhann et al. 1984; Evans et al. 1989), manifests as progressive dementia (McKhann et al. 1984) which is the result of abnormalities of neurons in multiple regions of the brain. The neuropathology of AD is characterized by the deposition of amyloid, cytoskeletal pathology in neurons, and death of nerve cells. Senile plaques, comprised of amyloid deposits in proximity to neurites, occur in the amygdala, hippocampus, and neocortex of cases of AD, older patients with Down's syndrome, and, to a lesser extent, aged primates of many species, including humans (Wisniewski and Terry 1973a,b; Wisniewski et al. 1973; Glenner and Wong 1984; Kemper 1984; Masters et al. 1985a,b; Struble et al. 1985; Selkoe et al. 1987; Rumble et al. 1989; Cork et al. 1990; Martin et al. 1991; Probst et al. 1991). Congophilic amyloid angiopathy, which occurs in each of these settings, is also seen in cases of hereditary cerebral hemorrhage with amyloidosis, Dutch type (HCHWA-D; Levy et al. 1990; Van Broeckhoven et al. 1990). In AD, subsets of neurons characteristically develop neurofibrillary tangles, abnormal neurites, and neuropil threads (Grundke-Iqbal et al. 1986; Brion 1990; Goedert et al. 1991; Lee et al. 1991). These fibrillary inclusions, comprised of insoluble paired helical filaments and 15-nm straight filaments, contain predominantly abnormally phosphorylated isoforms of tau (Brion 1990; Greenberg and Davies 1990; Goedert et al. 1991; Lee et al. 1991). These filaments, presumably generated by common mechanisms, interfere with the function of neurons (Grundke-Iqbal et al. 1986; Lee et al. 1991; Crowther et al. 1992; Goedert et al. 1992); eventually, these cells die (Kemper 1984; Arnold et al. 1991; Braak and Braak 1991). Clinical signs reflect disease in these populations of neurons that leads to deafferentation of targets.

Many lines of evidence suggest that amyloidogenesis plays a critical role in the development of these various manifestations of AD. $A\beta$ is an $\sim$ 4-kD peptide comprised of 11–15 amino acids of the transmembrane domain and 28 amino acids of the extracellular domain of APP type-I integral membrane glycoproteins (Kang et al. 1987; Kitaguchi et al. 1988; Ponte et al. 1988; Golde et al. 1990). The mechanisms of $A\beta$ formation, nucleation, and polymerization into fibrils are an active area of research (Jarrett and Lansbury 1993). Although $A\beta$ residues of 1–28, 12–28, 14–28, 16–28, 17–28, and 18–28, as well as $A\beta$ 1–40, spontaneously form fibrils in vitro (Wisniewski and Terry 1973b; Castaño et al. 1986; Gorevic et al. 1987; Fraser et al. 1992; Ghiso et al. 1993), the most fibrillogenic peptides are $A\beta$, 1–42, 43 (Jarrett and Lansbury 1993). The formation of amyloid is thought to be a nucleation-dependent phenomenon with the C-terminus being a critical determinant of the rate of amyloid formation (Jarrett et al. 1993; Jarrett and Lansbury 1993). Thus, Aβ 1–42 and/or Aβ 1–43, rather than Aβ 1–40, may be particularly important in amyloidogenesis (Jarrett and Lansbury 1993; Jarrett et al. 1993). In plaques, amyloid is often colocalized with other proteins, including α_1-antichymotrypsin (Abraham et al. 1989; Koo et al. 1991), apolipoprotein E (Apo E; Strittmatter et al. 1993), SP40, 40 (apolipo-protein J (Apo J); Ghiso et al. 1993), constituents of the complement cascade (McGeer et al. 1989; Johnson et al. 1992), etc. It has been speculated that Apo J may maintain Aβ in a soluble form (Ghiso et al. 1993), preventing the concentration of Aβ from achieving values critical for nucleation and fibril-logenesis. In contrast, the presence of two alleles of Apo E4, i.e., the major transporter of cholesterol (Mahley 1988), may influence Aβ sequestration and enhance amyloidogenesis (Corder et al. 1993; Saunders et al. 1993; Strittmatter et al. 1993).

To begin to model Aβ amyloidosis, we considered several factors implicated in the pathogeneses of this process: age (Delaére et al. 1993), trisomy 21 (Burger and Vogel 1973; Ball and Nuttal 1980; Giaccone et al. 1989; Mann and Esiri 1989; Rumble et al. 1989), and APP mutations (Chartier-Harlin et al. 1991; Goate et al. 1991; Murrell et al. 1991; Mullan et al. 1992). Our initial studies took advantage of the aged nonhuman primate as a model for age-associated Aβ amyloidogenesis; more recently, we have used YAC-ES cell technologies to generate transgenic mice that overexpress APP and may serve as a model for the amyloidogenesis that occurs in individuals with trisomy 21. In the future, information from genetic studies, including those documenting mutations in APP in FAD pedigrees and the presence of Apo E4 alleles in late-onset AD, will undoubtedly be used to model genetic influences that lead to AD (Table 1).

Biology of APP

Situated on the mid-portion of the long arm of human chromosome 21 (Kang et al. 1987), the human APP gene ($\sim$ 400 kb of DNA) is a member of a gene

Table 1. Alzheimer's disease.

Familial cases	$\sim$ 10%
Sporadic cases	Majority
Onset	FAD, mid life; sporadic, late life
Duration	8–12 years
Signs	Dementia
Chromosomal loci	21 + 14 (early-onset FAD); 19 (late-onset) FAD
Gene (chromosome)	APP (21) in some FAD families; Apo E4 (19) in late-onset cases
Selective vulnerability	Cortical, hippocampal, and cholinergic basal forebrain neurons
Cytoskeletal pathology	Neurofibrillary tangles; neurites; neuropil threads
Amyloid	Aβ deposits (parenchyma/vessels)
Death of neurons	Severe
Animal models	Aged nonhuman primates; APP transgenic mice; *in vivo* injection of Aβ

family that includes several APP homologues, termed amyloid precursor-like proteins (APLP; i.e., APLP1 and APLP2; Wasco et al. 1992, 1993; Slunt et al. 1994). The APP gene gives rise, by alternative splicing of APP pre-mRNA, to at least four transcripts that encode $A\beta$-containing glycoproteins (Kang et al. 1987; Kitaguchi et al. 1988; Ponte et al. 1988; Golde et al. 1990). APP, modified by the addition of both N- and O-linked carbohydrates and terminal sulfation events (Weidemann et al. 1989), appear at the cell surface where they may be cleaved by APP α-secretase at position 16 within $A\beta$ to release the ectodomain of APP (Esch et al. 1990; Sisodia et al. 1990; Anderson et al. 1991; Wang et al. 1991; Haass et al. 1992a; Sisodia 1992). APP can also be processed via another pathway, thought to involve endosomal-lysosomal systems, resulting in the production of a variety of C-terminal-containing fragments, some of which are potentially amyloidogenic (Golde et al. 1992; Haass et al. 1992a; Busciglio et al. 1993). Amyloid peptides, i.e., $A\beta$ 1–40 (~ 4 kD) and $A\beta$ 17–40 (~ 3 kD), are released into the media of primary cell cultures and cell lines (Haass et al. 1992b; Shoji et al. 1992; Busciglio et al. 1993) and into cerebrospinal fluid (Shoji et al. 1992; Seubert et al. 1993). These findings suggest that $A\beta$ may be released directly *in vivo*. However, these peptides may not reach sufficient concentration *in vivo* for nucleation, polymerization, and aggregation to occur (Jarrett and Lansbury 1993; Jarrett et al. 1993). The presence of the C-terminus of $A\beta$ is a significant determinant of the rate of $A\beta$ fibril formation, and it is likely that $A\beta$ 1–42, 43 is more fibrillogenic than $A\beta$ 1–40 and $A\beta$ 17–40. Thus, small amounts of $A\beta$ 1–42, 43 fibrils may serve as a nidus for amyloid formation (Jarrett and Lansbury 1993; Jarrett et al. 1993); subsequently, other $A\beta$-containing fragments of APP could aggregate at these sites.

Despite advances in our understanding of APP metabolism *in vitro*, much less is known regarding the biology of APP *in vivo*. APP transcripts/proteins are expressed in most neurons (Neve et al. 1988; Koo et al. 1990a; Martin et al. 1991; Sisodia et al. 1993), and APP are present in cell bodies, dendrites, axon hillocks, initial segments, and axons (Martin et al. 1991). Our studies in control animals have focused on aspects of the biology of APP in neurons in the peripheral and central nervous systems (CNS; Koo et al. 1990a,b; Sisodia et al. 1993).

In the dorsal root ganglia (DRG), we used reverse transcriptase-polymerase chain reaction to demonstrate that mRNA encoding APP-695 are expressed 10-fold in excess of transcripts encoding Kunitz-type serine protease inhibitors containing APP. *In situ* hybridization showed that APP-695 transcripts were localized principally in sensory neurons, whereas APP-751/770 transcripts were more conspicuous in non-neuronal cells (i.e., fibroblasts and Schwann cells; Sisodia et al. 1993). We labeled isolated DRG and nerve *in vitro* with [^{35}S]methionine and compared the APP species synthesized in the DRG or nerve (containing fibroblasts and Schwann cells but lacking neurons) with those synthesized in cultured cell lines transfected with either human APP-695 or -770 cDNA. The pattern of APP immunoprecipitated from DRG and nerve was consistent with the concept that APP-695 is predominantly synthesized in neurons, whereas APP-751/770 isoforms are synthesized by supporting cells of the sciatic nerve (Sisodia et al. 1993).

To analyze the *in vivo* transport of APP, double ligatures were placed on the sciatic nerve, and animals were sacrificed at various times thereafter (Koo et al. 1990b). The rates of accumulation of APP and acetylcholinesterase, a rapidly transported protein, were indistinguishable, an observation consistent with the idea that APP are carried by fast anterograde axonal transport. To test this idea more directly, $[^{35}S]$methionine was microinjected directly into the lumbar DRG, animals were sacrificed four hours following injection, and labeled APP were immunoprecipitated from the sciatic nerve and DRG (Sisodia et al. 1993). The most abundant APP species were the fully glycosylated ($\sim 120–125$ kD) forms of APP-695 that mature through the Golgi apparatus and are then transported anterogradely in axons, presumably as part of membranous vesicles that are translocated, via kinesin-mediated motors, along microtubules. Small amounts ($\sim 5\%$ of all transported full-length molecules) of glycosylated forms of APP-751/770 ($\sim 140–150$ kD) were also detected in nerve. A minor APP-related species of ~ 95 kD, not recognized by the C-terminal antibody, was also present in axons. Our present interpretations are that the ~ 95-kD product could be generated following axolemmal insertion of holo-APP, as occurs with other rapidly transported proteins (Griffin et al. 1981), or alternatively, could be a truncated species being carried in rapidly transported vesicles. Preliminary studies of pathways in the CNS are consistent with the idea that full-length APP species, particularly APP-695, are transported by CNS neurons. In distal axons and nerve terminals, APP appears to be processed to generate C-terminal fragments, several of which are potentially amyloidogenic (SS Sisodia, VE Koliatsos, and DL Price, personal observations). Ongoing efforts are designed to define details of the trafficking and processing of transported APP in the CNS. The roles of APP in the CNS are uncertain, but it has been hypothesized that APP may be important in cell-cell interactions and in synaptic functions (Schubert 1991). Recent studies suggest that a sequence in the APP cytoplasmic domain catalyzes GTP exchange with G_0, suggesting a role for APP as a G_0-coupled receptor (Nishimoto et al. 1993). The distributions and fates of transported APP isoforms in the CNS can be examined by *in vivo* labeling of APP, synthesized by specific populations of neurons, followed by the examination of APP processing in defined target fields. Similar approaches should prove very useful in the analysis of the biochemistry of amyloidogenesis in animals that show deposits of Aβ.

Animal Models

Aged Nonhuman Primates

Early in the third decade of life, *Macaca mulatta* develop age-associated impairments in performance on cognitive and memory tasks (Presty et al. 1987;

Bachevalier et al. 1991), and it is presumed that these impairments are related to brain abnormalities similar to those that occur in older humans and subjects with AD (Wisniewski and Terry 1973b; Bartus et al. 1978; Struble et al. 1982, 1985; Kitt et al. 1984; Davis 1985; Selkoe et al. 1987; Walker et al. 1987, 1990; Abraham et al. 1989; Wenk et al. 1989; Cork et al. 1990; Bachevalier et al. 1991; Martin et al. 1991). Because old animals develop amyloid and neurites (Wisniewski and Terry 1973b, Struble et al. 1982, 1985; Kitt et al. 1984; Selkoe et al. 1987; Walker et al. 1987, 1988, 1990; Abraham et al. 1989; Cork et al. 1990; Martin et al. 1991), these animals provide a model to examine AD-like abnormalities, including amyloidogenesis.

In the brains of these primates, small amounts of Aβ 1–40 (or fragments thereof) may be released normally throughout life (Golde et al. 1992; Haass et al. 1992a). However, young animals show no evidence of the Aβ deposition or fibril formation needed for nucleation and aggregation, presumably because levels of Aβ are below critical concentrations. However, when monkeys reach late middle life, Aβ begins to appear as diffuse deposits (Wisniewski and Terry 1973a,b; Struble et al. 1982, 1985; Selkoe et al. 1987; Walker et al. 1987, 1988, 1990; Abraham et al. 1989; Cork et al. 1990) perhaps, for reasons as yet unexplained, related to the increased levels of Aβ 1–40 or because of the presence of Aβ 1–42,43, which can provide a nidus for the deposition of Aβ 1–42,43, (Jarrett and Lansbury 1993; Jarrett et al. 1993). At these sites, we have detected enlarged neurites (Wisniewski and Terry 1973b; Struble et al. 1982, 1985; Selkoe et al. 1987; Walker et al. 1988; Cork et al. 1990) derived from a variety of transmitter systems (Kitt et al. 1984, 1985; Walker et al. 1987, 1988). Neurites accumulate membranous elements, degenerating mitochondria, and lysosomes; moreover, they may be enriched in APP, phosphorylated neurofilaments, transmitter markers, and synaptophysin (Martin et al. 1991). In individual plaques, APP- and synaptophysin-immunoreactive structures are often surrounded by a halo of distorted neuropil that, in adjacent sections, contains Aβ immunoreactivity; the proximity of APP-like immunoreactive neuronal perikarya and neurites within Aβ-containing plaques suggests that neurons and/or their processes can serve as a source for some of the deposited Aβ. These pathological events may be associated subsequently with synaptic disjunction (a potentially reversible process), followed by irreversible synaptic disconnection and deafferentation of targets, as has been suggested to occur in AD (DeKosky and Scheff 1990; Masliah et al. 1991; Terry et al. 1991). In the brains of aged animals, neurons are not the only potential source of Aβ; microglia and astrocytes are present in proximity to Aβ deposits and play roles in the synthesis/processing of APP or may influence the physical state of Aβ. Moreover, these cells may produce Aβ colocalizing proteins, including α_1-antichymotrypsin (Abraham et al. 1989; Koo et al. 1991), Apo E (Wisniewski and Frangione 1992; Corder et al. 1993; Saunders et al. 1993; Strittmatter et al. 1993), and SP40-40 (Apo J; Ghiso et al. 1993); these proteins may accelerate or retard amyloidogenesis. Finally, vascular cells may also contribute to Aβ amyloidogenesis. Significantly, aged rhesus and squirrel monkeys (*Saimiri sciureus*) show Aβ in the walls of meningeal and small cerebral vessels (Walker et al. 1987, 1990); preliminary studies of these animals suggest that some $A\beta$ may be derived from APP synthesized by vascular cells.

APP Transgenic Mice

Transgenic strategies are powerful tools to examine the causative links between the APP gene, its overexpression, the presence of mutations, and abnormalities in the brain. Moreover, these animals can be used to delineate the mechanisms that lead *in vivo* to amyloidogenesis and possibly other types of AD-related pathologies (Sisodia and Price 1992; Price and Sisodia, in press). Over the past several years, scientists have used transgenic approaches to try to produce animal models of AD (Quon et al. 1991; Lamb et al. 1993). However, with one possible exception (Quon et al. 1991), published reports of transgenic mice have not documented AD-type pathology convincingly (Sisodia and Price 1992; Price and Sisodia, in press). The difficulties in the work may reflect, in part, the problems encountered in trying to overexpress APP using conventional cDNA-based transgenic technologies.

Recently, we adopted a different strategy based on the idea that a more satisfactory level of expression might be achieved using the whole APP gene and based on the observation that individuals with Down's syndrome, who have an extra copy of chromosome 21 (and the APP gene), develop the histopathological hallmarks of AD, including amyloid deposits (Burger and Vogel 1973; Ball and Nuttal 1980; Glenner and Wong 1984; Masters et al. 1985a,b; Wisniewski et al. 1985; Giaccone et al. 1989; Mann and Esiri 1989; Rumble et al. 1989). If three copies of APP and increased levels of APP predispose to amyloidogenesis, then we hypothesized that transgenic mice overexpressing APP may mimic the trisomic APP dosage imbalance observed in individuals with Down's syndrome. To pursue this idea, a YAC carrying the human APP gene that contained an ~ 650 kb human DNA fragment was identified, purified, and introduced via lipid-mediated transfection into ES cells (Lamb et al. 1993). APP sequences were stably integrated, and they constitutively expressed APP mRNA and encoded polypeptides. These ES cells were used to generate chimeric mice; subsequent breeding disclosed that the human APP genomic sequences had been transmitted to the mouse germline. These sequences were transcribed actively in mouse tissue, the splicing pattern of human APP transcripts in transgenic mouse tissues mirrored the endogenous pattern of alternatively spliced mRNA, and the relative levels of human and mouse APP mRNA were similar. Using an antibody specific for human APP, Western analysis of this line of transgenic mice demonstrated levels of human APP expression in the brain and in various other organs. For example, in transgenic mouse brain, levels of human APP were $\sim 70\%$ of total APP. Finally, immunocytochemical studies with a human APP-specific antibody disclosed human APP immunoreactivity in neurons in the brain. As anticipated, two young animals did not show evidence of AD-type pathology. However, as occurs in individuals with trisomy 21, these transgenic animals may develop Aβ deposits in later adult life.

Another approach to model AD takes advantage of recent genetic studies linking mutations to FAD. More than 10 pedigrees of early-onset autosomal dominant FAD exhibit linkage to mutations of APP (Chartier-Harlin et al. 1991; Goate et al. 1991; Murrell et al. 1991). In these families, the valine residue at position 717 (of APP-770) is replaced by either isoleucine, phenylalanine, or glycine. In addition, two large, related, early-onset disease families from Sweden have a double mutation at codons 670 and 671 (of APP-770; Mullan et al. 1992), resulting in substitutions of the lysine-methionine dipeptide by asparagine-leucine. Neuropathological examination of a single case from one of the Swedish families disclosed the presence of senile plaques, neurofibrillary tangles, and congophilic angiopathy (B Winblad, personal communication). Moreover, cells transfected with cDNA encoding APP with this double mutation showed elevated levels of secreted Aβ-related peptides (Citron et al. 1992; Cai et al. 1993), whereas cells transfected with APP-717 mutations did not exhibit alterations in APP processing (Cai et al. 1993). The YAC-ES cell strategy can be used to introduce modified human APP that encode FAD mutations into the mouse germline and to determine whether the presence of these mutations predisposes to Aβ deposition and, possibly, the other brain abnormalities that occur in AD. This strategy provides a direct test of the significance of these APP gene mutations in the etiology/pathogenesis of FAD. Moreover, these mice produced by transgenic strategies should allow analyses of the sequential biochemical, cellular, and molecular pathologies characteristic of early-onset FAD.

Conclusions

Animal models are essential to analyze the biology of APP and to define the mechanisms of amyloidogenesis. Aged nonhuman primates are useful for examining the roles of age in the pathogenesis of these lesions, whereas transgenic mice, which have begun to show promise (Quon et al. 1991; Sisodia and Price 1992; Lamb et al. 1993), will be valuable for determining the roles of genetic and molecular processes that cause AD-type pathology (Price et al. in press). Finally, these models can be used to test therapeutic approaches designed to ameliorate age-related brain abnormalities that occur in humans with AD.

Acknowledgments. The authors thanks Drs. Mary Lou Voytko, Vassilis E. Koliatsos, Paul N. Hoffman, Linda C. Cork, and Cheryl A. Kitt for helpful discussions.

This work was supported by grants from the U.S. Public Health Service (NS AG 05146, NS, 20471, NS 07179) as well as the American Health Assistance Foundation, the Metropolitan Life Foundation, and The Robert L. & Clara G. Patterson Trust. Dr. Price is the recipient of a Leadership and Excellence in

Alzheimer's Disease (LEAD) award (AG 07914) and a Javits Neuroscience Investigator Award (NS 10580).

References

Abraham CR, Selkoe DJ, Potter H, Price DL, Cork LC (1989) α_1-antichymotrypsin is present together with the β-protein in monkey brain amyloid deposits. Neuroscience 32:715–720

Anderson JP, Esch FS, Keim PS, Sambamurti K, Lieberburg I, Robakis NK (1991) Exact cleavage site of Alzheimer amyloid precursor in neuronal PC-12 cells. Neurosci Lett 128:126–128

Arnold SE, Hyman BT, Flory, J. Damasio AR, Van Hoesen GW (1991) The topographical and neuroanatomical distribution of neurofibrillary tangles and neuritic plaques in the cerebral cortex of patients with Alzheimer's disease. Cereb Cortex 1:103–116

Bachevalier J, Landis LS, Walker LC, Brickson M, Mishkin M, Price DL, Cork LC (1991) Aged monkeys exhibit behavioral deficits indicative of widespread cerebral dysfunction. Neurobiol Aging 12:99–111

Ball MJ, Nuttal K (1980) Neurofibrillary tangles, granulovacuolar degeneration, and neuron loss in Down syndrome: quantitative comparison with Alzheimer dementia. Ann Neurol 7:462–465

Bartus RT, Fleming D, Johnson HR (1978) Aging in the rhesus monkey: debilitating effects on short-term memory. J Gerontol 33:858–871

Braak H, Braak E (1991) Neuropathological stageing of Alzheimer-related changes. Acta Neuropathol 82:239–259

Brion J-P (1990) Molecular pathology of Alzheimer amyloid and neurofibrillary tangles. Sem Neurosci 2:89–100

Burger PC, Vogel FS (1973) The development of the pathologic changes of Alzheimer's disease and senile dementia in patients with Down's syndrome. Am J Pathol 73:457–476

Busciglio J, Gabuzda DH, Matsudaira P, Yankner BA (1993) Generation of β-amyloid in the secretory pathway in neuronal and nonneuronal cells. Proc Natl Acad Sci USA 90: 2092–2096

Cai X-D, Golde TE, Younkin SG (1993) Release of excess amyloid β protein from a mutant amyloid β protein precursor. Science 259:514–516

Castaño EM, Ghiso J, Prelli F, Gorevic PD, Migheli A, Frangione B (1986) In vitro formation of amyloid fibrils from two synthetic peptides of different lengths homologous to Alzheimer's disease β-protein. Biochem Biophys Res Commun 141:782–789

Chartier-Harlin M-C, Crawford F, Houlden H, Warren A, Hughes D, Fidani L, Goate A, Rossor M, Roques P, Hardy J, Mullan M (1991) Early-onset Alzheimer's disease caused by mutations at codon 717 of the β-amyloid precursor protein gene. Nature 353:844–846

Citron M, Oltersdorf T, Haass C, McConlogue L, Hung AY, Seubert P, Vigo-Pelfrey C, Lieberburg, I, Selkoe DJ (1992) Mutation of the β-amyloid precursor protein in familial Alzheimer's disease increases β-protein production. Nature 360:672–674

Corder EH, Saunders AM, Strittmatter WJ, Schmechel DE, Gaskell PC, Small GW, Roses AD, Haines JL, Pericak-Vance MA (1993) Gene dose of apoliprotein-E type 4 allele and the risk of Alzheimer's disease in late onset families. Science 261:921–923

Cork LC, Masters C, Beyreuther K, Price DL (1990) Development of senile plaques. Relationships of neuronal abnormalities and amyloid deposits. Am J Pathol 137:1383–1392

Crowther RA, Olesen OF, Jakes R, Goedert M (1992) The microtubule binding repeats of tau protein assemble into filaments like those found in Alzheimer's disease, FEBS Lett. 309:199–202

Davis RT (1985) The effects of aging on the behavior of rhesus monkeys. In: Davis RT, Leathers CW (eds) Behavior and pathology of aging in rhesus monkeys. Monographs in Primatology, Vol. 8. New York, Alan R. Liss, pp 57–82

DeKosky ST, Scheff SW (1990) Synapse loss in frontal cortex biopsies in Alzheimer's disease: correlation with cognitive severity. Ann Neurol 27:457–463

Delaére P, He Y, Fayet G, Duyckaerts C, Hauw J-J (1993) βA4 deposits are constant in the brain of the oldest old: an immunocytochemical study of 20 French centenarians. Neurobiol Aging 14:191–194

Esch FS, Keim PS, Beattie EC, Blacher RW, Culwell AR, Oltersdor T, McClure D, Ward PJ (1990) Cleavage of amyloid β peptide during constitutive processing of its precursor. Science 248:1122–1124

Evans DA, Funkenstein HH, Albert MS, Scherr PA, Cook NR, Chown MJ, Hebert LE, Hennekens CH, Taylor JO (1989) Prevalence of Alzheimer's disease in a community population of older persons. Higher than previously reported. JAMA 262:2551–2556

Fraser PE, Nguyen JT, Inouye H, Surewicz WK, Selkoe DJ, Podlisny MB, Kirschner DA (1992) Fibril formation by primate, rodent, and Dutch-hemorrhagic analogues of Alzheimer amyloid β-protein. Biochemistry 31:10716–10723

Ghiso J, Matsubara E, Koudinov A, Choi-Miura NH, Tomita M, Wisniewski T, Frangione B (1993) The cerebrospinal-fluid soluble form of Alzheimer's amyloid beta is complexed to SP-40, 40 (apolipoprotein J), an inhibitor of the complement membrane-attack complex. Biochem J 293:27–30

Giaccone G, Tagliavini F, Linoli G, Bouras C, Frigerio L, Frangione B, Bugiani O (1989) Down patients: extracellular preamyloid deposits precede neuritic degeneration and senile plaques. Neurosci Lett 97:232–238

Glenner GG, Wong CW (1984) Alzheimer's disease: initial report of the purification and characterization of a novel cerebrovascular amyloid protein. Biochem Biophys Res Commun 120:885–890

Goate A, Chartier-Harlin M-C, Mullan M, Brown J, Crawford F, Fidani L, Giuffra L, Haynes A, Irving N, James L, Mant R, Newton P, Rooke K, Roques P, Talbot C, Pericak-Vance M, Roses A, Williamson R, Rossor M, Owen M, Hardy J (1991) Segregation of a missense mutation in the amyloid precursor protein gene with familial Alzheimer's disease. Nature 349:704–706

Goedert M, Sisodia SS, Price DL (1991) Neurofibrillary tangles and β-amyloid deposits in Alzheimer's disease. Curr Opin Neurobiol 1:441–447

Goedert M, Spillantini MG, Cairns NJ, Crowther RA (1992) Tau proteins of Alzheimer paired helical filaments: abnormal phosphorylation of all six brain isoforms. Neuron 8:159–168

Golde TE, Estus S, Usiak M, Younkin LH, Younkin SG (1990) Expression of β amyloid protein precursor mRNAs: recognition of novel alternatively spliced form and quantitation in Alzheimer's disease using PCR. Neuron 4:253–267

Golde TE, Estus S, Younkin LH, Selkoe DJ, Younkin SG (1992) Processing of the amyloid protein precursor to potentially amyloidogenic derivatives. Science 255:728–730

Gorevic PD, Castano EM, Sarma R, Frangione B (1987) Ten to fourteen residue peptides of Alzheimer's disease protein are sufficient for amyloid fibril formation and its characteristic X ray diffraction pattern. Biochem Biophys Res Commun 147:854–862

Greenberg SG, Davies P (1990) A preparation of Alzheimer paired helical filaments that displays distinct τ proteins by polyacrylamide gel electrophoresis. Proc Natl Acad Sci USA 87:5827–5831

Griffin JW, Price DL, Drachman DB, Morris J (1981) Incorporation of axonally transported glycoproteins into axolemma during nerve regeneration. J Cell Biol 88:205–214

Grundke-Iqbal I, Iqbal K, Quinlan M, Tung Y-C, Zaidi MS, Wisniewski HM (1986) Microtubule-associated protein tau. A component of Alzheimer paired helical filaments. J Biol Chem 261:6084–6089

Haass C, Koo EH, Mellon A, Hung AY, Selkoe DJ (1992a) Targeting of cell-surface β-amyloid precursor protein to lysosomes: alternative processing into amyloid-bearing fragments. Nature 357:500–503

Haass C, Schlossmacher MG, Hung AY, Vigo-Pelfrey C, Mellon A, Ostaszewski BL, Lieburg I, Koo EH, Schenk D, Teplow DB, Selkoe DJ (1992b) Amyloid β-peptide is produced by cultured cells during normal metabolism. Nature 359:322–325

Jarrett JT, Lansbury PT Jr (1993) Seeding "one-dimensional crystallization" of amyloid: a pathogenic mechanism in Alzheimer's disease and scrapie? Cell 73:1055–1058

Jarrett JT, Berger EP, Lansbury PT Jr (1993) The carboxy terminus of the β amyloid protein is critical for the seeding of amyloid formation: implications for the pathogenesis of Alzheimer's disease. Biochemistry 32:4693–4697

Johnson SA, Lampert-Etchells M, Pasinetti GM, Rozovsky I, Finch CE (1992) Complement mRNA in the mammalian brain: responses to Alzheimer's disease and experimental brain lesioning. Neurobiol Aging 13:641–648

Kang J, Lemaire H-G, Unterbeck A, Salbaum JM, Masters CL, Grzeschik K-H, Multhaup G, Beyreuther K, Müller-Hill B (1987) The precursor of Alzheimer's disease amyloid A4 protein resembles a cell-surface receptor. Nature 325:733–736

Kemper T (1984) Neuroanatomical and neuropathological changes in normal aging and in dementia. In: Albert ML (ed) Clinical neurology of aging. New York, Oxford University Press, pp 9–52

Kitaguchi N, Takahashi Y, Tokushima Y, Shiojiri S, Ito H (1988) Novel precursor of Alzheimer's disease amyloid protein shows protease inhibitory activity. Nature 331:530–532

Kitt CA, Price DL, Struble RG, Cork LC, Wainer BH, Becher MW, Mobley WC (1984) Evidence for cholinergic neurites in senile plaques. Science 226:1443–1445

Kitt CA, Struble RG, Cork LC, Mobley WC, Walker LC, Joh TH, Price DL (1985) Catecholaminergic neurites in senile plaques in prefrontal cortex of aged nonhuman primates. Neuroscience 16:691–699

Koo EH, Sisodia SS, Cork LC, Unterbeck A, Bayney RM, Price DL (1990a) Differential expression of amyloid precursor protein mRNAs in cases of Alzheimer's disease and in aged nonhuman primates. Neuron 2:97–104

Koo EH, Sisodia SS, Archer DR, Martin LJ, Weidemann A, Beyreuther K, Fischer P, Masters CL, Price DL (1990b) Precursor of amyloid protein in Alzheimer disease undergoes fast anterograde axonal transport. Proc Natl Acad Sci USA 87:1561–1565

Koo EH, Abraham CR, Potter H, Cork LC, Price DL (1991) Developmental expression of α_1-antichymotrypsin in brain may be related to astrogliosis. Neurobiol Aging 12:495–501

Lamb BT, Sisodia SS, Lawler AM, Slunt HH, Kitt CA, Kearns WG, Pearson PL, Price DL, Gearhart JD (1993) Introduction and expression of the 400 kb precursor amyloid protein gene in transgenic mice. Nature Genetics 5:22–30

Lee VM-Y, Balin BJ, Otvos L Jr, Trojanowski JQ (1991) A68: a major subunit of paired helical filaments and derivatized forms of normal tau. Science 251:675–678

Levy E, Carman MD, Fernandez-Madrid IJ, Power MD, Lieberburg I, van Duinen SG, Bots GTAM, Luyendijk W, Frangione B (1990) Mutation of the Alzheimer's disease amyloid gene in hereditary cerebral hemorrhage, Dutch type. Science 248:1124–1126

Mahley RW (1988) Apolipoprotein E: cholesterol transport protein with expanding role in cell biology. Science 240:622–630

Mann DMA, Esiri MM (1989) The pattern of acquisition of plaques and tangles in the brains of patients under 50 years of age with Down's syndrome. J Neurol Sci 89:169–179

Martin LJ, Sisodia SS, Koo EH, Cork LC, Dellovade TL, Weidemann A, Beyreuther K, Masters C, Price DL (1991) Amyloid precursor protein in aged nonhuman primates. Proc Natl Acad Sci USA 88:1461–1465

Masliah E, Hansen L, Albright T, Mallory M, Terry RD (1991) Immunoelectron microscopic study of synaptic pathology in Alzheimer's disease. Acta Neuropathol 81:428–433

Masters CL, Multhaup G, Simms G, Pottgiesser J, Martins RN, Beyreuther K (1985a) Neuronal origin of a cerebral amyloid: neurofibrillary tangles of Alzheimer's disease contain the same protein as the amyloid of plaque cores and blood vessels. EMBO J 4:2757–2763

Masters CL, Simms G, Weinman NA, Multhaup G, McDonald BL, Beyreuther K (1985b) Amyloid plaque core protein in Alzheimer disease and Down syndrome. Proc Natl Acad Sci USA 82:4245–4249

McGeer PL, Akiyama H, Itagaki S, McGeer EG (1989) Activation of the classical complement pathway in brain tissue of Alzheimer patients. Neurosci Lett 107:341–346

McKhann G, Drachman D, Folstein M, Katzman R, Price D, Stadlan EM (1984) Clinical diagnosis of Alzheimer's disease: report of the NINCDS-ADRDA Work Group under the auspices of Department of Health and Human Services Task Force on Alzheimer's Disease. Neurology 34:939–944

Mullan M, Crawford F, Axelman K, Houlden H, Lilius L, Winblad B, Lannfelt L (1992) A pathogenic mutation for probable Alzheimer's disease in the APP gene at the N-terminus of β-amyloid. Nature Genetics 1:345–347

Murrell J, Farlow M, Ghetti B, Benson MD (1991) A mutation in the amyloid precursor protein associated with hereditary Alzheimer's disease. Science 254:97–99

Neve RL, Finch EA, Dawes LR (1988) Expression of the Alzheimer amyloid precursor gene transcripts in the human brain. Neuron 1:669–677

Nishimoto I, Okamoto T, Matsuura Y, Takahashi S, Okamoto T, Murayama S, Ogata E (1993) Alzheimer amyloid protein precursor complexes with brain GTP-binding protein G_0. Nature 362:75–79

Ponte P, Gonzalez-DeWhitt P, Schilling J, Miller J, Hsu D, Greenberg B, Davis K, Wallace W, Lieburg I, Fuller F, Cordell B (1988) A new A4 amyloid mRNA contains a domain homologous to serine proteinase inhibitors. Nature 331:525–532

Presty SK, Bachevalier J, Walker LC, Struble RG, Price DL, Mishkin M, Cork LC (1987) Age differences in recognition memory of the rhesus monkey (Macaca mulatta). Neurobiol Aging 8:435–440

Price DL, Sisodia SS. Cellular and molecular biology of Alzheimer's diesase and animal models. Annu Rev Med, in press

Price DL, Martin LJ, Sisodia SS, Walker LC, Voytko ML, Wagster MV, Cork LC, Koliatsos VE: The aged nonhuman primate. A model for the behavioral and brain abnormalities occurring in aged human. In: Terry RD, Katzman R, and Bick KL (eds) Alzheimer disease. New York, Raven Press, in press

Probst A, Langui D, Ipsen S, Robakis N, Ulrich J (1991) Deposition of β/A4 protein along neuronal plasma membranes in diffuse senile plaques. Acta Neuropathol 83:21–29

Quon D, Wang Y, Catalano R, Scardina JM, Murakami K, Cordell B (1991) Formation of β-amyloid protein deposits in brains of transgenic mice. Nature 352:239–241

Rumble B, Retallack R, Hibich C, Simms G, Multhaup G, Martins R, Hockey A, Montgomery P, Beyreuther K, Masters CL (1989) Amyloid A4 protein and its precursor in Down's syndrome and Alzheimer's disease. N Engl J Med 320:1446–1452

Saunders AM, Strittmatter WJ, Schmechel D, St George-Hyslop PH, Pericak-Vance MA, Joo SH, Rosi BL, Gusella JF, Crapper-MacLachlan DR, Alberts MJ, Hulette C, Crain B, Goldgaber D, Roses AD (1993) Association of apolipoprotein E allele ε4 with late-onset familial and sporadic Alzheimer's disease. Neurology 43:1467–1472

Schubert D (1991) The possible role of adhesion in synaptic modification. Trends Neurosci 14:127–130

Selkoe DJ, Bell DS, Podlisny MB, Price DL, Cork LC (1987) Conservation of brain amyloid proteins in aged mammals and humans with Alzheimer's disease. Science 235:873–877

Seubert P, Oltersdorf T, Lee MG, Barbour R, Blomquist C, Davis DL, Bryant K, Fritz LC, Galasko D, Thal LJ, Lieburg I, Schenk DB (1993) Secretion of β-amyloid precursor protein cleaved at the amino terminus of the β-amyloid peptide. Nature 361:260–263

Shoji M, Golde TE, Ghiso J, Cheung TT, Estus S, Shaffer LM, Cai X-D, McKay DM, Tintner R, Frangione B, Younkin S (1992) Production of the Alzheimer amyloid β protein by normal proteolytic processing. Science 258:126–129

Sisodia SS (1992) β-amyloid precursor protein cleavage by a membrane-bound protease. Proc Natl Acad Sci USA 89:6075–6079

Sisodia SS, Price DL (1992) Amyloidogenesis in Alzheimer's disease: basic biology and animal models. Curr Opin Neurobiol 2:648–652

Sisodia SS, Koo EH, Beyreuther K, Unterbeck A, Price DL (1990) Evidence that β-amyloid protein in Alzheimer's disease is not derived by normal processing. Science 248:492–495

Sisodia SS, Koo EH, Hoffman PN, Perry G, Price DL (1993) Identification and transport of full-length amyloid precursor proteins in rat peripheral nervous system. J Neurosci 13:3136–3142

Slunt HH, Thinakaran G, Von Koch C, Lo ACY, Tanzi RE, Sisodia SS (1994) Expression of a ubiquitous, cross-reactive homologue of the mouse β-amyloid precursor protein (APP). J Biol Chem 269:2637–2644

Strittmatter WJ, Saunders AM, Schmechel D, Pericak-Vance M, Enghild J, Salvesen GS, Roses AD (1993) Apolipoprotein E: high-avidity binding to β-amyloid and increased frequency of type 4 allele in late-onset familial Alzheimer disease. Proc Natl Acad Sci USA 90:1977–1981

Struble RG, Cork LC, Whitehouse PJ, Price DL (1982) Cholinergic innervation in neuritic plaques. Science 216:413–415

Struble RG, Price DL Jr, Cork LC, Price DL (1985) Senile plaques in cortex of aged normal monkeys. Brain Res 361:267–275

Terry RD, Masliah E, Salmon DP, Butters N, DeTeresa R, Hill R, Hansen LA, Katzman R (1991) Physical basis of cognitive alterations in Alzheimer's disease: synapse loss is the major correlate of cognitive impairment. Ann Neurol 30:572–580

Van Broeckhoven C, Hann J, Bakker E, Hardy JA, Van Hul W, Wehnert A, Vegter-Van der Vlis M, Roos RAC (1990) Amyloid β protein precursor gene and hereditary cerebral hemorrhage with amyloidosis (Dutch). Science 248:1120–1126

Walker LC, Kitt CA, Cork LC, Struble RG, Dellovade TL, Price DL (1988) Multiple transmitter systems contribute neurites to individual senile plaques. J Neuropathol Exp Neurol 47:138–144

Walker LC, Kitt CA, Schwam E, Buckwald B, Garcia F, Sepinwall J, Price DL (1987) Senile plaques in aged squirrel monkeys. Neurobiol Aging 8:291–296

Walker LC, Masters C, Beyreuther K, Price DL (1990) Amyloid in the brains of aged squirrel monkeys. Acta Neuropathol 80:381–387

Wang R, Meschia JF, Cotter RJ, Sisodia SS (1991) Secretion of the $\beta/A4$ amyloid precursor protein. Identification of a cleavage site in cultured mammalian cells. J Biol Chem 266:16960–16964

Wasco W, Bupp K, Magendantz M, Gusella JF, Tanzi RE, Solomon F (1992) Identification of a mouse brain cDNA that encodes a protein related to the Alzheimer disease-associated amyloid-beta-protein precursor. Proc Natl Acad Sci USA 89:10758–10762

Wasco W, Gurubhagavatula S, Paradis Md, Romano DM, Sisodia SS, Hyman BT, Neve RL, Tanzi RE (1993) Isolation and characterization of APLP2 encoding a homologue of the Alzheimer's associated amyloid β protein precursor. Nature Genetics, 5:95–99

Weidemann A, König G, Bunke D, Fischer P, Salbaum JM, Masters CL, Beyreuther K (1989) Identification, biogenesis, and localization of precursors of Alzheimer's disease A4 amyloid protein. Cell 57:115–126

Wenk GL, Pierce DJ, Struble RG, Price DL, Cork LC (1989) Age-related changes in multiple neurotransmitter systems in the monkey brain. Neurobiol Aging 10:11–19

Wisniewski T, Frangione B (1992) Apolipoprotein E: a pathological chaperone protein in patients with cerebral and systemic amyloid. Neurosci Lett 135:235–238

Wisniewski HM, Terry RD (1973a) Morphology of the aging brain, human and animal. Prog Brain Res 40:167–186

Wisniewski HM, Terry RD (1973b) Reexamination of the pathogenesis of the senile plaque. In: Zimmerman HM (ed) Progress in neuropathology. Vol II New York, Grune & Stratton, pp 1–26

Wisniewski HM, Ghetti B, Terry RD (1973) Neuritic (senile) plaques and filamentous changes in aged rhesus monkeys. J Neuropathol Exp Neurol 32:566–584

Wisniewski KE, Wisniewski HM, and Wen GY (1985) Occurrence of neuropathological changes and dementia of Alzheimer's disease in Down's syndrome. Ann Neurol 17:278–282

The Roles of Zinc and Copper in the Function and Metabolism of the Amyloid Protein Precursor Superfamily

A. I. Bush*, W. Pettingell, and *R. E. Tanzi*

Summary

Abnormalities of zinc and copper homeostasis occur in Alzheimer's disease (AD), a dementia characterized by the aggregation of $A\beta$ in the brain, and in Down's syndrome (DS), a condition characterized by premature AD. The functional and conformational properties of amyloid protein precursor (APP) are influenced by specific zinc binding to a domain in the ectodomain which is homologous in other known members of the APP superfamily: amyloid precursor-like proteins 1 and 2 (APLP1 and APLP2), as well as drosophila APP-L. The finding of specific and saturable zinc binding to $A\beta$, the amyloidogenic catabolic product of APP, indicates that a physiological association between APP metabolism and brain zinc homeostasis is a possibility. Zinc binding to $A\beta$ results in a marked loss of $A\beta$ solubility *in vitro*, indicating that a small ($< 0.5 \, \mu M$) increase in interstitial Zn^{2+} concentration could accelerate $A\beta$ precipitation. Meanwhile, copper protects $A\beta$ from zinc-induced aggregation, stabilizing a soluble dimeric species. We propose that abnormalities of regional copper or zinc concentrations in the brains of patients with AD or DS may accelerate $A\beta$ amyloidosis in these conditions.

$A\beta$ and APP in Alzheimer's Disease

Our understanding of the molecular basis for the pathophysiology of Alzheimer's disease (AD) has advanced rapidly over the last decade. Much of that understanding has come from elaborating the role played by $A\beta$, the 4.3 kD peptide found to be the principal constituent of the cerebral amyloid deposits which are the pathological hallmarks of the disease (Masters et al. 1985; Glenner and Wong 1984). Considerable controversy exists as to whether $A\beta$ accumulation is itself neurotoxic, or whether $A\beta$ amyloidogenesis is an epiphenomenon of an alternative neuronal lesion. $A\beta$ is derived from the much larger amyloid

* Laboratory of Genetics and Aging, Neuroscience Center, Department of Neurology, Harvard Medical School, Massachusetts General Hospital East, Building 149, 13th Street, Charlestown, MA 02129, USA

C.L. Masters et al. (Eds.)
Amyloid Protein Precursor in Development,
Aging and Alzheimer's Disease
© Springer-Verlag Berlin Heidelberg 1994

protein precursor (APP; Kang et al. 1987; Tanzi et al. 1987), whose function is still uncertain. The cause of Alzheimer's disease remains elusive; however, the discovery of mutations of APP close to or within the $A\beta$ domain (Goate et al. 1991; Naruse et al. 1991; Murrell et al. 1991; Hendricks et al. 1992; Mullan et al. 1992) indicates that the metabolism of $A\beta$ and APP is likely to be intimately involved with the pathophysiology of this predominantly sporadic disease.

Most cases of AD are sporadic, with the proportion of familial AD (FAD) cases being $\approx 5\%$. AD invariably occurs in Down's syndrome (DS), where pathological changes, accelerated by some 30 years, are associated with increased APP mRNA (Tanzi et al. 1987) and protein levels (Rumble et al. 1989). The increased production of soluble $A\beta$ from human neuroblastoma cells transfected APP constructs (Cai et al. 1993; Citron et al. 1992) possessing the "Swedish" mutation (lys670-met671 to asp-leu; Mullan et al. 1992) indicates that sustained increases in extracellular $A\beta$ concentrations may be sufficient to cause $A\beta$ to precipitate into insoluble deposits. From studies of the solubility of the synthetic peptide $A\beta_{1-40}$, it is known that this supposedly normal secretion product (Shoji et al. 1992; Seubert et al. 1992; Haass et al. 1992; Busciglio et al. 1993), which is found in CSF (Shoji et al. 1992; Seubert et al. 1992), should remain soluble at concentrations up to 1 mg/ml (Burdick et al. 1992). Although it is not known whether DS is also accompanied by an increase in $A\beta$, soluble $A\beta$ in cerebrospinal fluid (CSF) has been reported as not being increased in sporadic AD cases (Shoji et al. 1992), indicating that sustained elevation of the interstitial $A\beta$ concentration is unlikely to be the cause of $A\beta$ precipitation in the brain in sporadic cases, and that other pathogenetic mechanisms are likely to be involved in inducing amyloid formation.

The amyloid protein precursors constitute a complex family of membrane-bound and soluble glycoproteins that are derived by alternate splicing of a gene on chromosome 21 yielding more than 10 isoforms, some of which contain a Kunitz-type protease inhibitory insert (KPI-APP; reviewed in Bush et al. 1993a). The description of two other highly homologous genes coding for amyloid precursor-like protein 1 (APLP1; Wasco et al. 1992), which maps to human chromosome 19 (Wasco et al. 1993a), and amyloid precursor-like protein 2 (APLP2; Wasco et al. 1993b), indicate that APP, APLP1 and APLP2 are members of a homologous superfamily whose products all carry a significantly negative charge at neutral pH (pI's of 4.5, 5.5 and 4.5, respectively).

The function of the APP superfamily is unknown, but because all members of the superfamily share strong homology of major domains (cysteine-rich amino terminus, zinc binding site, negatively charged mid-region, span the lipid bilayer once, short intracytoplasmic carboxyl terminus), they are likely to be functionally related. APLP1 and APLP2 lack the $A\beta$ domain, and hence could not be amyloidogenic.

Zinc has recently been implicated in the function of the APP superfamily (Bush et al. 1993b). A novel zinc binding site has been described in the ectodomain of the protein within exon five, at the end of the cysteine-rich region. This

```
APLP2  183 SYGMLLPCGVDQFHGLEYVCCPQTKDY
APLP1  185 GSGMLLPCGSDRFRGVEYVCCPPPATP
APPL   152 TFAMLLPCGISVFSGVEFVCCPKHFKT
APP    167 DYGMLLPCGIDKFRGVEFVCCPLAEES
```

Fig. 1. Homology of the zinc binding region of APP. The amyloid precursor-like protein 2 (APLP2) sequence (Wasco et al. 1993b) is compared with the homologous regions of APLP1 (Wasco et al. 1992), drosophila APPL (Rosen et al. 1989), and APP (Kang et al. 1987). The amino terminus residue position (numbers), zinc binding domain (bold), a portion of the synthetic zinc binding peptide (underlined), and amino acid identity (boxes) are indicated

domain is found in all known members of the APP superfamily as well as in the drosophila homolog, APP-L (Fig. 1). The affinity constant for binding is 750 nM, and binding to this site promotes the affinity of APP for heparin with an effect that saturates at 75 μM. A separate report demonstrated that zinc promoted the inhibition of coagulation factor XIa activity by KPI-APP with an effect which also saturated at 75 μM (Komiyama et al. 1992).

Prominent amongst the proposed functions for APP are its possible roles in cell adhesiveness (Shivers et al. 1988) and neurite outgrowth (Milward et al. 1992). Indeed the observation that APP is most greatly enriched in platelets and brain tissue (Bush et al. 1990) suggests that APP participates in tissue remodelling. It is intriguing that zinc, too, is most highly concentrated in the body in these two tissues (Baker et al. 1978; Frederickson 1989). APP is highly concentrated in vesicles in both of these tissues (Bush et al. 1990; Cole et al. 1990; Smith et al. 1990; Van Nostrand et al. 1990; Schlossmacher et al. 1992; Schubert et al. 1991). Although the co-localization of APP with zinc in these vesicles has yet to be demonstrated, zinc is actively taken up (Wolf et al. 1984; Wensink et al. 1988) and stored in synaptic vesicles in nerve terminals throughout the telencephalon (Ibata and Otsuka 1969; Perez-Clausell and Danscher 1985; Friedman and Price 1984). Zinc storage in vesicles in tissues like pancreatic β-cells, salivary secretory cells and pituitary gland is thought to function by stabilizing intravesicular proteins and endocrine peptides such as NGF and insulin (Frederickson et al. 1987). The effect of extracellular zinc upon platelet function is to increase platelet adhesiveness and aggregation (Heyns et al. 1985). The effect of zinc upon APP in increasing its affinity for heparin is reminiscent of this general effect. It will be interesting to determine whether extracellular zinc concentrations can modulate neurite outgrowth and neuronal or glial adhesiveness by modifying the affinity of APP or APLP for extracellular matrix elements. Because extracellular brain zinc levels may modulate the function of APP, an understanding of the homeostatic mechanisms governing the physiology of zinc could yield insights relevant to the pathophysiology of AD.

The Neurophysiology of Zinc Homeostasis

The regulation of brain zinc compartmentalization and transport is governed by very strict homeostatic mechanisms. Although zinc is essential for brain development and function, the mechanisms underlying brain zinc nutriture and metabolism are poorly understood. Zinc stores are so preserved in the brain that zinc malnutrition can be life-threatening without significantly depleting intracellular cerebral zinc reserves (Kasarkis 1984; O'Neal et al. 1970; Wallwork et al. 1983). However, the neuropsychological consequences of clinical zinc deficiency are well-documented and include impaired mentation and memory functions (Halas et al. 1983). The mechanisms that underlie the preservation of brain zinc in the event of clinically apparent deficiency are unclear. There is a pool of zinc interacting with the environment of the central nervous system which is responsive to nutritional events. This pool may be the only central nervous system compartment available for rapid exchange of zinc with plasma (Pullen et al. 1991). The uptake of zinc into the brain is accomplished by an unidentified active transport mechanism. Plasma zinc, which is mainly bound to albumin, does not easily transfer into the central nervous system, and most transfer is not passive (Pullen et al. 1991). The maximal accumulation of zinc into rat brain was shown to be only 0.5% of an intraperitoneal does and then subjected to a protracted intracerebral biological half-life in contrast to peripheral tissues (Kasarkis 1984). The blood-brain barrier and the choroid plexus appear to possess stringent means of protecting the brain from the passive zinc transfer which would be driven by the large gradient generated by the relative concentrations of zinc in plasma (20 μM; Davies et al. 1968) to CSF (0.15 μM; Frederickson 1989).

Zinc deficiency is associated with a significant elevation in brain copper levels (Wallwork et al. 1983), which could be an alternate explanation for the neuropsychological deficits seen in clinical zinc deficiency. The mechanism underlying the antagonistic homeostatic relationship between brain zinc and copper levels is not understood. Abnormal cerebral copper metabolism is associated with two major brain neurodegenerative disorders, Wilson's disease and Menkes' kinky hair disease, although the biochemical mechanism underlying the neurogeneration in these disorders is not known.

Curiously, zinc is neurotoxic in cell cultures in concentrations as low as 75 μM (Duncan et al. 1992), and higher concentrations may be irreversibly toxic during exposures as brief as 15 minutes (Choi et al. 1988). AMPA receptor activation potentiates zinc-induced neurotoxicity in neuronal cell cultures following even briefer (five-minute) exposure (Weiss et al. 1993). Assaf and Chung (1984) estimated that the peak extracellular concentration of zinc in the hippocampus rises to 300 μM during neurotransmission. Even higher concentrations might be expected at the synaptic cleft. Choi and coworkers proposed that this trans-synaptic movement of zinc may have a normal signalling function and may be involved in long-term potentiation (Weiss et al. 1989). However, because zinc can be rapidly neurotoxic at such high concentrations, active transport is likely to occur to remove the zinc from the interstitial space and to maintain homeostasis. The basis of this predicted homeostatic mechanism is still to be elucidated.

Zinc and Copper Homeostasis in Alzheimer's Disease

AD and DS are associated with abnormalities of zinc and copper metabolism. Changes reported in AD include decreased temporal lobe zinc levels (Wenstrup et al. 1990), elevated (80%) cerebrospinal fluid levels (Hershey et al. 1983), increased hepatic zinc with reduced zinc bound to metallothionein (Lui et al. 1990), a Zn^{2+}-modulated abnormality of APP in AD plasma (Bush et al. 1992), and decreased levels of astrocytic growth-inhibitory factor, a metallothionein-like protein which chelates zinc (Uchida et al. 1991). Clinical zinc deficiency is a common, pervasive yet cryptogenic phenomenon in DS (Franceschi et al. 1988), where it manifests as immune dysfunction (Bjorksten et al. 1980) and growth delay (Napolitano et al. 1990), and is associated with elevations of erythrocyte copper and superoxide dismutase activity (Mallet et al. 1979). Zinc has also been implicated in the pathogenesis of Guamanian amyotrophic lateral sclerosis/Parkinson's dementia complex, a disease also characterized by neurofibrillary tangles, where it has been demonstrated that flour made from cycads in the traditional Guamanian manner may introduce a dietary zinc dose which is 100-fold the recommended daily allowance (Duncan et al. 1992).

Serum and plasma levels of copper and zinc have been studied in several reports comparing Alzheimer's disease to control populations (Hicks et al. 1987). There appears to be no consensus on the nature of any differences, but estimations of blood zinc would be confounded by many variables which would make zinc levels inconsistent. Plasma zinc levels rise post-prandially (Pohit et al. 1981), and absorption is affected by the presence of various dietary elements such as proteins, fibre and sugars (Sandström et al. 1980), and is also subject to diurnal variation (McMaster et al. 1992). Hence, studies which do not control for such factors would be subject to greater variances.

No consistent trend has yet emerged in reports of abnormalities, if any, in copper levels or metabolism in AD or DS.

The hippocampus is the region of the brain which both contains the highest zinc concentrations (Frederickson et al. 1983) and is most severely and consistently affected by the pathological lesions of AD (Price et al. 1991). One of the prominent neurochemical deficits in AD is cholinergic deafferentation of the hippocampus. This has been shown experimentally also to raise the concentration of zinc in the region (Stewart et al. 1984).

```
- - +  -  -    +      --    +
DAEFRHDSGYEVHHQKLVFFAEDVGSNKGAIIGLMVGGVV
```

Fig. 2. Structure of Aβ. The amino acid sequence of $A\beta_{1-40}$ is shown. Charged residues are indicated. The obligatory zinc binding region (residues 6–28) is boxed. Histidine residues, implicated in zinc binding, are in bold

Zinc and Copper Bind to Aβ

Because of the associations between zinc, AD and APP, we studied the binding of Zn^{2+} to Aβ. The possibility of Aβ binding zinc is supported by the presence of three closely situated histidine residues and a cluster of negatively charged residues on the molecule (Fig. 2). The pI of the peptide is 5.5, indicating that, like all members of the APP superfamily, it is negatively charged at physiological pH.

Using $^{65}Zn^{2+}$ to probe immobilized peptide in a dot-blot system, Aβ was shown to manifest saturable and highly specific binding to zinc. Two classes of binding were evident, a high affinity ($K_D = 107$ nM) and a low affinity ($K_D = 5.2$ μM) binding association (Bush et al., in press). Using peptide mapping, the domain within the protein which is obligatory for zinc binding was shown to be a contiguous region within the frame of residues 6–28, requiring the α-secretase site at Lys16 (Esch et al. 1990; Sisodia et al. 1990) to be intact. Zinc binding was found to deteriorate with lower pH, indicating the involvement of histidine residues in the binding.

The binding of zinc at concentrations as low as 0.4 μM to Aβ induced a decrease in peptide solubility and an increase in Aβ adsorption to negatively charged surfaces. On size exclusion chromatography, Aβ was noted to migrate in monomeric, dimeric and polymeric (> 8 mer) forms. Copper prevented the adsorption of Aβ to negatively charged surfaces, and exclusively and specifically stabilized Aβ dimer formation in solution, reversing the effect of zinc. Other metal salts were unable to rescue Aβ at all, although some salts had partial effects on peptide precipitation. This behaviour indicted that Aβ may have a binding site for copper as well as zinc.

To confirm zinc and copper binding to Aβ, ^{125}I iodinated Aβ binding to zinc- and copper-charged chelating-Sepharose was studied. Whereas ^{125}I-Aβ was unable to bind to heparin-Sepharose or Q-Sepharose, significant binding of the labelled peptide to zinc- and copper-chelating-Sepharose was observed (Fig. 3). This chromatographic technique may now be exploited to purify Aβ from biological fluids.

Discussion

These findings demonstrate that APP possesses two novel zinc binding domains, one in the cysteine-rich ectodomain which modulates heparin affinity,

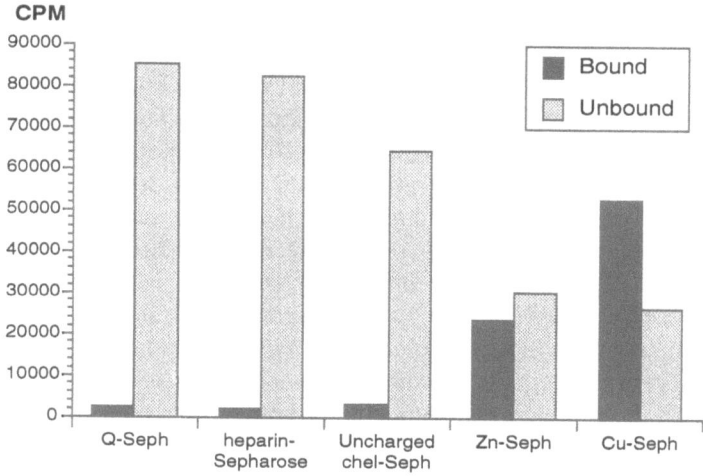

Fig. 3. Binding of ^{125}I-Aβ to chelating-Sepharose, Q-Sepharose and heparin-Sepharose. ^{125}I-Aβ (100 000 CPM, 1 nM) was adjusted to 1M NaCl, 50 mM Tris-HCl, pH 7.4 and loaded onto Pharmacia chelating-Sepharose (250 μl). The column was washed with equilibration buffer (3.25 ml) and then eluted with 50 mM EDTA. Alternatively, ^{125}I-Aβ (100 000 CPM, 1 nM) was adjusted to 150 mM NaCl, 50 mM Tris-HCl, pH 7.4 and loaded onto Pharmacia Q-Sepharose (250 μl) or heparin-Sepharose (in the presence of 0.1% BSA). The column was washed with equilibration buffer (3.25 ml) and then eluted with 2M NaCl. The bound and unbound counts were assayed as indicated. ^{125}I-Aβ bound only to copper- or zinc-charged chelating-Sepharose. The total recovery (bound plus unbound) from the zinc-chelating-Sepharose was reduced compared to uncharged chelating-Sepharose or copper-chelating-Sepharose, possibly due to zinc-induced precipitation of ^{125}I-Aβ on the column

and one within the Aβ domain itself. Both zinc binding motifs are novel in that they are not homologous to any known zinc binding domains on other proteins, although both sites contain residues that are favoured for zinc binding (cysteine and histidine). Nevertheless, both domains manifest strong and specific interaction with zinc. Although it is easy to imagine how extracellular zinc may play a role in the physiology of APP function by modifying its adhesiveness to extracellular matrix elements, the possible functions for Aβ are only beginning to be explored. Only recently has Aβ been demonstrated to be a soluble secretion product found in extracellular fluids (Shoji et al. 1992; Seubert et al. 1992; Haass et al. 1992; Busciglio et al. 1993). What roles zinc or copper may play in its normal physiology remain to be elucidated. Interestingly, a recent report stated that Aβ promotes neurite outgrowth by complexing with laminin and fibronectin in the extracellular matrix (Koo et al. 1993). Hence, both APP and Aβ appear to interact with the extracellular matrix to modulate cell adhesion. The possibility that zinc and copper are local environmental cofactors modulating this interaction merits investigation.

Our findings also indicate that polymerization and precipitation of secreted soluble forms of Aβ may be modulated by local concentrations of copper and zinc in the brain. Two forms of familial Aβ amyloidosis are caused by mutations of the APP gene within the zinc binding region of Aβ (Hendricks et al. 1992; Levy et al. 1990). It will be important in future studies to assess the zinc and copper binding properties of Aβ peptides containing these mutations.

Aβ accumulates most consistently in the hippocampus, where extreme fluctuations of zinc concentrations occur (0.15 to 300 μM; Frederickson 1989). Based on our findings, copper may function in such areas to stabilize Aβ as a soluble dimer in the presence of high zinc concentrations, e.g., during synaptic transmission (Assaf and Chung 1984; Howell et al. 1984; Xie and Smart 1991). Our results further indicate that abnormally high zinc or low copper concentrations could decrease the solubility of Aβ as well as favour high-order polymerization of the peptide. Zinc-induced precipitation of Aβ in the neuropil may, in turn, invoke a glial inflammatory response, free radical attack and oxidative cross-linking to ultimately form amyloid.

Aβ chelates zinc with such high affinity that reports that its introduction into neuronal cultures causes neurotoxicity (Yankner et al. 1990; Koh et al. 1990) might be explained by a disturbance of zinc homeostasis. Finally, the association of zinc with Aβ is intriguing in light of recent reports that APP functions as a metalloproteinase inhibitor (Miyazaki et al. 1993), and that zinc binds to APP, modulating heparin affinity (Bush et al. 1993). These observations indicate that both the function and processing of APP and Aβ may be modulated by zinc and copper levels in the local environment.

Acknowledgements. This work was supported by funds from the NIH, the American Health Assistance Foundation, a Harkness Fellowship, Commonwealth Fund of New York (AIB), and a French Foundation Fellowship (RET).

References

Assaf SY, Chung S-H (1984) Release of endogenous Zn^{2+} from brain tissue during activity. Nature 308:734–736

Baker RJ, McNeil JJ, Lander H (1978) Platelet metal levels in normal subjects determined by atomic absorption spectrophotometry. Thrombos Haemostas 39:360–365

Bjorksten B, Back O, Gustavson KH, Hallmans G, Hagglof B, Tarnvik A (1980) Zinc and immune function in Down's syndrome. Acta Paediatr Scand 69:183–187

Burdick D, Soreghan B, Kwon M, Kosmoski J, Knauer M, Henschen A, Yates J, Cotman C, Glabe C (1992) Assembly and aggregation properties of synthetic Alzheimer's A4/β amyloid peptide analogs. J Biol Chem 267:546–554

Busciglio J, Gabuzda DH, Matsudaira P, Yankner BA (1993) Generation of β-amyloid in the secretory pathway in neuronal and nonneuronal cells. Proc Natl Acad Sci USA 90:2092–2096

Bush AI, Martins RN, Rumble B, Moir R, Fuller S, Milward E, Currie J, Ames D, Weidemann A, Fischer P, Multhaup G, Beyreuther K, Masters CL (1990) The amyloid precursor protein of Alzheimer's disease is released by human platelets. J Biol Chem 265:15977–15983

Bush AI, Whyte S, Thomas LD, Williamson TG, Van Tiggelen CJ, Currie J, Small DH, Moir RD, Li Q-X, Rumble B, Mönning U, Beyreuther K, Masters CL (1992) An abnormality of plasma amyloid protein precursor in Alzheimer's disease. Ann Neurol 32:57–65

Bush AI, Beyreuther K, Masters CL (1993a) βA4 amyloid protein and its precursor in Alzheimer's disease. Pharmacol Ther 56:97–117

Bush AI, Multhaup G, Moir RD, Williamson TG, Small DH, Rumble B, Pollwein P, Beyreuther K, Masters CL (1993b) A novel zinc(II) binding site modulates the function of the βA4 amyloid protein precursor of Alzheimer's disease. J Biol Chem 268:16109–16112

Bush AI, Pettingell WH, Paradis MD, Tanzi RE (1994) Modulation of Aβ adhesiveness and secretase site cleavage by zinc. J Biol Chem, in press

Cai X-D, Golde TE, Younkin SG (1993) Release of excess amyloid β protein from a mutant amyloid β protein precursor. Science 259:514–516

Choi DW, Yokoyama M, Koh J (1988) Zinc neurotoxicity in cortical cell culture. Neuroscience 24:67–79

Citron M, Oltersdorf T, Haass C, McConlogue L, Hung AY, Seubert P, Vigo-Pelfrey C, Lieberburg I, Selkoe DJ (1992) Mutation of the β-amyloid precursor protein in familial Alzheimer's disease increases β-protein production. Nature 360:672–674

Cole GM, Galasko D, Shapiro IP, Saitoh T (1990) Stimulated platelets release amyloid β-protein precursor. Biochem Biophys Res Commun 170:288–295

Davies IJT, Musa M, Dormandy TL (1968) Measurements of plasma zinc. J Clin Pathol 21:359–365

Duncan MW, Marini AM, Watters R, Kopin IJ, Markey SP (1992) Zinc, a neurotoxin to cultured neurons, contaminates cycad flour prepared by traditional Guamanian methods. J Neurosci 12:1523–1537

Napolitano G, Palka G, Grimaldi S, Giuliani C, Laglia G, Calabrese G, Satta MA, Neri G, Monaco F (1990) Growth delay in Down syndrome and zinc sulphate supplementation. Am J Med Genet 7:63–65

Esch FS, Keim PS, Beattie EC, Blacher RW, Culwell AR, Oltersdorf T, McClure D, Ward PJ (1990) Cleavage of amyloid β peptide during constitutive processing of its precursor. Science 248:1122–1124.

Franceschi C, Chiricolo M, Licastro F, Zannotti M, Masi M, Mocchegiani E, Fabris N (1988) Oral zinc supplementation in Down's syndrome: restoration of thymic endocrine activity and of some immune defects. J Ment Defic Res 32:169–181

Frederickson CJ, Klitenick MA, Manton WI, Kirkpatrick JB (1983) Cytoarchitectonic distribution of zinc in the hippocampus of man and the rat. Brain Res 273:335–339

Frederickson CJ, Perez-Clausell J, Danscher G (1987) Zinc-containing 7S-NGF complex. Evidence from zinc histochemistry for localization in salivary secretory granules. J Histochem Cytochem 35:579–583

Frederickson CJ (1989) Neurobiology of zinc and zinc-containing neurons. Int Rev Neurobiol 31:145–328

Friedman B, Price JL (1984) Fiber systems in the olfactory bulb and cortex: a study in adult and developing rats, using the Timm method with the light and electron microscope. J Comp Neurol 223:88–109

Glenner GG, Wong CW (1984) Alzheimer's disease: initial report of the purification and characterization of a novel cerebrovascular amyloid protein. Biochem Biophys Res Commun 120:885–890

Goate A, Chartier-Harlin M, Mullan M, Brown J, Crawford F, Fidani L, Giuffra L, Haynes A, Irving N, James L, Mant R, Newton P, Rooke K, Roques P, Talbot C, Pericak-Vance M, Roses A, Williamson R, Rossor M, Owen M, Hardy J (1991) Segregation of a missense mutation in the amyloid precursor protein gene with familial Alzheimer's disease. Nature 349:704–706

Haass C, Schlossmacher MG, Hung AY, Vigo-Pelfrey C, Mellon A, Ostaszewski BL, Lieberburg I, Koo EH, Schenk D, Teplow DB, Selkoe DS (1992) Amyloid β-peptide is produced by cultured cells during normal metabolism. Nature 359:322–325

Halas ES, Eberhardt MJ, Diers MA, Sandstead HH (1983) Learning and memory impairment in adult rats due to severe zinc deficiency during lactation. Physiol Behav 30:371–381

Hendricks L, van Duijn CM, Cras P, Cruts M, van Hul W, van Harskamp F, Warren A, McInnis MG, Antonarakis SE, Martin J-J, Hofman A, van Broeckhoven C (1992). Presenile dementia and cerebral haemorrhage linked to a mutation at codon 692 of the β-amyloid precursor protein gene. Nature Genet 1:218–221

Hershey CO, Hershey LA, Varnes A, Vibhakar SD, Lavin P, Strain WH (1983) Cerebrospinal fluid trace element content in dementia: Clinical, radiologic, and pathologic correlations. Neurology 33:1350–1353

Heyns AduP, Eldor A, Yarom R, Marx G (1985) Zinc-induced platelet aggregation is mediated by the fibrinogen receptor and is not accompanied by release or by thromboxane synthesis. Blood 66:213–219

Hicks N, Brammer MJ, Hymas N, Levy R (1987) Platelet membrane properties in Alzheimer and multi-infarct dementias. Alzheimer Dis Assoc Disord 1:90–97

Howell GA, Welch MG, Frederickson CJ (1984) Stimulation-induced uptake and release of zinc in hippocampal slices. Nature 308:736–738

Ibata Y, Otsuka N (1969) Electron microscope demonstration of zinc in the hippocampal formation using Timm's sulfide-silver technique. J Histochem Cytochem 17:171–175

Kang J, Lemaire H, Unterbeck A, Salbaum JM, Masters CL, Grzeschik K, Multhaup G, Beyreuther K, Müller-Hill B (1987) The precursor of Alzheimer's disease amyloid A4 protein resembles a cell-surface receptor. Nature 325:733–736

Kasarkis EJ (1984) Zinc metabolism in normal and zinc-deficient rat brain. Exp Neurol 85:114–127

Koh J, Yang LL, Cotman CW (1990) β-amyloid protein increases the vulnerability of cultured cortical neurons to excitotoxic damage. Brain Res 533:315–320

Komiyama Y, Murakami T, Egawa H, Okubo S, Yasunaga K, Murata K (1992) Purification of factor XIa inhibitor from human platelets. Thromb Res 66:397–408

Koo EH, Park L, Selkoe DJ (1993) Amyloid β-protein as a substrate interacts with extracellular matrix to promote neurite outgrowth. Proc Natl Acad Sci USA 90:4748–4752

Levy E, Carman MD, Fernandez-Madrid IJ, Power MD, Lieberburg I, Van Duinen SG, Bots GTAM, Luyendijk W, Frangione B (1990) Mutation of the Alzheimer's disease amyloid gene in hereditary cerebral hemorrhage, Dutch type. Science 248:1124–1126

Lui E, Fisman M, Wong C, Diaz F (1990) Metals and the liver in Alzheimer's disease: an investigation of hepatic zinc, copper, cadmium, and metallothionein. J Am Geriatr Soc 38:633–639

Mallet B, Poulet P, Ayme S, Mattei MG, Mattei JF, Rebuffel P (1979) Erythrocyte copper levels in children with trisomy 21. J Ment Defic Res 23:219–225

Masters CL, Simms G, Weinman NA, Multhaup G, McDonald BL, Beyreuther K (1985) Amyloid plaque core protein in Alzheimer disease and Down syndrome. Proc Natl Acad Sci USA 82:4245–4249

McMaster D, McCrum E, Patterson CC, Kerr MMcF, O'Reilly D, Evans AE, Love AHG (1992) Serum copper and zinc in randon samples of the population of Northern Ireland. Am J Clin Nutr 56:440–446

Milward EA, Papadopoulos R, Fuller SJ, Moir RD, Small D, Beyreuther K, Masters CL (1992) The amyloid protein precursor of Alzheimer's disease is a mediator of the effects of nerve growth factor on neurite outgrowth. Neuron 9:129–137

Miyazaki K, Hasegawa M, Funahashi K, Umeda M (1993) A metalloproteinase inhibitor domain in Alzheimer amyloid protein precursor. Nature 362:839–841

Mullan M, Crawford F, Axelman K, Houlden H, Lilius L, Winblad W, Lannfelt L (1992) A pathogenic mutation for probable Alzheimer's disease in the N-terminus of β-amyloid. Nature Genet 1:345–347

Murrell J, Farlow M, Ghetti B, Benson MD (1991) A mutation in the amyloid precursor protein associated with hereditary Alzheimer disease. Science 254:97–99

Napolitano G, Palka G, Grimaldi S, Giuliani C, Laglia G, Calabrese G, Satta MA, Neri G, Monaco F (1990) Growth delay in Down syndrome and zinc sulphate supplementation. Am J Med Genet 7:63–65

Naruse S, Igarashi S, Kobayashi J, Aoki K, Kaneko K, Inuzuka T, Shimizu T, Iihara K, Kojima T, Miyatake T, Tsuji S (1991) Mis-sense mutation Val-Ile in exon 17 of amyloid precursor protein gene in Japanese familial Alzheimer's disease. Lancet 337:978–979

O'Neal RM, Pla GW, Fox MRS, Gibson FS, Fry BE (1970) Effect of zinc deficiency and restricted feeding on protein and ribonucleic acid metabolism of rat brain. J Nutr 100:491–497

Perez-Clausell J, Danscher G (1985) Intravesicular localization of zinc in rat telencephalic boutons. A histochemical study. Brain Res 337:91–98

Pohit J, Saha KC, Pal B (1981) A zinc tolerance test. Clinica Chimica Acta 114:279–281

Price JL, Davis PB, Morris JC, White DL (1991) The distribution of tangles, plaques and related immunohistochemical markers in healthy aging and Alzheimer's disease. Neurobiol Aging 12:295–312

Pullen RGL, Franklin PA, Hall GH (1991) ^{65}Zn Uptake from blood into brain in the rat. J Neurochem 56:485–489

Rosen DR, Martin-Morris L, Luo L, White K (1989) A drosophila gene encoding a protein resembling the human β-amyloid protein precursor. Proc Acad Sci USA 86:2478–2482

Rumble B, Retallack R, Hilbich C, Simms G, Multhaup G, Martins R, Hockey A, Montgomery P, Beyreuther K, Masters CL (1989) Amyloid A4 protein and its precursor in Down's syndrome and Alzheimer's disease. New Engl J Med 320:1446–1452

Sandström B, Arvidsson B, Cederblad A, Björn-Rasmussen E (1980) Zinc absorption from composite meals. 1. The significance of wheat extraction rate, zinc, calcium, and protein content in meals based on bread. Am J Clin Nutr 33:739–745

Schlossmacher MG, Ostaszewski BL, Hecker LI, Celi A, Haass C, Chin D, Lieberburg I, Furie BC, Furie B, Selkoe DJ (1992) Detection of distinct isoform patterns of the β-amyloid precursor protein in human platelets and lymphocytes. Neurobiol Aging 13:421–434

Schubert W, Prior R, Weidemann A, Dircksen H, Multhaup G, Masters CL, Beyreuther K (1991) Localization of βA4 precursor protein at central and peripheral synaptic sites. Brain Res 563:184–194

Seubert P, Vigo-Pelfrey C, Esch F, Lee M, Dovey H, Davis D, Sinha S, Schlossmacher M, Whaley J, Swindlehurst C, McCormack R, Wolfert R, Selkoe D, Lieberberg I, Schenk D (1992) Isolation and quantification of soluble Alzheimer's β-peptide from biological fluids. Nature 359:325–327

Shivers BD, Hilbich C, Multhaup G, Salbaum M, Beyreuther K, Seeburg PH (1988) Alzheimer's disease amyloidogenic glycoprotein: expression pattern in rat brain suggests role in cell contact. EMBO J 7:1365–1370

Shoji M, Golde TE, Ghiso J, Cheung TT, Estus S, Shaffer LM, Cai X-D, McKay DM, Tintner R, Frangione B, Younkin SG (1992) Production of the Alzheimer amyloid β protein by normal proteolytic processing. Science 258:126–129

Sisodia SS, Koo EH, Beyreuther K, Unterbeck A, Price DL (1990) Evidence that β-amyloid protein in Alzheimer's disease is not derived by normal processing. Science 248:492–495

Smith RP, Higuchi DA, Broze GJ Jr (1990) Platelet coagulation factor XIa-inhibitor, a form of Alzheimer amyloid precursor protein. Science 248:1126–1128

Stewart GR, Frederickson CJ, Howell GA, Gage FH (1984) Cholinergic denervation-induced increase of chelatable zinc in mossy-fiber region of the hippocampal formation. Brain Res 290:43–51

Tanzi RE, Gusella JF, Watkins PC, Bruns GAP, St George-Hyslop P, van Keuren ML, Patterson D, Pagan S, Kurnit DM, Neve RL (1987) Amyloid β protein gene: cDNA, mRNA distribution and genetic linkage near the Alzheimer locus. Science 235:880–884

Uchida Y, Takio K, Titani K, Ihara Y, Tomonaga M (1991) The growth-inhibitory factor that is deficient in the Alzheimer's disease brain is a 68-amino acid metallothionein-like protein. Neuron 7:337–347

Van Nostrand WE, Schmaier AH, Farrow JS, Cunningham DD (1990) Protease nexin-II (amyloid β-protein precursor): a platelet α-granule protein. Science 248:745–748

Wallwork JC, Milne DB, Sims RL, Sandstead HH (1983) Severe zinc deficiency: effects on the distribution of nine elements (potassium, phosphorus, sodium, magnesium, calcium, iron, zinc, copper, and manganese) in regions of the rat brain. J Nutr 113:1895–1905

Wasco W, Bupp K, Magendantz M, Gusella JF, Tanzi RE, Solomon F (1992) Identification of a mouse brain cDNA that encodes a protein related to the Alzheimer disease-associated β precursor protein. Proc Natl Acad Sci USA 89:10758–10762

Wasco W, Brook JD, Tanzi RE (1993a) The amyloid precursor-like protein (APLP) gene maps to the long arm of human chromosome 19. Genomics 15:238–239

Wasco W, Gurubhagavatula S, Paradis Md, Romano D, Sisodia SS, Hyman BT, Neve RL, Tanzi RE (1993b) Isolation and characterization of the human APLP2 gene encoding a homologue of the Alzheimer's associated amyloid β protein precursor. Nature Genet 5:95–100

Weiss JH, Koh J, Christine CW, Choi DW (1989) Zinc and LTP. Nature 338:212

Weiss JH, Hartley DM, Koh J, Choi DW (1993) AMPA receptor activation potentiates zinc neurotoxicity. Neuron 10:43–49

Wensink J, Molenaar AJ, Woroniecka UD, Van Den Hamer CJ (1988) Zinc uptake into synaptosomes. J Neurochem 50:783–789

Wenstrup D, Ehmann WD, Markesbery WR (1990) Trace element imbalances in isolated subcellular fractions of Alzheimer's disease brains. Brain Res 533:125–131

Wolf G, Scutte M, Römhild W (1984) Uptake and subcellular distribution of ^{65}zinc in brain structures during the postnatal development of the rat. Neurosci Lett 51:277–280

Xie X, Smart TG (1991) A physiological role for endogenous zinc in rat hippocampal synaptic neurotransmission. Nature 349:521–524

Yankner BA, Duffy LK, Kirschner DA (1990) Neurotrophic and neurotoxic effects of amyloid β protein: reversal by tachykinin neuropeptides. Science 250:279–282

The Diverse Molecular Nature of Inherited Alzheimer's Disease

R. E. Tanzi*, D. Romano, S. Gaston, A. Crowley, A. I. Bush, J. Peppercorn, M. Paradis, W. Pettingell, S. Gurubhagavatula, D. Kovacs, J. Haines, P. St George-Hyslop, and *W. Wasco*

Summary

Alzheimer's diseases (AD) is a major health problem which will continue to intensify in magnitude as the elderly in the population continue to increase in number. The age at which AD strikes is variable, ranging from the fourth to tenth decades, with the greatest proportion of cases occurring in the seventh and eighth decades. A genetic component of this disorder has been strongly indicated by family and survey studies, as well as life table analyses (reviewed in St George-Hyslop et al. 1989). Genetic linkage and association studies of kindreds displaying evidence for familial AD (FAD) have led to the localization of gene defects responsible for this genetically heterogeneous disorder on chromosomes 14, 19 and 21. In a small set of FAD kindreds, mutations have been found in the amyloid beta protein precursor (APP) gene. Yet, the available data indicate that the identity of the genes responsible for the majority of late-onset (> 65 years) as well as early-onset inherited AD remain unknown. Powerful and novel advances in the methodology available for performing genetic linkage analyses on genetically complex disorders have made it feasible to scan the entire human genome in a relatively fast and easy manner for the purpose of localizing the genes responsible for, or predisposing to, inherited AD. Here we describe progress on attempts to further localize and identify various FAD gene defects throughout the genome, with special emphasis on the major early-onset gene defect residing on the long arm of chromosome 14.

Genetic Heterogeneity of Familial Alzheimer Disease

FAD has been shown by epidemiology studies to be inherited in an autosomal dominant fashion with age-dependent penetrance (Breitner et al. 1988; Mohs et al. 1987). Farrer et al. (1991) demonstrated strong evidence for the segregation of at least one major FAD gene based on the study of segregation of the disorder in

---

* Laboratory of Genetics and Aging, Neuroscience Center, Department of Neurology, Harvard Medical School, Massachusetts General Hospital East, Building 149, 13th Street, Charlestown, MA 02129, USA

C.L. Masters et al. (Eds.)
Amyloid Protein Precursor in Development,
Aging and Alzheimer's Disease
© Springer-Verlag Berlin Heidelberg 1994

over 230 families specifically ascertained according to strict diagnostic criteria. In that study, heterozygote transmission of the "major gene" was found to be greater than 50%, suggesting that there are at least two more genes responsible for FAD. In a small proportion of families with early-onset, FAD, the gene defect has been linked to chromosome 21 (St George-Hyslop et al. 1987). While these findings were later confirmed by Goate et al. (1989), others obtained negative results with chromosome 21 using specific sets of FAD pedigrees (Schellenberg et al. 1988; Pericak-Vance et al. 1991a) one of these groups obtained evidence for linkage of late-onset FAD to markers on chromosome 19 (Pericak-Vance et al. 1991a); however, many other early- and late-onset FAD kindreds still remained unlinked to either chromosome 21 or 19 (Pericak-Vance et al. 1991). These findings suggesting the existence of genetic heterogeneity in FAD were later confirmed in a large, international, collaborative study of 48 early- and late-onset FAD kindreds (St George-Hyslop et al. 1990).

In a recent set of reports, it has become clear that a major gene defect for early-onset FAD resides on chromosome 14 (Schellenberg et al. 1992a; St George-Hyslop et al. 1992; Van Broeckhoven et al. 1992; Mullan et al. 1992b). While the gene defect in 70–90% of early-onset FAD kindreds may turn out to be linked to the chromosome 14 locus, no late-onset FAD pedigrees tested to date have provided evidence for linkage (Schellenberg et al. 1992a; St George-Hyslop et al. 1992; Van Broeckhoven et al. 1992; Mullan et al. 1992b). Additionally, no late-onset FAD families have been shown to contain APP mutations.

The location of a gene involved with late-onset FAD has been established on chromosome 19 (Pericak-Vance et al. 1991a,b). More recently, in support of the existence of an FAD locus on chromosome 19, significant allelic association of late-onset FAD and some sporadic AD cases with the ApoE4 allele of the gene encoding apoliploprotein E has been reported (Strittmatter et al. 1993). This finding serves to confirm previous reports of allelic association of late onset FAD with the apoliploprotein C gene which resides in close proximity to the ApoE gene (Schellenberg et al. 1987, 1992b). Meanwhile, linkage studies employing the Affected Pedigrees Member (APM; Weeks and Lange 1988) method indicate that a proportion of FAD late-onset pedigrees demonstrate linkage with chromosome 19 markers in the vicinity of ApoE. This finding raises the possibility that the linkage observed with chromosome 19 is actually a reflection of allelic association with the ApoE/ApoCII cluster, since the APM method does not distinguish between linkage and association. It is presently difficult to determine the precise percentage of late-onset FAD associated with chromosome 19 locus. The allele frequency of the APOE-4 allele is only about 16% in an age-matched set of controls, but approximately 50% in late-onset FAD cases. Since the APOE4 allele appears in normal aged individuals, it probably does not represent the sole, causative gene defect. Its effect could result from a biological susceptibility analogous to that of the HLA loci in diabetes, or could result from being in linkage disequilibrium with an as-of-yet unidentified gene defect either elsewhere in the APOE gene or in a nearby gene.

It is important to note that an allelic association is indicative of linkage disequilibrium between the gene or marker tested and the locus of interest. Linkage disequilibrium data primarily lend information as to *where* the gene defect resides as opposed to *what* the gene actually is. The strong allelic association reported for APOE4 and a large subset of late-onset FAD suggest three distinct possibilities with regard to the identity of the gene defect on chromosome 19. Essentially, the late onset FAD gene defect on chromosome 19 is either 1) APOE4 itself, 2) a gene defect in APOE other than the APOE4 variant, or 3) a defect in a gene other than APOE, but which resides physically quite close (e.g., within one megabase) to APOE.

Recently, a protein whose predicted 653 amino acid sequence is 42% identical and 64% similar to APP has been isolated. This amyloid precursor-like protein (APLP) contains many domains similar to those in APP and resembles APP in overall structure (Wasco et al. 1992). The gene encoding APLP has been mapped to the proximal long arm of chromosome 19 in the same general vicinity as the putative late onset FAD gene defect (Wasco et al. 1993a). Given the significant homology of this gene to APP, we are actively exploring the possibility that APLP may represent a gene defect responsible for a late-onset form of FAD on chromosome 19. We have also isolated and mapped a second APLP, APLP2, to chromosome 11 (Wasco et al. 1993b). Genetic linkage, single-stranded conformational polymorphism (SSCP) and sequence analysis are currently underway for both the APLP and APLP2 genes.

APP Gene Mutations in FAD

The neuropathological lesions associated with AD, especially the senile plaques (SP), have provided critical clues toward delineating the genetic etiology of this disorder. The amyloid cores of SP are made primarily of Aβ, a 39–43 amino acid peptide (Glenner and Wong 1984) derived from a much larger precursor protein (APP; Goldgaber et al. 1987; Kang et al. 1987; Robakis et al. 1987; Tanzi et al. 1987a). The APP gene is localized on chromosome 21 in the same vicinity as a locus for FAD (Tanzi et al. 1987a). In 1987, when APP was directly tested for linkage to FAD in the same four pedigrees that were used to show linkage of FAD to DNA markers on chromosome 21, at least one obligate crossover event was detected in each pedigree, suggesting that APP was not tightly linked FAD in these as well as other families (Tanzi et al. 1987b; Van Broeckhoven et al. 1987).

Further genetic based-studies of the APP gene in FAD were later prompted by the findings that FAD is a genetically heterogeneous disorder (thus, the APP gene could still represent the gene defect in some pedigrees; Tanzi et al. 1991; Tanzi 1991) and that a mutation near the βA4 region of APP (exon 17) is responsible for hereditary cerebral hemorrhage with amyloidosis-Dutch type (Levy et al. 1990). In 1991, Hardy and colleagues sequenced exon 17 of APP in patients from a chromosome 21-linked FAD pedigree that exhibited no crossovers with APP, and a missense mutation causing an amino acid substitution Val → Ile at codon APP717 was found in affected individuals in two separate pedigrees (Goate et al. 1991). Meanwhile, the mutation was absent in hundreds of healthy control individuals (Goate et al. 1991; our unpublished findings), implying that this change is not simply a rare polymorphism in APP but could actually represent an etiologic gene defect.

Recently, several other FAD-associated mutations in APP have also been found, including two additional changes in codon 717 (Val → Phe, Murrell et al. 1991; and Val → Gly, Chartier-Harlin et al. 1991), one at codon 692 (Ala → Gly, Hendriks et al. 1992), and a double mutant at the N-terminus of Aβ (Mullan et al. 1992a). As a result of these findings it has become extremely important to assess the extent to which APP mutations are associated with FAD. It has been reported that approximately 3% of FAD pedigrees assessed harbor the known APP717 mutations (Tanzi et al. 1992). In this same study, a large set of pedigrees was also assessed for other mutations in exons 16 and 17 (encoding the Aβ domain) of the APP gene, and none were found (Tanzi et al. 1992). Overall, these data in combination with the existence of largely negative genetic linkage between APP and FAD (Tanzi et al. 1987b, 1992; Van Broeckhoven et al. 1987; Schellenberg et al. 1991a,b) indicate that the major portion of FAD (> 95%) cases do not involve mutations in the APP gene.

Chromosome 14 and FAD

The increase in the number of FAD pedigrees that are now available for genetic linkage analysis and the emergence of highly informative simple sequence repeat (SSR; Weber and May 1989) markers have made it considerably easier to scan the total human genome for additional FAD loci. Using SSR technology, several laboratories have recently discovered a major FAD gene defect on chromosome 14 in the vicinity of the markers *D14S43* and *D14S53* which map to the region 14q24 (Schellenberg et al. 1992a; St George-Hyslop et al. 1992; Van Broeckhoven et al. 1992; Mullan et al. 1992b). In our data set, the combined FAD pedigrees tested yielded a highly significant peak lod score of + 23.4 in the vicinity of above two markers. This is indicative of the existence of a major FAD locus on chromosome 14 which appears to be tightly linked to the early-onset FAD pedigrees.

In our original analysis of FAD and chromosome 14, eight genetic markers spanning the long arm of chromosome 14 were tested in 21 FAD pedigrees (St George-Hyslop et al. 1992). While five of the markers yielded no significant scores, the remaining three markers, spanning a 12 cM region on the central portion of chromosome 14q, yielded highly significant two point lod scores (*D14S43, D4S53, D4S55*; St George-Hyslop et al. 1992). The highest individual score obtained was 6.99 (at $\Theta = 0$) with *D14S43* in the pedigree FAD3. The overall lod score across all families exceeded 20 for *D14S53*, 11 for *D14S53* and 6 for *D14S53*. Multipoint analysis with the former two markers yielded a maximum score of 23.4, 5cM distal to *D14S43*, with a secondary peak of 23.17 5cM proximal to *D14S43*. Thus, this initial analysis provided overwhelming support for a chromosome 14 locus in FAD, but could not precisely localize it relative to the two most informative markers. The latter is due to different families being informative for one or the other, but not both of the markers. We have now typed a total of 12 genetic markers from the linked region of the long arm of chromosome 14 in 30 well-characterized FAD pedigrees. Multipoint analysis of FAD pedigrees 1–30 with *D14S43*, *D14S53* and a third DNA marker, *D14S42*, which resides proximal to *D14S43*, yielded a maximum lod score of 20.00 with a recombination fraction of 0.01 proximal to *D14S43*, positioning the FAD gene very close to this marker. In addition to the above three markers, we have also typed nine additional markers from the linked 14q24.3 region, the current best order of which is: *D14S55-D14S53-D14S59-D14S61-FOS-D14S76-D14S43-D14S71-D14S77-D14S57-D14S63-D14S52*.

The average spacing among these 12 markers is approximately 1 centimorgan. Although the computer-based linkage analysis (two-point and multipoint) is still being performed on this data set, visual analysis and haplotype construction of genotypes obtained thus far with these markers suggest that the FAD gene resides within the *D14S43-D14S71-D14S77-D14S57-D14S63* cluster but could be anywhere between *D14S53* and *D14S63* (Fig. 1). This minimal candidate region is now being confirmed by searching for additional recombinants. It is also being directly targeted for attempts to generate additional microsatellite polymorphisms to test for linkage disequilibrium, and for physical mapping/cloning experiments.

The general region of chromosome 14 (14q24.3) that demonstrates genetic linkage to FAD includes a number of candidate genes. Two particularly interesting candidate genes are the FOS oncogene and a member of the 70 kd heat shock protein (HSP70) family. The APP promotor contains the AP-1 transcriptional element which interacts with FOS-JUN complexes to modulate transcriptional regulation. A breakdown in this regulation could result in overexpression of APP and propagate a situation similar to that which occurs in Down syndrome patients, where increased expression of APP (due to trisomy 21) appears to result in accelerated amyloid formation. With respect to *HSP70*, this family of proteins function, among other things, as molecular chaperones (Pelham 1986). *HSP70* molecules might bind APP or the βA4 peptide and serve to assure proper proteolysis/compartmentilization of APP and prevent amyloid formation. We have recently cloned the chromosome 14 HSP70 gene and preliminary mapping of this gene does not place it in the minimal candidate region.

The entire coding region of the *FOS* oncogene has been sequenced in chromosome 14-linked FAD patients and no potentially pathogenic differences were found (St George-Hyslop et al., in press) Additionally, the promotor of the *APP* gene, including the AP1 transcription element that is recognized by FOS-JUN complexes, was found to contain no pathogenic mutations. However, in both *FOS* and the *APP* promotor, polymorphisms were found. These

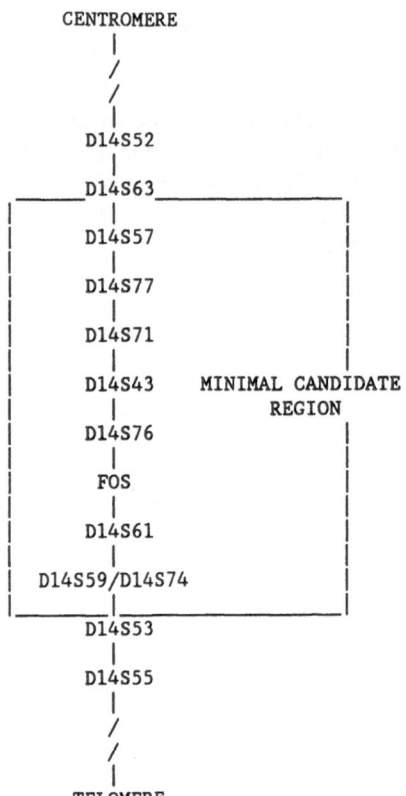

Fig. 1. Minimal candidate region of the FAD gene defect chromosome on 14q24.3

included a silent third position T → C mutation in exon 2 of *FOS* and a C → G substitution at -209 bp in the promotor of *APP*. Neither of these substitutions was specific to FAD. We are currently analyzing the 5′ and 3′ untranslated regions of cFOS, since abnormal expression of this gene could presumably result in cell death. Finally although both FOS and *HSP70* represent reasonable gene candidates. it is entirely likely that the chromosome 14 FAD locus is a novel gene which may or may not play a direct role in amyloid formation.

In an attempt to further localize the gene defect on chromosome 14, we are currently physically mapping and cloning the region around *D14S43*. To this end, we have screened the CEPH (Centre d'Etude du Polymorphisme Humain, Paris) yeast artificial chromosome (YAC) library by polymerase chain reaction (PCR) and have identified or isolated more than 30 YAC clones for *D14S74*, *D14S61*, *D14S76*, *D14S43*, *D14S71*, *D14S77*, *D14S57*, *FOS*, and *HSP70*. The largest YACs obtained contain multiple markers, including one with *D14S43-D14S71-D14S77* (approximately 1 megabase in size) and one containing at least *FOS-D14S76-D14S61* (600 Kb). A complete YAC contig of the minimal candidate region is now under construction.

To obtain expressed sequences from this region, we have begun to isolate individual exons by "exon-trapping." For this purpose, we initially use the YAC

DNA (isolated by pulse-field gel electrophoresis) to screen cosmids from a flow-sorted chromosome 14-specific cosmid library provided by the Los Alamos National Laboratory. The library consists of approximately 17,000 cosmids in 175 96-well dishes representing 148 genome equivalents of chromosome 14. Individual clones are grown in 96-well dishes and are transferred to gridded nylon filters using a BIOMEK robot and specially customized software. Then, using the YACs spanning the minimal candidate region as a hybridization probe, the cosmids from the region are identified and used to "trap" exons (Buckler et al. 1991). This technique, termed exon amplification, has very stringent criteria for capturing an exon, since both 5' and 3' splice sites are required. A typical experiment on a single cosmid yields an average of three trapped exons. The trapped exon products are usually single-copy, making them exceptional hybridization probes, and average 100–150 bp, making them ideally suited for generation by PCR. Thus, in addition to being a rapid means to screen cDNA libraries for genes in a region of interest, the cloned exons are also ideal reagents for physical mapping and YAC walking.

The eventual identification of the chromosome 14 gene defect underlying early-onset FAD as well as the late-onset FAD gene defects should provide a tremendous step forward in both furthering our understanding of the etiology of AD and ultimately leading to the development of novel means of therapeutically intervening with this devastating neurological disorder.

References

Breitner JCS, Silverman JM, Mohs RC, Davis KL (1988) Familial aggregation in Alzheimer's disease: Comparison of risk among relatives of early- and late-onset cases and among male and female relatives in successive relatives. Neurology 38:207–212.

Buckler AJ, Chang DD, Graw SL, Brook JD, Haber DA, Sharp PA, Housman DE (1991) Exon amplification: a strategy to isolate mammalian genes based on RNA splicing. Proc Natl Acad Sci U.S.A. 88:4005–4009

Chartier-Harlin M-C, Crawford F, Houlden H, Warren A, Hughes D, Fidani L, Goate A, Rossor M, Roques P, Hardy J, Mullan M (1991) Early-onset Alzheimer's disease caused by mutations at codon 717 of the β-amyloid precursor protein gene. Nature 353:884–846

Farrer LA, Myers RH, Connor L, Cupples A, Growdon JH (1991) Segregation analysis reveals evidence for a major gene for Alzheimer's disease. Am J Hum Genet 48:1026–1033.

Glenner GG, Wong CW (1984) Alzheimer's disease: initial report of the purification and characterization of a novel cerebrovascular amyloid protein. Biochem Biophys Res Commun 120:885–890

Goate AM, Haynes AR, Owen MJ, Farrall M, James LA, Lai LYC, Mullan MJ, Roques P, Rossor MN, Williamson R, Hardy J (1989) Predisposing locus for Alzheimer's disease on chromosome 21, Lancet 18:352–355

Goate AM, Chartier-Harlin MC, Mullan MC, Brown J, Crawford F, Fidani L, Guiffra A, Haynes A, Irving N, James L, Mant R, Newton P, Rooke K, Roques P. Talbot C, Pericak-Vance M, Roses A, Williamson R, Rossor M, Owen M, Hardy J (1991) Segregation of a missense mutation in the amyloid precursor protein gene with familial Alzheimer's disease. Nature 349:704–706

Goldgaber D, Lerman JI, McBride OW, Saffiotti U, Gajdusek DC (1987) Characterization and chromosomal localization of a cDNA encoding brain amyloid of fibril protein. Science 235:877–880

Hendriks L, van Duijn CM, Cras P, Cruts M, Van Hul W, van Harskamp F, Warren A, McInnis MG, Antonarakis SE, Martin J-J, Hofman A, Van Broeckhoven C. (1992) Presenile dementia and cerebral haemorrhage linked to a mutation at codon 692 of the β-amyloid precursor protein gene. Nature Gent 1:218–221

Kang J, Lemaire HG, Unterbeck A, Salbaum J, Masters L, Grzeschik KH, Multhaup G, Beyreuther K, Müller-Hill B (1987) The precursor of Alzheimer's disease amyloid A4 protein resembles a cell-surface receptor. Nature 325:733–736

Levy E, Carman MD, Fernandez-Madrid IJ, Powder MD, Lieberburg I, Sjoerd G, Van Duinen SG, Bots GTAM, Luyendijk W, Frangione B (1990) Mutation of Alzheimer's disease amyloid gene in hereditary cerebral hemorrhage, Dutch type. Science 248:1124–1126

Mohs RC, Breitner JCS, Silverman JM, Davis KL (1987) Alzheimer's disease: morbid risk among first degree relatives approximates 50% by age 90. Arch Gen Psychiat 44:405–408

Mullan M, Crawford F, Axelman K, Houlden H, Lilius L, Winblad W, Lannfelt L (1992a) A pathogenic mutation for probable Alzheimer's disease in the N-terminus of β-amyloid. Nature Genetics 1:345–347

Mullan M, Houlden H, Windelspecht M, Fidani L, Lombardi C, Diaz P, Rossor M, Crook R, Hardy J, Crawford F (1992b) A locus for familial Alzheimer's disease on the long arm of chromosome 14, proximal to the alpha-1-antichymotrypsin gene. Nature Genet 2:340–342

Murrell J, Farlow M, Ghetti B, Benson M (1991) A mutation in the amyloid precursor protein associated with hereditary Alzheimer's disease Science 254:97–99

Pelham HR (1986) Speculations on the functions of the major heat shock and glucose-regulated proteins. Cell 46:959–961

Pericak-Vance MA, Bebout JL, Gaskell PC, Yamaoka LH, Hung W-Y, Alberts MJ, Walker AP, Bartlett RJ, Haynes CA, Welst KA, Earl NL, Heymark A, Clark CM, Roses AD (1991a) Linkage studies in familial Alzheimer's disease: evidence for chromosome 19 linkage. Am J Hum Genet 48:1034–1050

Pericak-Vance MA, Haines JL, St. George-Hyslop PH, Bebout J, Haynes C, Tanzi R, Yamaoka L, Gusella, JF, Roses AD (1991b) Joint linkage analysis of chromosomes 19 and 21 in familial Alzheimer Disease. Am J Human Genet 49:355A

Robakis NK, Ramakrishna N, Wolfe G, Wisniewski HM (1987) Molecular cloning and characterization of a cDNA encoding the cerebrovascular and the neuritic plaque amyloid peptides. Proc Nat Acad Sci USA 84:4190–4194

St George-Hyslop PH, Tanzi RE, Polinsky RJ, Haines JL, Nee L, Watkins PC, Myers RH, Feldman RG, Pollen D, Drachman D, Growdon J, Bruni A, Foncin J-F, Salmon D, Frommelt P, Amaducci L, Sorbi S, Piacentini S, Stewart GD, Hobbs WJ, Connealy PM, Gusella JF (1987) The genetic defect causing familial Alzheimer's disease maps on chromosome 21. Science 235:885–889

St George-Hyslop PM, Myers RH, Haines JL, Farrer LA, Tanzi RE, Abe K, James MF, Conneally PM, Polinsky RJ, Gusella JF (1989) Familial Alzheimer's disease: progress and problems. Neurobiol Aging 10:417–425

St George-Hyslop PH, Haines JL, Farrer LA, Polinsky R, Van Broeckhoven C, Goate A, Crapper McLachlan DR, Orr H, Bruni AC, Sorbi S, Rainero I, Foncin J-F, Pollen D, Cantu JM, Tupler R, Voskresenskaya N, Mayeux R, Growdon J, Nee L, Backhovens H, Martin JJ, Rossor M, Owen MJ, Mullan M, Percy ME, Karlinsky H, Rich S, Heston L, Montes M, Mortilla M, Nacmias N, Vaula G, Gusella JF, Hardy JA (1990) Genetic linkage studies suggest that Alheimer's disease is not a single homogeneous entity. Nature 347:194–197

St George-Hyslop PH, Haines J, Rogaev E, Mortilla M, Vaula G, Pericak-Vance M, Foncin J-F, Montesi M, Bruni A, Sorbi S, Rainero I, Pinessi L, Pollen D, Polinsky R, Nee L, Kennedy J, Macciardi F, Rogaeva E, Liang Y, Alexandrova N, Lukiw W, Schlumpf K, Tanzi R, Tsuda T, Farrer L, Cantu J-M, Duara R, Amaducci L, Bergamini L, Gusella J, Roses A, Crapper-McLachlan D (1992) Genetic evidence for a novel familial Alzheimer's disease locus on chromosome 14, Nature Genet 2:330–334

Schellenberg GD, Deeb SS, Boehnke ML, Bryant EM, Martin GM, Lampe TH, Bird TD (1987) Association of apolipoprotein CII allele with familial dementia of the Alzheimer type. J Neurogenet 4:97–108

Schellenberg GD, Bird TD, Wijsman EM, Moore DK, Boehnke M, Bryant EM, Lampe TH, Nochlin D, Sumi SM, Deeb SS, Beyreuther K, Martin GM (1988) Absence of linkage of chromosome 21q21 markers to familial Alzheimer's disease. Science 241:1507–1510

Schellenberg GD, Pericak-Vance MA, Wijsman EM, Moore DK, Gaskell PC, Yamaoka LA, Bebout JL (1991a) Linkage analysis of familial Alzheimer's disease using chromosome 21 markers. Am J Human Genet 48:563–583

Schellenberg GD, Anderson L, O'Dahl S, Wijsman E, Sadovnik AD, Ball MJ, Larson EB, Kukull WA, Martin GM, Roses AD, Bird TD (1991b) APP717, APP693, and PRIP mutations are rare in Alzheimer's disease. Am J Human Genet 49:511–517

Schellenberg GD, Bird TD, Wijsman EM, Orr HT, Anderson L, Nemens E, White JA, Bonnycastle L, Weber JL, Alonso ME, Potter H, Heston LL, Martin J (1992a) Genetic linkage evidence for a familial Alzheimer's disease locus on chromosome 14. Science 258:668–671

Schellenberg GD, Boehnke M, Wisjman EM, Moore DK, Martin GM, Bird TD (1992b) Genetic association and linkage analysis of the apolipoprotein CII locus and familial Alzheimer's disease. Ann Neurol 31:223–227

Strittmatter WJ, Saunders AM, Schnechel D, Pericak-Vance M, Enghild J, Salvesen G, Roses AD (1993) Apolipoprotein E: High avidity binding to β-amyloid and increased frequency of type 4 allele in late-onset familial Alzheimer disease. Proc Natl Acad Sci USA 90:1977–1981

Tanzi RE, Genetic linkage studies of human neurodegenerative disorders. Gurr Opinions Neurobiol (1991) 1:455–461

Tanzi RE, Gusella JF, Watkins PC, Bruns GA, St George-Hyslop P, VanKeuren ML, Patterson SP, Pagan S, Kurnit DM, Neve RL (1987a) Amyloid beta protein gene: cDNA, mRNA distribution, and genetic linkage near the Alzheimer locus. Science 235:880–884

Tanzi RE, St George-Hyslop PH, Haines JL, Polinsky RJ, Nee L, Foncin J-F, Neve RL, McClatchy AI, Conneally PM, Gusella JF (1987b) The genetic defect in familial Alzheimer's disease is not tightly linked to the amyloid β-protein gene. Nature 329:156–157

Tanzi RE, St George-Hyslop PH, Gusella JF (1991) Molecular genetics of Alzheimer disease amyloid. J Biol Chem 266:20579–20582

Tanzi RE, Vaula G, Romano DM, Mortilla M, Huang TL, Tupler RG, Wasco W, Hyman BT, Haines JL, Jenkins BJ, Kalaitsidaki M, Warren AC, McInnis MG, Antonarakis SE, Karlinsky H, Percy ME, Connor L, Growdon J, Crapper-Mclanchlan DR, Gusella JF, St George-Hyslop PH (1992) Assessment of amyloid β protein precursor gene mutations in a large set of familial and sporadic Alzheimer disease cases. Am J Human Genet 51:273–282

Van Broeckhoven C, Genthe CA, Vandenberghe B, Horstemke B, Backhovens P, Raeymaekers P, Van Hul W, Wehnert A, Gheuens J, Cras P, Bruyland M, Martin JJ, Salbaum M, Multhaup G, Masters CL, Beyreuther K, Gurling HMD, Mullan MJ, Holland A, Barton A, Irving N, Williamson R, Richards SJ, Hardy JA (1987) Failure of familial Alzheimer's disease to segregate with the A-4 amyloid gene in several European families. Nature 329:153–155

Van Broeckhoven C, Backhovens H, Cruts M, De Winter G, Bruyland M, Cras P, Martin J-J (1992) Mapping of a gene predisposing to early-onset Alzheimer's disease to chromosome 14q24.3, Nature Genet 2:334–339

Wasco W, Bupp K, Magendantz M, Gusella J, Tanzi RE, Solomon F (1992) Identification of a mouse brain cDNA that encodes a protein related to the Alzheimer-associated amyloid β precursor protein. Proc Natl Acad Sci USA 87:2405–2408

Wasco W, Brook JD, Gusella JF, Housman DE, Tanzi RE (1993a) The amyloid Precursor-like protein gene maps to the long arm of chromosome 19. Genomics 15:237–239

Wasco W, Gurubhagavatula S, Paradis Md, Romano DM, Sisodia S, Hyman BT, Neve RL, Tanzi RE (1993b) Isolation and characterization of the human APLP2 gene encoding a homologue of the Alzheimer's associated amyloid β protein precursor. Nature Genet 5:95–100

Weber JL, May PE (1989) Abundant class of human DNA polymorphisms which can be typed by the polymerase chain reaction. Am J Human Genet 44:388–396

Weeks D, Lange K, (1988) The affected pedigree member method of linkage analysis. Am J Human Genet 42:315–326

Genetic Variability and Alzheimer's Disease

J. Hardy, M. Mullan, F. Crawford, K. Duff, R. Crook, P. Diaz, C. Bennett,
H. Houlden, L. Fidani, A. Goate, M. Parfitt, P. Roques, M. Rossor,
and M.-C. Chartier-Harlin*

Molecular genetic analyses of pedigrees multiply affected by Alzheimer's disease
(AD) have revealed that some cases of the disease are caused by mutations in the
β-amyloid precursor protein (APP) gene and others are caused by a lesion on
chromosome 14. In this chapter we shall discuss the nature of genetic variants in
APP and their biochemical and clinical phenotypes, and progress towards
identifying the chromosome 14 lesion.

APP Mutations and their Biochemical and Clinical Phenotypes

It is now clear that mutations in the β-amyloid precursor protein (APP) gene
cause two well-defined phenotypes. These are hereditary cerebral hemorrhage
with amyloidosis (Dutch; HCHWA-D; APP693 Glu → Gln; Levy et al. 1990)
and AD (APP717Val → Ile; Goate et al. 1991; APP717Val → Phe; Murrell et al.
1991; APP717Val → Gly; Chartier-Harlin et al. 1991a,b; APP670/1Lys/Met →
Asn/Leu; Mullan et al. 1992a. In addition, other mutations are either associated
with disorders with intermediate phenotypes (APP692Ala → Gly; Hendriks et
al. 1992) or are not clearly associated with any phenotype. This latter category
includes APP713 Ala → Val (found in a familial schizophrenic, but with no
segregation information; Jones et al. 1992); APP713 Ala → Thr (found in a case
of familial AD, but did not segregate with disease; Carter et al. 1992); APP693
Glu → Gly (found in a case of familial AD, but did not segregate with disease;
Kamino et al. 1992) and APP673 Ala → Thr (found in a control case who died of
a stroke at age 65; Peacock et al. 1993). Both genetic data (Tanzi et al. 1992;
Kamino et al. 1992; Mullan et al. 1992a) and sequence data (ibid., Chartier
Harlin et al. 1991a; Crawford et al. 1991; Fidani et al. 1992) indicate that it is
unlikely that mutations in other parts of the APP gene are associated which
beta-amyloidopathies (see Fig. 1 for a diagram of the mutations).

These data clearly demonstrate that the position and nature of mutations in
the APP gene alter the clinical phenotype. To a large extent, they are the

* Suncoast Alzheimer's Disease Research Group, Department of Psychiatry, University of South
Florida, Tampa, FL 33613 USA

C.L. Masters et al. (Eds.)
Amyloid Protein Precursor in Development,
Aging and Alzheimer's Disease
© Springer-Verlag Berlin Heidelberg 1994

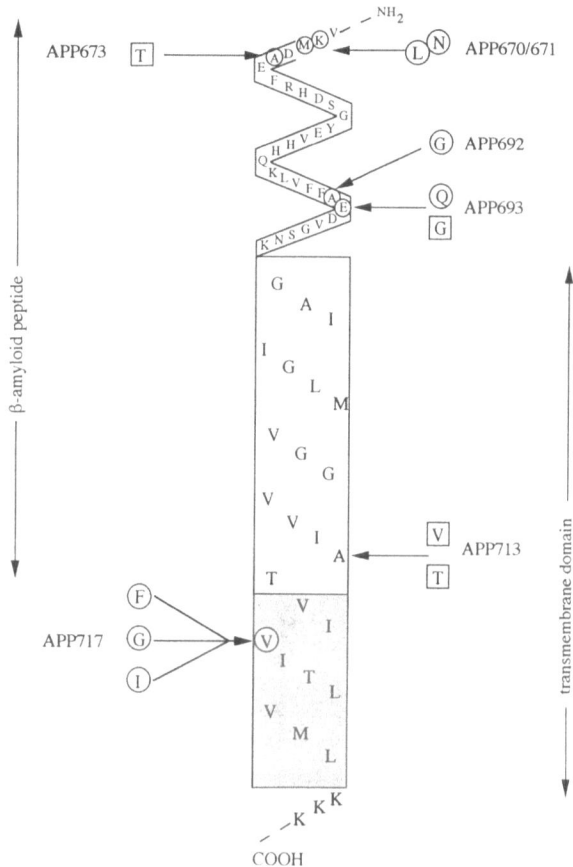

Fig. 1. Diagram of APP mutations modified from Goate et al. (1991) and Kang et al. (1987). Circles indicate mutation causes Alzheimer's disease or cerebral angiopathy. Squares indicate pathogenic status is unclear

intellectual underpinning of the amyloid cascade hypothesis for AD (Glenner and Murphy 1989; Selkoe 1991; Hardy and Allsop 1991; Hardy and Higgins 1992). It is presumed the pathogenic mutations affect the phenotype by increasing the rate of β-amyloid deposition; however, there is little information concerning the nature of the alteration(s) of the biochemical phenotype of the mutations. Only two pieces of data are available. First, Wisniewski and colleagues (1991) showed that APP693 Glu → Gln decreases the solubility of β-amyloid. Second, Citron and Cai and colleagues (Citron et al. 1992; Cai et al. 1993) have shown that the APP670/1 mutation increases the proportion of APP metabolized to β-amyloid (see below). These observations directly suggest biochemical mechanisms underlying beta-amyloid deposition in cases with these mutations and, perhaps, the subtle mechanistic differences underlie the differing phenotypes of the APP670/1 variant and APP693 Glu → Gln variant.

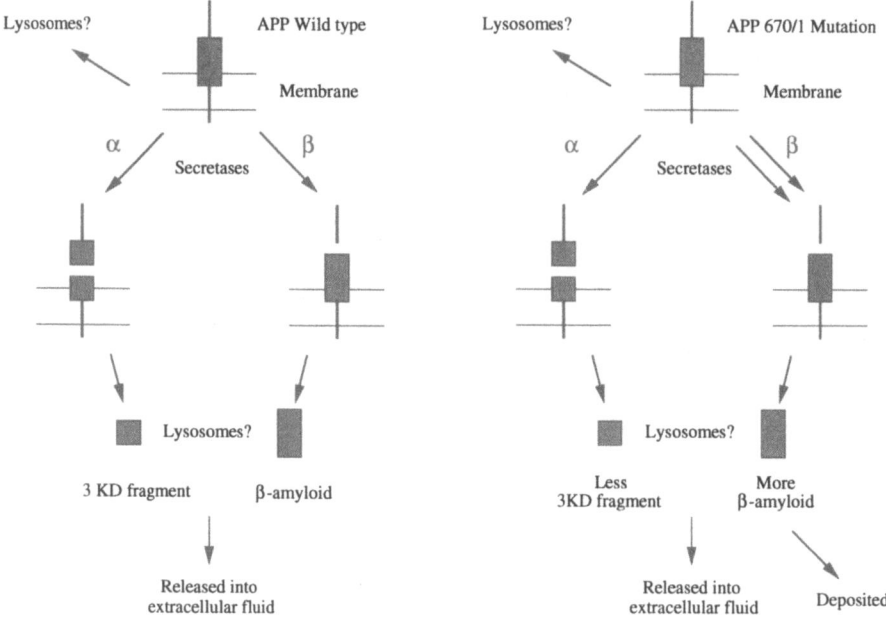

Fig. 2. Possible schemes of APP metabolism derived from several sources in the reference list

APP metabolism is complex and, at present, incompletely defined. Undoubtedly, there are several different fates for the APP molecule, and APP metabolism occurs at different sites within the cell (see Fig. 2 for a scheme). Furthermore, data from CSF studies seem to indicate that different transcripts of APP have different metabolic fates (Kennedy et al. 1993) and that APP695 (Kang et al. 1987) is the principle source of β-amyloid in vivo.

The best defined pathway for APP metabolism is the "secretase" pathway (more recently defined as the α-secretase pathway; Esch et al. 1990; Anderson et al. 1991). This pathway involves cleavage of the APP molecule between lysine (at APP687) and leucine (at APP688). α-secretase cleavage is incompatible with beta-amyloid formation. However, a 3kD derivative of β-amyloid is a product of APP metabolism and is believed to be derived from this cleavage pathway (see Fig. 2). The specificity of α-secretase has been extensively studied (Sisodia 1992). It has a broad specificity and apparently requires only that the conformation of the region around the cleavage site is alpha-helical.

Another pathway of APP metabolism is the endosomal-lysosomal pathway (Estus et al. 1992; Golde et al. 1992; Haass et al. 1992). This pathway involves cleavage at or around the N-terminal of β-amyloid and yields C-terminal derivatives of APP that contain the entire β-amyloid fragment. The derivatives of APP formed by this process are potentially amyloidogenic. The precise relationship between this metabolic pathway and the "β-secretase" pathway outlined below remains unclear, as does the role (if any) of this pathway in amyloidogenesis.

β-amyloid has recently been shown to be a normal product of cellular metabolism (Haass et al. 1992; Seubert et al. 1992; Shoji et al. 1992), although it is not clear whether this β-amyloid is derived from the C-terminal fragment produced by the endosomal lysosomal system or not. The cleavages involved in the production of β-amyloid must occur between Met671 and Asp672 at the N-terminal and closer to the C-terminal than Val711. The position of the cleavage at the N-terminal side (β-secretase cleavage) can be assigned with certainty, since N-terminal derivatives of APP finishing at Met671 have been identified (Seubert et al. 1993). Thus the β-secretase cleavage is exactly at the site of the APP670/1 mutation. With this background, it is perhaps unsurprising that the APP670/1 mutation facilitates this cleavage and β-amyloidogenesis (see Fig. 2).

The precise position of the amyloidogenic cleavage at the C-terminal remains unclear. One possibility is that the liberating cleavage is just on the cytoplasmic side of the membrane and is followed by carboxypeptidase nibbling of the fragment to produce soluble β-amyloid. Despite the fact that the APP717 mutations were found before the APP670/1 mutation, their mode of pathogenesis is less clear. The limited published information (Cai et al. 1993) suggests that they do not alter the rate of β-amyloid formation in the same way as does the APP670/1 variant. These mutations are just outside the ill-defined C-terminus of β-amyloid. One possibility is that these mutations are pathogenic because they inhibit the C-terminal nibbling and cause longer, less soluble β-amyloid to be produced and then deposited (see Fig. 2). This hypothesis would most comfortably fit with the notion that β-amyloid deposition initiates the disease pathogenesis (Hardy and Mullan, 1992).

The biochemical effects of the four mutations which are not clearly associated with any phenotype (APP713 Ala → Val; Jones et al. 1992; APP713Ala → Thr; Carter et al. 1992; APP693Glu → Gly; Kamino et al. 1992 and APP673Ala → Thr; Peacock et al. 1993) have not been assessed. Each of these mutations has been found in a single individual, making it impossible to be definitive about causation in the way that occurrence and cosegregation allow definitive statements about APP693Glu → Gln (Van Broeckhoven et al. 1990) and the APP717 mutations. Perhaps, however, it is significant that none of these variants has been found in a well proband. One possible explanation is that these variants contribute to pathogenesis. If this is the case, one would expect their effects on APP metabolism to be similar to, but less pronounced than, the pathogenic variants.

One notable feature of the pathogenic APP mutations is that the vast majority of cases with these mutations develop the disease in their late 40s to 60 years of age (Goate et al. 1991; Hardy et al. 1991; Naruse et al. 1991; Chartier Harlin et al. 1991b; Murrell et al. 1991; Yoshioka et al. 1991; Fidani et al. 1992; Mullan et al. 1992a,b). No families with an age of onset below 45 years has been reported to have an APP mutation; equally, no family with an age of onset of more than 60 years has been found to have an APP mutation (Table 1).

Table 1. Age of onset of familial Alzheimer's disease correlated with genetic aetiology[a, b, c]

	Age of onset			
	30–39	40–49	50–59	> 60
APP mutations				
Tampa/London Group	0	0	6	0
Boston/Toronto Group	0	0	2	0
Seattle Group	0	0	0	0
Antwerp Group	0	0	0	0
Total	0	0	8	0
No APP mutations				
Tampa/London Group	5	4	5	1
Boston/Toronto Group	0	5	5	19
Seattle Group	0	8	1	49
Antwerp Group	2	0	0	0
Total	7	17	11	69
Chromosome 14 linked				
Tampa/London Group	0	2	0	0
Boston/Toronto Group	0	6	1	0
Seattle Group	0	2	0	0
Antwerp Group	2	0	0	0
Total	2	10	1	0

[a] One family, Flo10, was scored by Tanzi and colleagues (1992) as not having an APP mutation. This has recently been re-evaluated and does indeed have APP717Val → Ile. This information is included in this table.

[b] Two families have been analysed by both the Boston/Toronto group and the Seattle group. These are SNW (Seattle) which is FAD3 (Boston/Toronto) and 603. Both these families are counted, arbitrarily, in the Boston/Toronto series. Data from the Volga German families has not been included. A family with a mutation at APP693Glu → Gly which did not segregate with disease is also not included.

[c] A lod score of > 1 is arbitrarily used as defining ch14 linkage. This will almost certainly underestimate the number of families with mutations at the ch14 locus. Therefore it would be misleading to compare the numbers of ch14 families with APP families. However, the age distribution of onsets is unlikely to be skewed.

Chromosome 14 and Alzheimer's Disease

The realisation that AD was genetically heterogeneous (Schellenberg et al. 1988; St George Hyslop et al. 1990), with some families with cosegregation of mutations in APP and disease (see above) but many families in which specific alleles of APP did not cosegregate with disease (Van Broeckhoven et al. 1987; Tanzi et al. 1987), strongly suggested that there must be at least one other locus. *A priori*, searching for other loci was a daunting task because of the possibility of multiple other loci confounding the genetic analysis. However, Schellenberg and colleagues (1992) found very good evidence for genetic linkage to markers on the long arm of chromosome 14. This result was rapidly confirmed by all the other major groups carrying out genetic analysis of families with early onset AD (St George Hyslop et al. 1992; Van Broeckhoven et al. 1992; Mullan et al. 1992b). From the combined data, it is clear that the majority of families with early onset AD have mutations at the chromosome 14 locus, though there is some evidence for residual heterogeneity (see especially Schellenberg et al. 1992). It is most likely that the chromosome 14 gene encodes a protein intimately connected with APP metabolism; indeed the nature of this gene is a sensitive test of the amyloid cascade hypothesis.

One bizarre and unexpected consequence of the identification of a chromosome 14 linkage for AD is that those families which originally showed evidence for genetic linkage to chromosome 21 markers (St George Hyslop et al. 1987) now show much stronger evidence for linkage to chromosome 14 markers (St George Hyslop et al. 1992). Thus, it seems that the original linkage report was obtained by chance but, fortuitously, was close to an area of true linkage in other AD families (Goate et al. 1989, 1991).

The families which have shown unambiguous evidence for genetic linkage to chromosome 14 markers have all had an age of onset of less than 50 years and thus, as a group, are significantly younger than those with APP mutations. There is, however, likely to be some overlap. This observation further strengthens the notion that, alone of the clinical features, age of onset is a useful discriminator of etiology (Table 1).

The nature of the locus on chromosome 14 is likely to be elucidated in one of three ways: 1) there are two "candidate genes" which map into approximately the right area; these are a heat shock gene and a c-fos gene. These are both candidate genes because they alter APP expression (Goldgaber et al. 1989; Abe et al. 1991); 2) a new candidate gene (a secretase?) might be cloned and localised into the correct region then found to have mutations in AD families; and, 3) positional cloning (aided by the Genome Project) might yield candidate genes and then pathogenic mutations.

It is difficult, if not impossible, to gauge how long it will take to identify this second locus. The fact that all major groups agree upon its approximate location, together with the speed of the Human Genome Project, suggests that its identification may come sooner rather than later.

Acknowledgements. This chapter is dedicated with thanks to Prof. Bob Williamson for his support and help over the years. Work carried out in the authors' labs was funded by the MRC, Research into Ageing, the MHF, NATO and by private donors.

References

Abe K, St George Hyslop PH, Tanzi RE, Kogure K (1991) Induction of amyloid precursor protein mRNA after heat shock in cultured human lymphoblastoid cells. Neurosci Letts 125:169–171

Anderson JP, Esch FS, Keim PS, Sambamurti K, Lieberburg I, Robakis NK (1991) Exact cleavage site of Alzheimer amyloid precursor in neuronal PC-12 cells. Neurosci Lett 128:126–128

Cai, XD, Golde TE, Younkin SG (1993) Excess amyloid β protein is released from a mutant amyloid β protein precursor linked to familial Alzheimer's disease. Science 259:514–516

Carter DA, Desmarais E, Bellis M, Campion D, Clerget-Darpoux F, Bryce A, Agid Y, Jaillard-Serradt A, Mallet J (1992) More missense in amyloid gene. Nature Genet 2:255–256

Chartier Harlin MC, Crawford F, Hamandi K, Mullan M, Goate A, Backhovens H, Martin JJ, Van Broeckhoven C (1991a) Screening for the β-amyloid precursor protein mutation (APP:Val → Ile) in extended pedigrees with early onset Alzheimer's disease. Neurosci Letts 129:134–135

Chartier Harlin MC, Crawford F, Houlden H, Warren A, Hughes D, Fidani L, Goate A, Rossor M, Roques P, Hardy J, Mullan M (1991b) Early onset Alzheimer's disease caused by mutations at codon 717 of the β-amyloid precursor protein gene. Nature 353:844–846

Citron M, Oltersdorf T, Haass C, McConlogue L, Hung AY, Seubert P, Vigo-Pelfrey C, Lieberburg I, Selkoe DJ (1992) Mutation of the β amyloid precursor protein in familial Alzheimer's disease causes increased β-amyloid production. Nature 360:672–674

Crawford F, Hardy J, Mullan M, Goate A, Hughes D, Fidani L, Roques P, Rossor M, Chartier-Harlin MC (1991) Sequencing of exons 16 and 17 of the β-amyloid precursor protein gene in families with early onset Alzheimer's disease fails to reveal mutations in the β-amyloid sequence. Neurosci Lett 133:1–2

Esch FS, Keim PS, Beattie EC, Blacher RW, Culwell, AR, Oltersdorf T, McClure D, Ward PJ (1990) Cleavage of amyloid β peptide during constitutive processing of its precursor. Science 248:1122–1124

Estus S, Golde TE, Kunishita T, Blades D, Lowery D, Eisen M, Usiak M, Qu X, Tabira T, Greenberg BD, Younkin SG (1992) Potentially amyloidogenic, carboxyl terminal derivatives of the amyloid protein precursor. Science 255:726–728

Fidani L, Rooke K, Chartier-Harlin MC, Hughes D, Tanzi R, Mullan M, Roques P, Rossor M, Hardy J, Goate A (1992) Screening for mutations in the open reading frame and promoter of the β-amyloid precursor protein gene in familial Alzheimer's disease; identification of a further family with APP717 Val → Ile. Hum Mol Genet 1:165–168

Glenner GG, Murphy MA (1989) Amyloidosis of the nervous system. J Neurol Sci 94:1–28

Goate A, Chartier Harlin MC, Mullan M, Brown J, Crawford F, Fidani L, Giuffra L, Haynes A, Irving N, James L, Mant R, Newton P, Rooke K, Roques P, Talbot C, Pericak-Vance M, Roses A, Williamson R, Rossor M, Owen M, Hardy J (1991) Segregation of a missense mutation in the amyloid precursor protein gene with familial Alzheimer's disease. Nature 349:704–706

Goate AM, Haynes AR, Owen MJ, Farrall M, James LA, Lai LY, Mullan MJ, Roques P, Rossor MN, Williamson R, Hardy JA (1989) Predisposing locus for Alzheimer's disease on chromosome 21. Lancet 1:352–355

Golde TE, Estus S, Younkin LH, Selkoe DJ, Younkin SG (1992) Processing of the amyloid protein precursor to potentially amyloidogenic fragments. Science 255:728–730

Goldgaber D, Harris HW, Hla T, Maciag T, Donnell RJ, Jacobsen JS, Vitek MP, Gadjusek DC (1989) Interleukin 1 regulates synthesis of amyloid β-protein precursor mRNA in human endothelial cells. Proc Natl Acad Sci USA 86:7606–7610

Haass C, Koo EH, Mellon A, Hung AY, Selkoe DJ (1992) Targeting of cell-surface β-amyloid precursor protein to lysosomes;; alternative processing into amyloid-bearing fragments. Nature 357:500–503

Haass C, Schlossmacher MG, Hung AY, Vigo-Pelfrey C, Mellon A, Ostaszewski BL, Lieberburg I, Koo EH, Schenk D, Teplow DB, Selkoe DJ (1992) Amyloid β peptide is produced by cultured cells during normal metabolism. Nature 359:322–325

Hardy J, Allsop D (1991) Amyloid deposition as the central event in the aetiology of Alzheimer's disease. Trends Pharmacol 12:383–388

Hardy J, Mullan M, Chartier Harlin MC, Brown J, Goate A, Rossor M, Collinge J, Roberts G, Luthert P, Lantos P, Naruse S, Kaneko K, Tsuji S, Miyatake T, Shimizu T, Kojima T, Nakano I, Yoshioka K, Sakaki Y, Miki T, Katsuya T, Ogihara T, Roses A, Pericak-Vance M, Haan J, Roos R, Lucotte G, David F (1991) Molecular classification of Alzheimer's disease. Lancet 337:1342–1343

Hardy J, Mullan M (1992) Alzheimer's disease: in search of the soluble. Nature 358:268–269

Hardy JA, Higgins GA (1992) Alzheimer's disease: the amyloid cascade hypothesis. Science 256:184–185

Hendriks L, van Duijn CM, Cras P, Cruts M, Van Hul W, van Harskamp F, Marin JJ, Hofman A, Van Broeckhoven C (1992) Presenile dementia and cerebral haemorrhage caused by a mutation at codon 692 of the β amyloid precursor protein gene. Nature Genet 1:218–221

Jones CT, Morris S, Yates CM, Moffoot A, Sharpe C, Brock DJH, St.Clair D (1992) Mutation in codon 713 of the beta-amyloid precursor protein gene presenting with schizophrenia. Nature Genet 1:306–309

Kamino K, Orr HT, Payami H, Wijsman E, Alonso ME, Pulst S, Anderson L, O'dahl S, Nemens E, White J, Sadovnick AD, Ball MJ, Kaye J, Warren A, McInnis M, Antonorakis S, Korenberg J, Sharma V, Kukull W, Larson E, Heston LL, Martin GM, Bird TD, Schellenberg GD (1992) Linkage and mutational analysis of familial Alzheimer's disease kindreds for the APP gene region. Am J Hum Genet 51:998–1014

Kang J, Lemaire HG, Unterbeck A, Salbaum JM, Masters CL, Grzeschik KH, Multhaup G, Beyreuther K, Müller Hill B (1987) The precursor of Alzheimer's disease amyloid A4 protein resembles a cell-surface receptor. Nature 325:733–736

Kennedy H, Kametani F, Allsop D (1993) Only Kunitz-inhibitor-containing isoforms of secreted Alzheimer amyloid precursor protein show amyloid immunoreactivity in normal cerebrospinal fluid. Neurodegen 1:59–64

Levy E, Carman MD, Fernandez Madrid IJ, Power MD, Lieberburg I, van Duinen SG, Bots GT, Luyendijk W, Frangione B (1990) Mutation of the Alzheimer's disease amyloid gene in hereditary cerebral hemorrhage, Dutch type. Science 248:1124–1126

Mullan M, Crawford F, Axelman K, Houlden H, Lilius L, Winblad B, Lannfelt L (1992a) A new mutation in APP demonstrates that pathogenic mutations for probable Alzheimer's disease frame the β amyloid sequence. Nature Genet 1:345–347

Mullan M, Houlden H, Windelspecht M, Fidani L, Lombardi C, Diaz P, Rossor M, Crook R, Hardy J, Duff K, Crawford F (1992b) A locus for familial early onset Alzheimer's disease on the long arm of chromosome 14 proximal to the α1 antichymotrypsin gene. Nature Genet 2:340–342

Murrell J, Farlow M, Ghetti B, Benson M (1991) A mutation in the amyloid precursor protein associated with hereditary Alzheimer's disease. Science 254:97–99

Naruse S, Igarashi S, Kobayashi H, Aoki K, Inuzuka T, Kaneko K, Shimizu T, Iihara K, Kojima T, Miyatake T, Tsuji S (1991) Mis-sense mutation Val → Ile in exon 17 of amyloid precursor protein gene in Japanese familial Alzheimer's disease. Lancet 337:978–979

Peacock ML, Warren JT, Roses AD, Fink JK (1993) Novel polymorphism in the A4 region of amyloid precursor protein gene in patient without Alzheimer's disease. Neurology 43:1254–1256

Schellenberg GD, Bird TD, Wijsman EM, Moore DK, Boehnke M, Bryant EM, Lampe TH, Nochlin D, Sumi SM, Deeb SS, Beyreuther K, Martin GM (1988) Absence of linkage of chromosome 21q21 markers to familial Alzheimer's disease. Science 241:1507–1510

Schellenberg GD, Bird T, Wijsman E, Orr H, Anderson L, Nemens L, White J, Heston L, Martin GM (1992) Genetic linkage evidence for a familial Alzheimer's disease locus on chromosome 14. Science 258:668–671

Selkoe DJ (1991) The molecular pathology of Alzheimer's disease. Neuron 6:487–491

Seubert P, Vigo-Pelfrey C, Esch F, Lee M, Dovey H, Davis D, Sinha S, Whaley J, Swindlehurst C, McCormack R, Wolfert R, Selkoe D, Lieberburg I, Schenk D (1992) Isolation and quantification of soluble Alzheimer's β peptide in biological fluids. Nature 359:325–329

Seubert P, Oltersdorf T, Lee MG, Barbour R, Blomquist C, Davis DL, Bryant K, Fritz LC, Galasko D, Thal LJ, Lieberburg I, Schenk DB (1993) Secretion of β-amyloid precursor protein cleaved at the amino terminus of the β-amyloid peptide. Nature 361:260–263

Shoji M, Golde TE, Cheung TT, Ghiso K. Shaffer LM, Cai XD, Tintner RD, Frangione B, Younkin SG (1992) Normal processing produces the Alzheimer amyloid β protein. Science 258:126–129

Sisodia SS (1992) β amyloid precursor protein cleavage by a membrane-bound protease. Proc Natl Acad Sci USA 89:6075–6079

St George Hyslop PH, Tanzi RE, Polinsky RJ, Haines JL, Nee L, Watkins PC, Myers RH, Feldman RG, Pollen D, Drachman D, Growdon J, Bruni A, Foncin J-F, Salmon D, Frommelt P, Amaducci L, Sorbi S, Piacentini S, Stewart GD, Hobbs WJ, Conneally PM, Gusella JF (1987) The genetic defect causing familial Alzheimer's disease maps on chromosome 21. Science 235:885–890

St George Hyslop PH, Haines JL, Farrer LA, Polinsky R, Van Broeckhoven C, Goate A, McLachlan DR, Orr H, Bruni AC, Sorbi S, Rainero I, Foncin J-F, Pollen D, Cantu JM, Tupler R, Voskersenskaya N, Mayeux R, Growdon J, Fried VA, Myers RH, Nee L, Backhoven H, Martin JJ, Rossor M, Owen MJ, Mullan M, Percy ME, Karlinski H, Rich S, Heston L, Montesi M, Mortilla M, Nacmias N, Gusella JF, Hardy JA (1990) Genetic linkage studies suggest that Alzheimer's disease is not a single homogeneous disorder. FAD Collaborative Study Group. Nature 347:194–197

St George Hyslop PH, Haines J, Rogaev E, Mortilla M, Vaula G, Pericak-Vance M, Foncin JF, Montesi A, Bruni S, Sorbi S, Rainero I, Pinessi L, Pollen D, Polinsky R, Nee L, Kennedy J, Macciardi F, Rogaeva E, Liang Y, Alexandrova N, Lukiw W, Schlump K, Tanzi R, Tsuda T, Farrer L, Cantu JM, Duara R, Amaducci L, Bergamini L, Gusella J, Roses A, Crapper McLachlan D (1992) Genetic evidence for a novel familial Alzheimer's disease locus on chromosome 14. Nature Genet 2:330–334

Tanzi RE, St George Hyslop PH, Haines JL, Polinsky RJ, Nee L, Foncin JF, Neve RL, McClatchey AI, Conneally PM, Gusella JF (1987) The genetic defect in familial Alzheimer's disease is not tightly linked to the amyloid β protein gene. Nature 329:156–157

Tanzi RE, Vaula G, Romano D, Mortilla M, Huang TL, Tupler RG, Wasco W, Hyman BT, Haines JL, Jenkins B, Kalaitsidaki M, Warren AC, McInnis MC, Antonarakis SE, Karlinsky H, Percy M, Connor L, Growdon J, Crapper McLachlan DR, Gusella JF, St George Hyslop PH (1992) Assessment of amyloid β protein gene mutations in a large set of familial and sporadic Alzheimer disease cases. Am J Hum Genet 51:273–282

Van Broeckhoven C, Genthe AM, Vandenberghe A, Horsthemke B, Backhovens H, Raeymaekers P, Van Hul W, Wehnert A, Gheuens J, Cras P, Bruyland M, Martin JJ, Salbaum M, Multhaup G, Masters CL, Beyreuther K, Gurling HMD, Mullan MJ, Holland A, Barton A, Irving N, Williamson R, Richards SJ, Hardy JA (1987) Failure of familial Alzheimer's disease of segregate with the A4-amyloid gene in several European families Nature 329:153–155

Van Broeckhoven C, Haan J, Bakker E, Hardy JA, Van Hul W, Wehnert A, Vegter Van der Vlis M, Roos RA (1990) Amyloid beta protein precursor gene and hereditary cerebral hemorrhage with amyloidosis (Dutch). Science 248:1120–1122

Van Broeckhoven C, Backhovens H, Cruts M, De Winter G, Bruyland M, Cras P (1992) Mapping of a gene predisposing to early-onset Alzheimer's disease to Chromosome 14q24.3. Nature Genet 2:335–339

Wisniewski T, Ghiso J, Frangione B (1991) Peptides homologous to the amyloid protein of Alzheimer's disease containing a glutamine for glutamic acid substitution have accelerated amyloid fibril formation. Biochem Biophys Res Commun 179:1247–1254

Yoshioka K, Miki T, Katsuya T, Ogihara T, Sakaki Y (1991) The 717Val $\rightarrow$ Ile substitution in amyloid precursor protein is associated with familial Alzheimer's disease regardless of ethnic groups. Biochem Biophys Res Commun 178:1141–1146

Genetic Defects in Early Onset Alzheimer's Disease and Related Disorders

L. Hendriks*, C. Van Broeckhoven,
and *the Alzheimer's Disease Research Group*

Summary

There is sufficient evidence that genes play an important role in the aetiology of Alzheimer's disease (AD). In families with patients with an early onset of AD (EOAD) before the age of 65 years, the disease segregates as an autosomal dominant trait. Molecular genetic techniques have been applied to these families and hitherto two different genetic loci have been identified. One is the amyloid precursor protein (APP) gene on chromosome 21q21.2. In a few EOAD families mutations in APP at codons 717 and 670/671 have been detected. APP mutations have also been identified in AD-related disorders. A mutations at codon 693 in APP causes hereditary cerebral haemorrhages with amyloidosis Dutch type (HCHWA-D). In a family segregating both presenile dementia of the AD type and cerebral haemorrhages, a mutation was identified at codon 692 of APP. A second locus was identified on chromosome 14q24.3, which seems to be responsible for EOAD in 70% of the families. The chromosome 14 EOAD gene has not been identified yet.

Introduction

Alzheimer's disease (AD) is a neurodegenerative disorder of the central nervous system and the major cause of senile dementia in the developed countries. Neuropathologically the disease is characterized by the progressive deposition of βA4 amyloid, a proteolysis product of a larger amyloid precursor protein (APP), in the parenchyma as "senile" plaques (SPs) and in the walls of the blood vessels of primarily the hippocampus and cerebral cortex. In addition, the intracellular neurofibrillary tangle, consisting mainly of abnormally phosphorylated, microtubuli-associated protein tau, is a typical lesion in brains of AD patients. The aetiology of AD is complex and the primary causes of the disease have not yet been resolved. However, it has been recognized that genetic

* Laboratory of Neurogenetics, Born Bunge Foundation, University of Antwerp (UIA), Department of Biochemistry, 2610 Antwerp, Belgium

C.L. Masters et al. (Eds.)
Amyloid Protein Precursor in Development, Aging and Alzheimer's Disease
© Springer-Verlag Berlin Heidelberg 1994

factors play an important role in the pathogenesis of AD. Although most AD patients are sporadic cases, familial aggregation has been observed in about 40% of the patients. In some families the inheritance pattern of AD is clearly autosomal dominant. The patients in these families most often have an early onset of AD (EOAD) before the age of 65 years. So far, using molecular genetic techniques, two separate genetic loci have been identified in EOAD families: one on chromosome 21, i.e., the amyloid precursor protein (APP) gene localized on 21q21.2, and a second on chromosome 14 localized on 14q24.3. In the latter case the gene itself has not yet been identified.

Chromosome 21

The idea that chromosome 21 may be carrying a gene for AD came from the observation in aged Down's syndrome (trisomy 21) patients of a brain pathology very similar to that of AD patients (Wisniewski et al. 1988). Two findings eventually led to the detection of the gene mutations that are most likely responsible for AD in some EOAD families, i.e., linkage with DNA markers located on proximal 21q (St George-Hyslop et al. 1987, 1990) and the localization of the APP gene close to these DNA-markers (Kang et al. 1987; Tanzi et al. 1987). The mutations were found in the APP gene in exons 16 and 17 coding for the βA4 amyloid (e.g., Goate et al. 1991). βA4 amyloid is a 4 kD proteolysis product of APP and is the major constituent of the SPs. APP is a membrane-bound glycoprotein encoded by a gene comprising 18 exons and localized in 21q21.2. Three major isoforms of APP are produced by alternative splicing of two exons: APP770 (Tanzi et al. 1988; Kitaguchi et al. 1988) and APP751 (Ponte et al. 1988), containing a Kunitz protease inhibitor domain, and APP695 (Kang et al. 1987). Although many functions have been proposed for APP, its real function is unknown. APP is processed through different proteolytic pathways. The major pathway is a secretory pathway which cleaves APP extracelluarly within the βA4 amyloid portion at condon 687 (α-secretase clip side; Esch et al. 1990). The extracellular part of APP is secreted and, if it contains the Kunitz inhibitor domain, is homologous to the protease inhibitor nexin-II (Oltersdorf et al. 1989; Van Nostrand et al. 1989). Since this secretory pathway does not produce intact βA4 amyloid, it is non-amyloidogenic and thus not responsible for AD pathology. A second pathway, a lysosomal/endosomal pathway, produces βA4 amyloid containing carboxyl-terminal derivatives of APP (Estus et al. 1992; Golde et al. 1992; Haass et al. 1992a). It has also been shown that a second secretory pathway that secretes βA4 amyloid must exist (Seubert et al. 1993). These amyloidogenic pathways exist not only in AD patients but also in normal individuals, since βA4 amyloid was detected in media of cultured cells during normal metabolism and in cerebrospinal fluid of normal controls (Haass et al. 1992b; Seubert et al. 1992; Shoji et al. 1992). However, the proteolytic enzymes involved in the different APP pathways have not yet been isolated.

The mutations in the APP gene in familial EOAD patients change amino acids at codon 717 of APP (codon numbering according to APP770 isoform), i.e., Val to Ile (Goate et al. 1991), Val to Phe (Murrell et al. 1991) and Val to Gly (Chartier-Harlin et al. 1991), and at codons 670/671 Lys to Asn and Met to Leu (Mullan et al. 1992a). Only the APP 717 (Val to Ile) mutation has been observed in distinct EOAD families of different ethnic backgrounds and it is, therefore, the most common APP mutation in AD. In the majority of the EOAD families with mutations in the APP gene, the mean age at onset is between 50 and 60 years.

Mutations in the APP gene have also been described in AD-related disorders. In patients with hereditary cerebral haemorrhage with amyloidosis-Dutch type (HCHWA-D), a mutation at codon 693 (Glu to Gln) was observed (Levy et al. 1990). HCHWA-D is a rare, autosomal dominant disease occurring in four families living in two coastal villages in the Netherlands. The disease is characterized by recurrent strokes due to extensive βA4 amyloid deposition in the cerebral blood vessel walls. The first stroke occurs between the ages of 45 and 60 years, and 50% of the patients die (Luyendijk et al. 1988; Haan et al. 1989). There are indications that, in patients who survive their first stroke, a progressive dementia develops that is similar to multi-infarct dementia (Haan et al. 1990a, b). HCHWA-D has been referred to as the vascular form of AD because of its predominant vascular involvement, and also since, in HCHWA-D patients, the neuronal cell population seems not to be involved because neither dystrophic neurites nor neurofibrillary tangles were detected (van Duinen et al. 1987).

We described a family with patients with probable EOAD according to NINCDS criteria and patients with cerebral haemorrhages due to cerebral amyloid angiopathy (Hendriks et al. 1992). The mean age at onset for all patients was 45.7 ± 7.3 years. No signs of dementia were detected in the patients with cerebral haemorrhages prior to their stroke. Histopathological analysis of brain biopsy material obtained at brain surgery of one of these patients indicated that the cerebral haemorrhage was the consequence of βA4 amyloid deposition in the blood vessel walls. Parenchymal βA4 amyloid deposits surrounded by dystrophic neurites were also present, but no neurofibrillary tangles could be observed. However, it remains to be seen if these patients will develop clinical signs of dementia which may be accompanied by the appearance of neurofibrillary tangles. In the patients with probable EOAD, there were no indications of major strokes prior to or during the dementia. At present, no autopsy data are available on these patients that might confirm the diagnosis of AD based on the presence of both SPs and neurofibrillary tangles. A mutation was found in the APP gene at codon 692 (Ala to Gly) in patients suffering from a cerebral haemorrhage and patients with probable EOAD. Since the current information on the function and processing of APP is only fragmentary, it is difficult to understand how one mutation can lead to two different phenotypes. However, it is also possible that, secondary to the APP692 mutation, other factors, genetic and/or environmental, are involved that are responsible for one or both phenotypes.

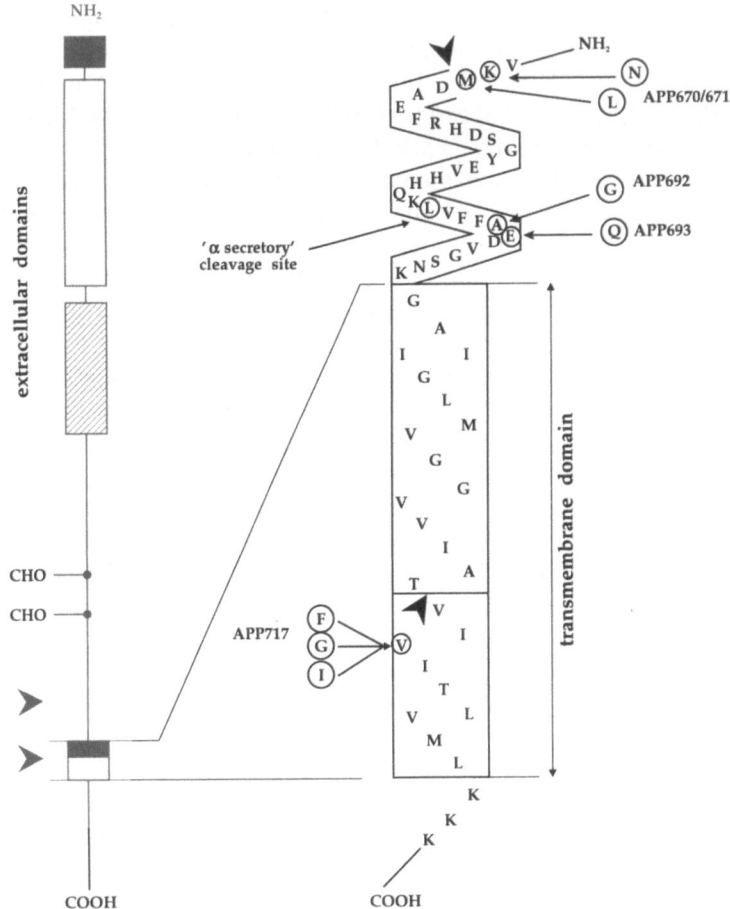

Fig. 1. Mutations in APP. Proposed domain structure of APP as a cell-surface glycoprotein (Kang et al. 1987): black box, signal sequence; open box, cysteine-rich domain; hatched box, highly negatively charged domain (45% Asp and Glu residues); filled circles, N-glycosylation sites. The βA4 amyloid is between the arrowheads with its amino acid sequence. The amino acid substitutions involving the different APP mutations are shown

The EOAD mutations, APP717 and APP670/671, are located outside the βA4 amyloid sequence, with APP717 close to the carboxyl-terminal clipping side within the transmembrane domain and APP670/671 near the amino-terminal clipping side within the extracellular part of APP (Fig. 1). In contrast, the APP692 and APP693 mutations are located inside the βA4 amyloid sequence, close to the α-secretase clipping side. It is not yet known, however, how mutations in APP may be responsible for the pathology seen in AD and AD-related disorders. It was shown that the double mutation APP670/671 provokes an overproduction of βA4 amyloid in the medium of cell cultures transfected with an APP cDNA bearing this mutation (Cai et al. 1993; Citron et al. 1992). In this case upregulation of the βA4 amyloid secretion might be responsible for the acceleration of the cerebral amyloid deposition causing AD. In APP717 (Val to Ile) cDNA transfected cell cultures, no differences were detected in the βA4 amyloid secretion (Cai et al. 1993). It is possible that in the APP717 mutations longer βA4 amyloid peptides are produced which are more amyloidogenic. In vitro experiments using synthetic βA4 amyloid peptides have shown that the 42 amino acids containing βA4 amyloid peptide polymerize more rapidly into amyloid fibrils than the more common form of βA4 amyloid of 40 amino acids (Jarrett et al. 1993). Also synthetic βA4 amyloid peptides containing the APP693 mutation showed accelerated fibril formation (Wisniewski et al. 1991). Hitherto no effects of the APP692 mutation on the βA4 amyloid formation have been described. We have used site directed mutagenesis to introduce the APP692 as well as the APP693 and APP670/671 mutations in the human APP cDNA (Deng and Nicholoff 1992), and we are currently investigating their influence on the βA4 amyloid production in transfected COS cell cultures.

Chromosome 14

Mutations in the APP gene have been found in only a small proportion (approximately 5%) of the EOAD families. In most EOAD families linkage with chromosome 21 was excluded and no mutation could be detected in the APP gene (Schellenberg et al. 1988; Kamino et al. 1992). These families became the subject of a genome search, and linkage was found with markers on chromosome 14 (Schellenberg et al. 1992; St George-Hyslop et al. 1992; Van Broeckhoven et al. 1992; Mullan et al. 1992b). We have been using two extended Belgian families, AD/A and AD/B, with EOAD. Both families have been studied intensively by neurologists and neuropathologists at the Born Bunge Foundation (Antwerp, Belgium). The clinical and pathological characteristics of the disease in the families are consistent with classical AD, although with an extremely early mean age of onset of 35.1 ± 4.8 years in family AD/A and 34.7 ± 3.0 years in family AD/B (Martin et al. 1991). Linkage analysis with DNA polymorphisms in the APP gene demonstrated recombinations with EOAD, excluding the APP gene as the site of mutation in these two families (Van Broeckhoven et al. 1987). This finding was in part confirmed by sequencing exons 16 and 17 of the APP gene revealing no mutations. Linkage analysis with DNA markers localized at regular distances along the 21q arm excluded linkage with chromosome 21, with the exception of a region around the marker D21S13 ($z_{max} = 2.20$ at $\Theta = 0.05$; Van Broeckhoven et al. 1992). However, since highly negative lod scores were obtained with markers closely flanking D21S13, we decided that it was highly unlikely that an EOAD gene resided in this region. Therefore, we started a genome search using highly polymorphic short tandem repeat (STR) markers with a well-defined subchromosomal localization and

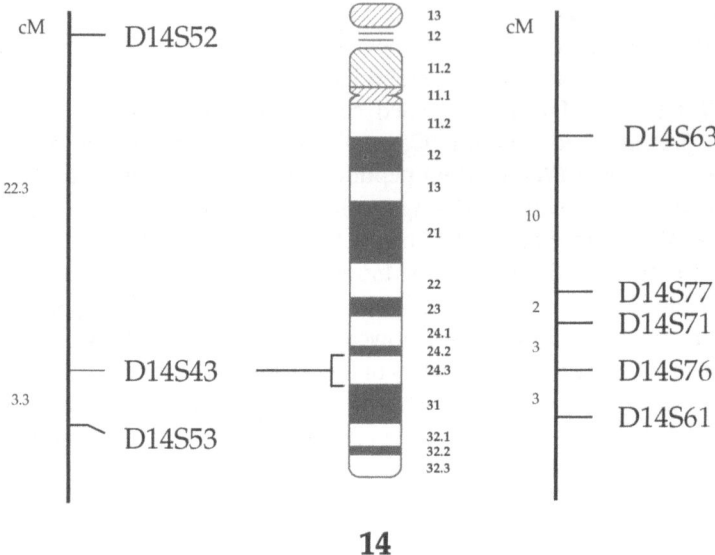

Fig. 2. Genetic maps of the chromosome 14q24.3 region according to the NIH/CEPH collaborative mapping group (1992; left) and to Genethon (Weissenbach et al. 1992; right)

a heterozygosity of minimal 70%. When the 10th marker, D14S43 localized in 14q24.3, was tested a conclusive lod score (z_{max} = 13.25 at Θ = 0) was obtained (Van Broeckhoven et al. 1992). Additional STR markers were tested and the EOAD gene was initially mapped between the markers D14S42 and D14S53 which are, respectively, centromeric and telomeric of the D14S43 (NIH/CEPH Collaborative Research Group 1992). However, new genetic mapping information has indicated that the position of D14S42 on the genetic map centromeric of D14S43 was wrong and that in fact this marker is located telomeric of D14S53 (communicated by the Cooperative Human Linkage Center, Iowa, USA). Our physical mapping data using yeast artificial chromosomes (YACs) support the new genetic position of D14S42 (data not published). Therefore, the closest flanking markers for the EOAD gene on the NIH/CEPH genetic map of chromosome 14 are centromeric D14S52 and telomeric D14S53 and the size of the candidate region is around 25 cM (Fig. 2).

However, we also showed in families AD/A and AD/B that two previously unmapped markers, D14S57 and D14S59, are closely linked to EOAD, with D14S57 most likely localized centromeric of D14S43 and D14S59 located telomeric at distances of 7 and 1 cM, respectively. New STR markers localized in the 14q24.3 region became available through the French human genome mapping effort at Genethon (Evry, France; Weissenbach et al. 1992). Linkage studies in families AD/A and AD/B showed no recombinants between EOAD and the markers D14S77 (z_{max} = 10.82, Θ = 0.0), D14S71 (z_{max} = 5.92, Θ = 0.0) and

D14S76 ($z_{max} = 8.66$, $\Theta = 0.0$; Fig. 2). Recombinants were detected, with the markers D14S63 ($z_{max} = 3.92$ at $\Theta = 0.10$) and D14S61 ($z_{max} = 5.91$ at $\Theta = 0.07$) delineating the candidate region for the EOAD gene to a region of 18 cM on the Genethon map (Fig. 2). However, although both the NIH/CEPH and Genethon maps are based on genotype information obtained in the CEPH reference pedigrees, no published genetic map is available yet that merges the information of all markers. Also, no mapping data of D14S57 and D14S59 in the CEPH references pedigrees have been published.

Our preliminary YAC mapping data support the following order for the linked markers: telomere–(D14S63, D14S57)–(D14S71, D14S43)–D14S76–D14S61–D14S59–D14S53–centromere. Therefore, the closest flanking marker of the EOAD gene on the telomeric side is D14S61. On the centromeric side the closest flanking marker is not exactly known since we have not yet been able to resolve the order of the markers D14S63 and D14S57. However, since both these markers are contained within the same YAC, the candidate region for the EOAD gene is essentially the region of 18 cM between D14S63 and D14S61. Since on average a genetic distance of 1 cM corresponds with a physical distance of 1 million base pairs, the region that contains the EOAD gene is still large and it will be necessary to test additional markers in order to narrow down the candidate region.

Another possible way to get to the EOAD gene more quickly is to look for known genes localized in the candidate region. If it is accepted that βA4 amyloid deposition is crucial to the AD pathogenesis, two genes localized on 14q24.3 are of particular interest, i.e., the proto oncogene c-Fos (FOS) and the 70 kD heat shock protein (HSPA2). FOS is a transcriptional activator and mutations in this protein might upregulate the APP transcription leading to overproduction of APP and, consequently, to βA4 amyloid deposition. HSPA2, which is a molecular chaperone, might be responsible for a shift in the cellular balance between the different proteolytic pathways of APP towards the production of higher amounts of βA4 amyloid. We are now analyzing cosegregation of these two genes with EOAD as well as determining their complete nucleotide sequence in patients. It remains possible, however, that the gene on chromosome 14 does not interfere with APP metabolism. There are more EOAD families with linkage evidence to chromosome 14 than there are families with a mutation in the APP gene, suggesting that the chromosome 14 gene is a major cause of EOAD. Preliminary estimates indicate that about 70% of EOAD cases carry the chromosome 14 defect. Interestingly, the mean age of onset of EOAD in the chromosome 14-linked families is below the age of 50 years, whereas the mean onset age is above 50 years in the families with mutations in the APP gene. This may imply that the mean age at onset of the disease could be used as a discriminator in the identification of EOAD families with a genetic defect on chromosome 14 or chromosome 21. However, it has to be kept in mind that the genetics of EOAD is complicated by the fact that EOAD families have been identified that do not show linkage to either chromosome 14 or the APP gene.

References

Cai X-D, Golde TE, Younkin SG (1993) Release of excess amyloid β protein from a mutant amyloid β protein precursor. Science 259:514–516

Chartier-Harlin M-C, Crawford F, Houlden H, Warren A, Hughes D, Fidani L, Goate A, Rossor M, Roques P, Hardy J, Mullan M (1991) Early-onset Alzheimer's disease caused by mutations at codon 717 of the β-amyloid precursor protein gene. Nature 353:844–846

Citron M, Oltersdorf T, Haass C, McConlogue L, Hing AY, Seubert P, Vigo-Pelfrey C, Lieberburg I, Selkoe DJ (1992) Mutation of the β-amyloid precursor protein in familial Alzheimer's disease increases β-protein production. Nature 360:672–674

Deng WP, Nickoloff JA (1992) Site directed mutagenesis of virtually any plasmid by eliminating a unique side. Anal Biochem 200:81–88

Esch FS, Keim PS, Beattie EC, Blacher RW, Culwell AR, Oltersdorf T, McClure D, Ward PJ (1990) Cleavage of amyloid β peptide during constitutive processing of its precursor. Science 248:1122–1124

Estus S, Golde TE, Kunishita T, Blades D, Lowery D, Eisen M, Udiak M, Qu X, Tabira T, Greenberg BD, Younkin SG (1992) Potentially amyloidogenic, carboxyl-terminal derivatives of the amyloid protein percursor. Science 255:726–728

Goate A, Chartier-Harlin MC, Mullan M, Brown J, Crawford F, Fidani L, Giuffra L, Haynes A, Irving N, James L, Mant R, Newton P, Rooke K, Roques P. Talbot C, Pericak-Vance M, Roses A, Williamson R, Rossor M, Owen M, Hardy J (1991) Segregation of a missense mutation in the amyloid precursor protein gene with familial Alzheimer's disease. Nature 349:704–706

Golde T, Estus S, Younkin LH, Selkoe DJ, Younkin SG (1992) Processing of the amyloid protein precursor to potentially amyloidogenic derivatives. Science 255:728–730

Haan J, Roos RAC, Briet PE, Herpers MJHM, Luyendijk W, Bots GTAM (1989) Hereditary cerebral haemorrhage with amyloidosis of the Dutch type. Clin Neurol Neurosurg 81:285–290

Haan J, Algra Pr, Roos RAC (1990a) Hereditary cerebral hemorrhage with amyloidosis-Dutch type: clinical and CT analysis of 24 cases. Arch Neurol 47:649–653

Haan J, Lanser JBK, Zijderveld I, Van Der Does IGF, Roos RAC (1990b) Dementia in hereditary cerebral hemorrhage with amyloidosis-Dutch type. Arch Neurol 47:956–968

Haass C, Koo EH, Mellon A, Hung AY, Selkoe DJ (1992a) Targeting of cell-surface β-amyloid precursor protein to lysosomes: alternative processing into amyloid-bearing fragments. Nature 357:500–503

Haass C, Schlossmacher MG, Hung AY, Vigo-Pelfrey C, Mellon A, Ostaszewski BL, Lieberburg I, Koo EH, Schenk D, Teplow DB, Selkoe DJ (1992b) Amyloid β-peptide is produced by cultured cells during normal metabolism. Nature 359:322–327

Hendriks L, van Duijn C, Cras P, Cruts M, Van Hul W, van Harskamp F, Warren A, McInnis M, Antonarakis SE, Martin JJ, Hofman A, Van Broeckhoven C (1992) Presenile dementia and cerebral haemorrhage linked to a mutation at codon 692 of the β-amyloid precursor protein gene. Nature Genet 1:218–221

Jarrett JT, Berger EP, Lansbury PT Jr (1993) The carboxy terminus of the β amyloid protein is critical for the seeding of amyloid formation: implications for the pathogenesis of Alzheimer's disease. Biochemistry 32:4693–4697

Kamino K, Orr HT, Payami H, Wijsman ZM, Alonso MA, Pulst SM, Anderson L, O'dahl S, Nemens E, White JA, Sandovnick AD, Ball MJ, Kaye J. Warren A, McInnis M, Antonarakis SE, Korenberg JR, Sharma V, Kukull W, Larson E, Heston LL, Martin GM, Bird TD, Schellenberg GD (1992) Linkage and mutational analysis of familial Alzheimer disease kindreds for the APP gene region. Am J Human Genet 51:998–1014

Kang J, Lemaire HG, Unterbeck A, Salbaum JM, Masters CL, Grzeschik KH, Multhaup G, Beyreuther K, Müller-Hill B (1987) The precursor of Alzheimer's disease amyloid A4 protein resembles a cell-surface receptor. Nature 325:733–736

Kitaguchi N, Takahashi Y, Tokushima Y, Shiojiri S, Ito H (1988) Novel precursor of Alzheimer's disease amyloid protein shows protease inhibitory activity. Nature 331:530–532

Levy E, Carman M, Fernandez-Madrid IJ, Power M, Lieberburg I, van Duinen S, Bots G, Luyendijk W, Frangione B (1990) Mutation of the Alzheimer's disease amyloid gene in hereditary cerebral haemorrhage, Dutch type. Science 248:1124–1126

Luyendijk W, Bots GTAM, Vegter-Van Der Vlis M, Went LN, Frangione B (1988) Hereditary cerebral haemorrhage caused by cortical amyloid angiopathy. J Neurol Sci 85:267–280

Martin J-J, Gheuens J, Bruyland M, Cras P, Vandenberghe A, Masters CL, Beyreuther K, Dom R, Ceuterick C, Lübke U, Van Heuverswijn H, De Winter G, Van Broeckhoven C (1991) Early-onset Alzheimer's disease in 2 large Belgian families. Neurology 41:62–68

Mullan M, Crawford F, Axelman K, Houlden H, Lilius L, Winblad B, Lannfelt L (1992a) A pathogenic mutation for probable Alzheimer's disease in the APP gene at the N-terminus of β-amyloid. Nature Genet 1:345–347

Mullan M, Houlden H, Windelspecht M, Fidani L, Lombardi C, Diaz P, Rossor M, Crook R, Hardy J, Duff K, Crawford F (1992b) A locus for familial early-onset Alzheimer's disease on the long arm of chromosome 14, proximal to the α1-antichymotrypsin gene. Nature Genet 2:340–342

Murrell J, Farlow M, Ghetti B, Benson M (1991) A mutation in the amyloid precursor protein associated with hereditary Alzheimer's disease. Science 254:97–99

NIH/CEPH Collaborative Mapping Group (1992) A comprehensive genetic linkage map of the human genome. Science 258:67–86

Oltersdorf T, Fritz LC, Schenk DB, Lieberburg I, Johnson-Wood, Beattie EC, Ward PJ, Blacher RW, Dovey HF, Sinha S (1989) The secreted form of the Alzheimer's amyloid precursor protein with the Kunitz domain is protease nexin-II; Nature 341:144–147

Ponte P, DeWhitt PG, Schilling J, Miller J, Hsu D, Greenberg B, Davis K, Wallace W, Lieberburg I, Fuller F, Cordell B (1988) A new A4 amyloid mRNA contains a domain homologous to serine proteinase inhibitors. Nature 331:525–527

Schellenberg GD, Bird TD, Wijsman EM, Moore DK, Boehnke M, Bryant EM, Lampe TH, Nochlin D, Sumi SM, Deeb SS, Beyreuther K, Martin GM (1988) Absence of linkage of chromosome 21q21 markers to familial Alzheimer's disease. Science 241:1507–1510

Schellenberg GD, Bird TD, Wijsman EM, Orr HT, Anderson L, Nemens E, White JA, Bonnycastle L, Weber JL, Alonso ME, Potter H, Heston LL, Martin HG (1992) Genetic linkage evidence for a familial Alzheimer's disease locus on chromosome 14. Science 258:668–671

Seubert P, Vigo-Pelfrey C, Esch F, Lee M, Dovey H, Davis D, Sinha S, Schlossmacher M, Whaley J, Swindlehurst C, McCormack R, Wolfert R, Selkoe D, Lieberburg I, Schenk D (1992) Isolation and quantification of soluble Alzheimer's β-peptide from biological fluids. Nature 359:325–327

Seubert P, Oltersdorf T, Lee MG, Barbour R, Blomquist C, Davis DL, Bryant K, Fritz LC, Galasko D, Thal LJ, Lieberburg I, Schenk DB (1993) Secretion of β-amyloid precursor protein cleaved at the amino terminus of the β-amyloid peptide. Nature 361:260–263

Shoji M, Golde TE, Ghiso J, Cheung TT, Estus S, Shaffer LM, Cai X-D, McKay DM, Tintner R, Frangione B, Younkin SG (1992) Production of the Alzheimer's amyloid β protein by normal proteolytic processing. Science 258:126–129

St George-Hyslop PH, Tanzi RE, Polinsky RJ, Haines JL, Nee L, Watkins PC, Myers RH, Feldman RG, Pollen D, Drachman D, Growdon J, Bruni A, Foncin J-F, Salmon D, Frommelt P, Amaducci L, Sorbi S, Piacentini S, Stewart GD, Hobbs WJ, Conneally PM, Gusella JF (1987) The genetic defect causing familial Alzheimer's disease maps on chromosome 21. Science 235:885–890

St George-Hyslop PH, Haines JL, Farrer LA, Polinsky R, Van Broeckhoven C, Goate A, McLachlan DRC, Orr H, Bruni AC, Sorbi S, Rainero I, Foncin J-F, Pollen D, Cantu J-M, Tupler R, Voskresenskaya N, Mayeux R, Growdon J, Fried VA, Myers RH, Nee L, Backhovens H, Martin J-J, Rossor M, Owen MJ, Mullan M, Percy ME, Karlinsky H, Rich S, Heston L, Montesi M, Mortilla M, Nacmias N, Gusella JF, Hardy JA and other members of the FAD collaborative study group (1990) Genetic linkage studies suggest that Alzheimer's disease is not a single homogeneous disorder. Nature 347:194–197

St George-Hyslop PH, Haines J, Rogaev E, Mortilla M, Vaula G, Pericak-Vance M, Foncin JF, Montesi M, Bruni A, Sorbi S, Rainero I, Pinessi L, Pollen D, Polinsky R, Nee L, Kennedy J, Macciardi F, Rogaeva E, Liang Y, Alexandrova N, Lukiw W, Schlumpf K, Tanzi R, Tsuda T, Farrer L, Cantu JM, Duara R, Amaducci L, Bergamini L, Gusella J, Roses A, McLachlan DC (1992) Genetic evidence for a novel familial Alzheimer's disease locus on chromosome 14q24.3. Nature Genet 2: 335–339

Tanzi RE, Gusella JF, Watkins PC, Bruns GAP, St George-Hyslop P, Van Keuren ML, Patterson SP, Pagan S, Kurnit DM, Neve RL (1987) Amyloid β protein gene: cDNA, mRNA distribution, and genetic linkage near the Alzheimer locus. Science 235: 880–884

Tanzi RE, McClatchey AI, Lamperti ED, Villa-Komaroff L, Gusella JF, Neve RL (1988) Protease inhibitor domain encoded by an amyloid protein precursor mRNA associated with Alzheimer's disease. Nature 331: 528–530

Van Broeckhoven C, Genthe AM, Vandenberghe A, Horsthemke B, Backhovens H, Raeymaekers P, Van Hul W, Wehnert A, Gheuens J, Cras P, Bruyland M, Martin J-J, Salbaum M, Multhaup G, Master CL, Beyreuther K, Gurling HMD, Mullan MJ, Holland A, Barton A, Irving N, Williamson R, Richards SJ, Hardy J (1987) Failure of familial Alzheimer's disease to segregate with the A4-amyloid gene in several European families. Nature 329: 153–155

Van Broeckhoven C, Backhovens H, Cruts M, De Winter G, Bruyland M, Cras P, Martin J-J (1992) Mapping of a gene predisposing to early-onset Alzheimer's disease to chromosome 14q24.3. Nature Genet 2: 335–339

van Duinen SG, Castaño EM, Prelli F, Bots GTAB, Luyendijk W, Frangione B (1987) Hereditary cerebral hemorrhage with amyloidosis in patients of Dutch origin is related to Alzheimer disease. Proc Natl Acad Sci USA 84: 5991–5994

Van Nostrand WE, Wagner SL, Suzuki M, Choi BH, Farrow JS, Geddes JW, Cotman CW, Cunningham DD (1989) Protease nexin-II, a potent anti-chymotrypsin, shows identity to amyloid β-protein precursor. Nature 341: 546–549

Weissenbach J, Gyapay F, Dib C, Vignal A, Morisette J, Millasseau P, Vaysseix G, Lathrop M (1992) A second-generation linkage map of the human genome. Nature 359: 794–801

Wisniewski HM, Rabe A, Wisniewski KE (1988) Neuropathology and dementia in people with Down's syndrome In: Davies P, Finch C (eds) Molecular neuropathology of aging. Banbury report. Cold Spring Harbor Laboratory, NY, pp 399–413

Wisniewski T, Ghiso J, Frangione B (1991) Peptides homologous to the amyloid protein of Alzheimer's disease containing a glutamine for glutamic acid substitution have accelerated amyloid fibril formation. Biochem Biophys Res Commun 179: 1247–1254

APP Gene Mutations in Familial Alzheimer's Disease in Sweden

L. Lannfelt*, N. Bogdanovic, J. Johnston, and *R. Cowburn*

Summary

The last few years have seen considerable advances in understanding the pathogenesis of Alzheimer's disease (AD). In 1992, we identified a double mutation in exon 16 of the amyloid precursor protein (APP) gene in two large Swedish AD families that results in a double amino acid substitution at codons 670 and 671. A follow-up genealogical study of these two Swedish 670/671 families has indicated that they are related to a common founder. We recently performed a two-point linkage analysis of this extended pedigree and obtained a lod score of 7.62 at zero recombination. Furthermore, following the death of a demented carrier from this family, we obtained pathological confirmation of the clinical diagnosis of AD in this family. The discovery of the Swedish 670/671 mutation has provided strong evidence that the expression of an altered APP can cause AD and has significantly strengthened the case for the amyloid hypothesis of AD.

Introduction

Alzheimer's disease (AD) is a progressive neurodegenerative disorder for which there are three well-recognised risk factors, namely heredity, Down's syndrome and old age. AD is characterised neuropathologically by the accumulation of neuritic plaques and neurofibrillary tangles as well as by cerebrovascular amyloid deposition and neuronal cell loss. The major component of neuritic plaques and cerebrovascular amyloid is a 39–43 amino acid peptide, termed β-amyloid, which is derived from a larger precursor protein (APP), localised on chromosome 21 (Glenner and Wong 1984). Increasing evidence has led to the hypothesis that an abnormal deposition of β-amyloid initiates the pathological cascade that causes Alzheimer's disease (Hardy and Allsop 1991), as Downs syndrome individuals inevitably develop Alzheimer's disease pathology by the fifth decade as a consequence of an extra copy of the APP gene on chromosome

* Alzheimer's Disease Research Centre, Department of Geriatric Medicine, Huddinge University Hospital, The Karolinska Institute, 14186 Huddinge, Sweden

C.L. Masters et al. (Eds.)
Amyloid Protein Precursor in Development,
Aging and Alzheimer's Disease
© Springer-Verlag Berlin Heidelberg 1994

```
Asn Leu
 ↑  ↑
Lys Met│Asp Ala Glu Phe Arg His Asp Ser Gly Tyr Glu Val His His Gln Lys Leu Val Phe Phe
670 671│


Ala Glu Asp Val Gly Ser Asn Lys Gly Ala Ile Ile Gly Leu Met Val Gly Gly Val Val│Ile Ala Thr

            Ile
             ↑ 717
Val Ile Val
         ↓  ↓
        Gly  Phe
```

Fig. 1. The 40 amino acid residues constituting the β-amyloid amino acid sequence is within the dotted vertical lines, with the codon 670/671 mutations and the codon 717 mutations framing the sequence

21. The central importance of the β-amyloid protein in the pathogenesis of AD has also been strengthened considerably by the identification of mutations in the APP gene that cosegregate with the disease in a number of autosomal dominant AD families. In this chapter, we will describe the background for these developments, with an emphasis on the Swedish APP 670/671 mutation.

Pathogenic Point Mutations in the APP Gene

In 1991, Hardy and co-workers (Goate et al. 1991) identified an English AD family in which the disease cosegregated with chromosome 21 DNA markers. They sequenced the region of the APP gene encoding the β-amyloid peptide and identified a pathogenic point mutation in exon 17. This mutation at codon 717 occurs C-terminal of the β-amyloid fragment and results in an amino acid substitution of valine to isoleucine (Fig. 1). Since then, two other pathogenic point mutations at codon 717 have been identified in other AD families (Chartier-Harlin et al. 1991; Murrell et al. 1991) that result in amino acid substitutions of valine to either glycine or phenylalanine.

The Swedish APP 670/671 Double Mutation

Recently, we identified a double mutation in codon 670/671 of the APP gene in two large Swedish families with early onset familial AD where the disease has an autosomal dominant pattern of inheritance (Mullan et al. 1992a). The mutation co-segregates with the disorder and consists of two base pair transversions (G → T, A → C) in exon 16 of the APP gene. The mutation produces both a lysine to asparagine substitution at codon 670 and a methionine to leucine substitution at codon 671. These substitutions occur N-terminal of β-amyloid at the proposed endosomal/lysosomal cleavage site for APP (Beyreuther and

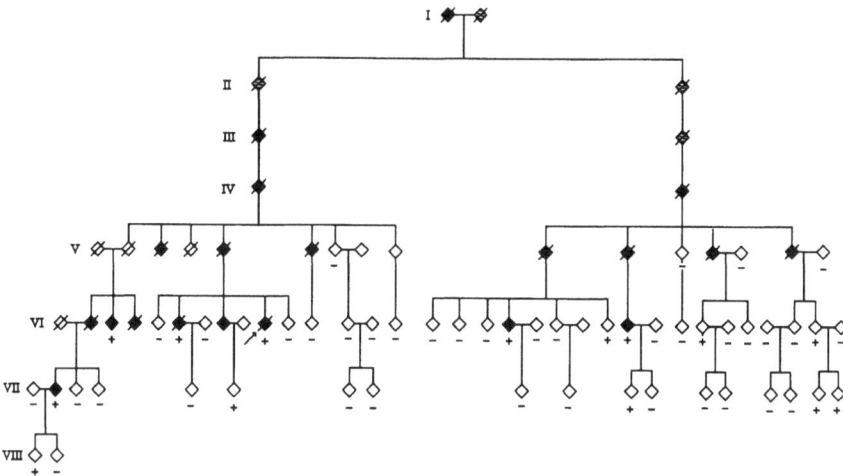

Fig. 2. Disguised and simplified pedigree of the Swedish family with an APP 670/671 mutation showing segregation of the mutation, where + denotes presence and − denotes absence of the mutation. Symbols with a diagonal line represent deceased individuals. Affected individuals are shown as ◆, healthy individuals as ◇ and individuals where clinical information is incomplete as ⬦. Index case, where autopsy has been made, is indicated by an arrow

Masters 1991). The importance of the Swedish APP 670/671 double mutation for the amyloid hypothesis of AD has become evident from recent studies in which the mutations were transfected into cell lines and were shown to result in a greatly enhanced production of β-amyloid, compared to both wild type cells and cells transfected with codon 717 APP mutations (Citron et al. 1992; Cai et al. 1993). Moreover, of the two mutations, the 671 methionine to leucine substitution was sufficient to produce this effect. Taken together, these data have provided a direct link between the familial AD genotype and the clinicopathological genotype of the disorder, although we remain a long way from determining exactly how these APP mutations work to cause AD.

Since our original identification of the Swedish 670/671 families we have carried out genealogical investigations in which we have traced the ancestors back eight generations and have shown that both families are related to a common founder in 1745 (Fig. 2). Subsequent two-point linkage analysis of the extended pedigree has given us a lod score of 7.62 at zero recombination (Table 1). This finding, together with our estimation of 100% penetrance in this family, indicates that the Swedish APP 670/671 mutation is sufficient in itself to cause AD and that the mutation carriers will most likely develop the disease.

The median age of onset in the Swedish 670/671 family is 54 years, with the latest onset age that we have been able to document being 61 years. In individuals with the mutation, death occurs around 60 years of age, and no diseased individual has lived past the age of 69. We are interested in why the

Table 1. Lod scores: APP 670/671 mutation versus AD

	Recombination fraction						
	0.00	0.05	0.10	0.15	0.20	0.30	0.40
Lod scores	7.62	7.00	6.34	5.66	4.95	3.43	1.77

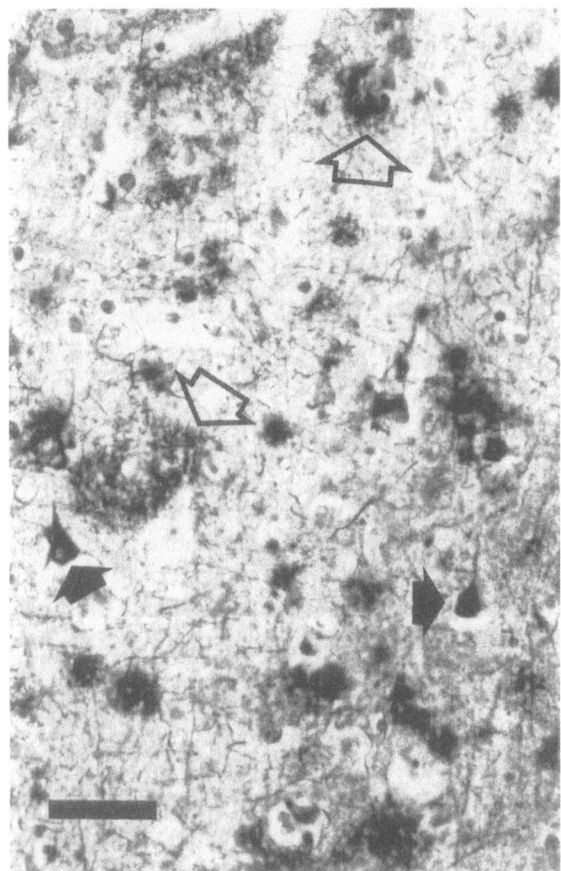

Fig. 3. Silver-impregnated paraffin section (Bielschowsky) through the cortex of supramarginal gyrus showing neurofibrillary tangles in pyramidal cell bodies (solid arrows) and abundance of senile plaques (open arrows) throughout layer III. Bar = 50 μm

Swedish family shows a diverse age of onset for the disease and we are currently investigating factors that may be important.

An important recent finding concerning the significance of the Swedish APP 670/671 mutation has come from the death of a demented carrier from the family. Pathological investigation of the brain of this individual has confirmed the clinical diagnosis of AD for the family. Figure 3 shows the abundance of silver-stained neuritic plaques and neurofibrillary tangles in the cortex of the supramarginal gyrus from this individual. Of the other brain regions that we have studied from this individual, we have found large numbers of neuritic plaques throughout the cortex as well as in the nucleus basalis, hippocampus and cerebellum. Abundant neurofibrillary tangles, but not Lewy bodies, were seen in the hippocampus and cortex.

Screening for the Swedish mutation is easy since the $G \rightarrow T$ transversion in codon 670 removes a MboII restriction site. Using PCR and MboII restriction enzyme digestion we have screened for the APP 670/671 mutation in sufferers from 46 other Swedish families with AD (Lannfelt et al. 1993a). The mutation was found only in the family previously reported and not in the other families that we have identified. Moreover, we have also screened for this and other APP gene mutations in our familial cases through direct sequencing of exons 16 and 17 and by SSCP. Using this approach we have been unable to find either previously reported or novel APP gene mutations in any of our family material (Johnston et al. 1993), thus indicating that APP mutations are a rare cause of familial AD in Sweden.

The ease of screening for the Swedish APP 670/671 mutation has also meant that we are able to perform presymptomatic testing for family individuals at risk of developing the disorder. Three individuals have so far asked for information about their status, and we are building up medical and psychological competence for taking care of them.

Search for new AD Genes

The realisation that APP mutations are a rare cause of familial AD in Sweden (Lannfelt et al. 1993a; Johnston et al. 1993), together with the knowledge that the disease is genetically heterogeneous, has stimulated us to look for new AD genes in our Swedish family material. Following the reports of chromosome 14 linkage in several early onset AD families (Schellenberg et al. 1992; St. George-Hyslop et al. 1992; Mullan et al. 1992b; Van Broeckhoven et al. 1992), we have screened our families with five chromosome 14 microsatellite markers. In both our early and late onset families we found significantly negative lod scores, indicating a lack of linkage to chromosome 14 (Lannfelt et al. 1993b). Significantly negative lod scores were also obtained for the chromosome 21 marker D21S210 closely linked to the APP gene, in both early and late onset families. These data, taken together with that demonstrating chromosome 19 linkage in late onset AD families (Pericak Vance et al. 1991), indicate that there may be at least five genes involved in the aetiology of AD, namely the APP and perhaps another gene on chromosome 21, genes on chromosome 14 and 19 and a gene elsewhere in the genome. The goal for the future will be to identify these genes and to determine whether they cause AD by affecting expression and metabolism of APP. This remains the "acid test" of the amyloid hypothesis of AD (Hardy 1992).

References

Beyreuther K, Masters C (1991) Amyloid precursor protein (APP) and βA4 amyloid in the etiology of Alzheimer's disease: precursor-product relationship in the derangement of neuronal function. Brain Pathol 1:241–251

Cai X-D, Golde TE, Younkin SM (1993) Release of excess amyloid β protein precursor. Science 259:514–516

Chartier-Harlin M-C, Crawford F, Houlden H, Warren A, Hughes D, Fidani L, Goate A, Rossor M, Roques P, Hardy J, Mullan M (1991) Early-onset Alzheimer's disease caused by mutations at codon 717 of the β-amyloid precursor protein gene. Nature 353:844–846

Citron M, Oltersdorf T, Haass C, McConlogue L, Hung AY, Seubert P, Vigo-Pelfrey C, Lieberburg I, Selkoe D (1992) Mutation of the β-amyloid precursor protein in familial Alzheimer's disease increases β-protein production. Nature 360:672–674

Glenner GG, Wong CW (1984) Alzheimer's disease: Initial report of the purification and characterization of a novel cerebrovascular amyloid protein. Biochem Biophys Res Commun 120:885–890

Goate A, Chartier-Harlin M-C, Mullan M, Brown J, Crawford F, Fidani L, Giuffra L, Haynes A, Irving N, James L, Mant R, Newton P, Rooke K, Roques P, Talbot C, Pericak-Vance M, Roses A, Williamson R, Rossor M, Owen M, Hardy J (1991) Segregation of a missense mutation in the amyloid precursor protein gene with familial Alzheimer's disease. Nature 349:704–706

Hardy J (1992) The genetics of Alzheimer's Disease. Neurosci Facts 3:365

Hardy J, Allsop D (1991) Amyloid deposition as the central event in the aetiology of Alzheimer's disease. Trends Phamacol 12:383–388

Johnston J, Lilius L, Axelman K, Cowburn R, Viitanen M, Winblad B, Lannfelt L (1993) Sequencing of exons 16 and 17 of the β-amyloid precursor protein gene tails to identify new mutations in Swedish Alzheimer's disease patients. Hum Mol Genet 2:1045–1046

Lannfelt L, Viitanen M, Johansson K, Axelman K, Lilius L, Almqvist E, Winblad, B (1993a) Low frequency of the APP 670/671 mutation in familial Alzheimer's disease in Sweden. Neurosci Lett 153:85–87a

Lannfelt L, Lilius L, Appelgren H, Axelman K, Forsell C, Liu L, Johansson K, Graff C (1993b) No linkage to chromosome 14 in Swedish Alzheimer's disease families. Nature Genet 4:218–219b

Mullan M, Crawford F, Axelman K, Houlden H, Lilius L, Winblad B, Lannfelt L (1992a) A pathogenic mutation for probable Alzheimer's disease in the APP gene at the N-terminus of β-amyloid. Nature Genet 1:345–347a

Mullan M, Houlden H, Windelspecht M, Fidani L, Lombardi C, Diaz P, Rossor M, Crook R, Hardy J, Duff K, Crawford F (1992b) A locus for familial early onset Alzheimer's disease on the long arm of chromosome 14, proximal to α₁-antichymotrypsin. Nature Genet 2:340–342

Murrell J, Farlow M, Ghetti B, Benson MD (1991) A mutation in the amyloid precursor protein associated with hereditary Alzheimer's disease. Science 254:97–99

Pericak-Vance MA, Bebout JL, Gaskell PC, Yamaoka LH, Hung WY, Alberts MJ, Walker AP, Bartlett RJ, Haynes CA, Welsh KA, Earl NL, Heyman A, Clark CM, Roses AD (1991) Linkage studies in familial Alzheimer's disease: Evidence for chromosome 19 linkage. Am J Human Genet 48:1034–1050

Schellenberg GD, Bird TD, Wijsman EM, Orr HT, Anderson L, Nemens E, White JA, Bonnycastle L, Weber JL, Alonso ME, Potter H, Heston LL, Martin GM (1992) Genetic linkage evidence for familial Alzheimer's disease locus on chromosome 14. Science 258:668–671

Selkoe DJ (1991) The molecular pathology Alzheimer's disease. Neuron 6:487–498
St George-Hyslop P, Haines J, Rogaev E, Mortilla M, Vaula G, Pericak-Vance M, Foncin J-F, Montesi M, Bruni A, Sorbi S, Rainero I, Pinessi L, Pollen D, Polinsky R, Nee L, Kennedy J, Macciardi F, Rogaeva E, Liang Y, Alexandrova N, Lukiwi W, Schlumpf K, Tanzi R, Tsuda T, Farrer L, Cantu J-M, Duara R, Amaducci L, Bergamini L, Gusella J, Roses A, Crapper McLachlan D (1992) Genetic evidence for a novel familial Alzheimer's disease locus on chromosome 14. Nature Genet 2:330–334
Van Broeckhoven C, Backhovens H, Cruts M, De Winter G, Bruyland M, Cras P, Martin J-J (1992) Mapping of a gene predisposing to early-onset Alzheimer's disease to chromosome 14q24.3. Nature Genet 2:335–339

Aging, Energy and Alzheimer's Disease

*A. C. Bowling** and *M. F. Beal*

Summary

The most important risk factor for Alzheimer's disease (AD) is increasing age. However, the mechanism by which increasing age contributes to an increase in risk is unknown. One possibility is that a decline in oxidative phosphorylation may occur due to progressive impairment of mitochondrial function. Mitochondrial DNA is particularly susceptible to oxidative damage due to its lack of protective histones, its limited repair mechanisms, and its close relationship to the inner mitochondrial membrane, where free radicals are generated. Consistent with these findings, we and others have found progressive increases in mitochondrial deletions with normal aging in human postmortem brain tissue. The increase in deletions is most marked in the putamen, whereas the cerebellum, which has a lower metabolic rate, shows fewer deletions. We also made direct measurements of oxidative damage to both mitochondrial and nuclear DNA in human postmortem brain tissue. We measured the amounts of 8-hydroxy-2-deoxyguanosine, one of approximately 20 modified bases which occur following oxidative damage to DNA. These measurements showed progressive increases in oxidative damage to both nuclear and mitochondrial DNA with aging in human brain. A key issue is whether these changes are accompanied by any functional changes. Prior studies showed a progressive decrease in mitochondrial complex I and complex IV activity with normal aging in human muscle biopsies. We examined the activity of the mitochondrial oxidative phosphorylation enzymes in cortical tissue of 20 rhesus monkeys across the life span of this species. These studies showed a progressive decline in complex I and complex IV activity with normal aging, yet complex II–III and complex V activities were unaffected. This finding is consistent with the observation that several functionally important complex I and complex IV subunits are encoded by mitochondrial DNA, whereas complex II–III subunits are mostly encoded by nuclear DNA. In collaborative studies, we found a small number of point mutations in mitochondrial DNA in Alzheimer's disease patients, which may exacerbate age-related declines in activity of mitochondrial enzymes. We

---

* Neurology Service, Neurochemistry Laboratory, Massachusetts General Hospital, Boston, MA 02114, USA

C.L. Masters et al. (Eds.)
Amyloid Protein Precursor in Development,
Aging and Alzheimer's Disease
© Springer-Verlag Berlin Heidelberg 1994

hypothesize that such declines in mitochondrial enzyme activity may facilitate excitotoxicity or other pathologic processes. In the context of AD, impaired mitochondrial function may lead to increased generation of free radicals, which may oxidize β-amyloid and enhance its aggregation. This may also produce a form of β-amyloid which is neurotoxic. We have examined the effects of intracortical injections of β-amyloid or control peptides in both young and old rhesus monkeys. Although β-amyloid was not toxic in young monkeys, it produced neurotoxic effects in old monkeys. Age-related declines in energy metabolism may therefore serve as an important risk factor for amyloid deposition and toxicity in AD.

Introduction

The most important risk factor for Alzheimer's disease (AD) is advancing age. The incidence and prevalence of AD increase steeply with age after age 60, with one study showing a prevalence of 47% in patients over age 85 (Evans et al. 1989). One theory to account for the age-dependent onset of degenerative diseases such as AD is that mitochondrial dysfunction may hasten neuronal death (Linnane et al. 1989; Miquel 1991; Wallace 1992). It has been proposed that the accumulation of mitochondrial genome mutations during life results in a progressive impairment of oxidative phosphorylation. The rate of mutations in mitochondrial DNA is about ten times greater than that in chromosomal DNA (Linnane et al. 1989). A high rate of mutation has been suggested by extensive restriction fragment polymorphism among individual human beings (Brown et al. 1979). Furthermore, mutations in mitochondrial DNA are more likely to have functional consequences since mitochondrial DNA has no non-coding sequences, except for a small segment involved in the replication of mitochondrial DNA.

Age-Associated Changes in Mitochondrial Function

Mitochondria in different tissues exhibit different sizes, shapes, and densities (Wallace 1986). Each mitochondrion consists of an outer membrane, an inner membrane, and the matrix, which is the space enclosed by the inner membrane. The tricarboxylic acid cycle occurs in the matrix, whereas oxidative phosphorylation occurs on the inner membrane. Five different protein complexes catalyze oxidative phosphorylation: complex I (NADH: ubiquinone oxidoreductase), complex II (succinate: ubiquinol oxidoreductase), complex III (ubiquinol: cytochrome c oxidoreductase), complex IV (cytochrome c oxidase), and complex V (ATP synthase). The electron transport chain consists of complexes I, II, III, and IV. Each mitochondrion also contains mitochondrial DNA, which is a circular molecule that encodes for 22 tRNA molecules, two rRNA molecules, and 13 polypeptides, including seven complex I subunits, one complex III subunit, three complex IV subunits, and two complex V subunits. The remaining subunits of the oxidative phosphorylation system are encoded by nuclear DNA.

Previous studies in brain as well as other tissues have indicated that there may be an age-related impairment of mitochondrial energy metabolism. In rat brain, aging has been associated with reduced respiratory activity in intact mitochondria (Harmon et al. 1987) and reduced complex IV activity (Curti et al. 1990). In aged rat muscle, one study demonstrated reduced activities of complexes I and IV and no change in complex II–III activity (Torii et al. 1992). In humans, previous studies have shown reduced state 3 and state 4 respiration in liver mitochondria (Yen et al. 1989), increased numbers of complex IV-deficient myocytes in skeletal and cardiac muscle (Muller-Hocker 1989), and reduced activities of several electron transport chain complexes in skeletal muscle mitochondria (Trounce et al. 1989; Cooper et al. 1992).

Due to the lack of information regarding age-associated changes in oxidative phosphorylation in brain tissue from primates, we examined the activities of the enzymes that catalyze oxidative phosphorylation in frontoparietal cortex of 20 rhesus monkeys with a wide range of ages (5–34 years old; Bowling et al. 1993). These studies demonstrated a significant negative correlation of enzyme activity with age for complexes I and IV; no significant age-associated changes in activity were observed for complexes II–III and V. The activities of complexes I and IV were both reduced by 22% in the oldest monkeys (30.7 $\pm$ 0.9 years) relative to the youngest monkeys (6.9 $\pm$ 0.9 years).

Free Radicals, Oxidative Damage, and Mitochondrial Function

One possible mechanism by which mitochondrial energy metabolism may become impaired is through free radical-induced oxidative damage. Mitochondrial oxidative phosphorylation generates most of the free radicals in the cell, and mitochondrial DNA is particularly susceptible to oxidative damage (Richter et al. 1988). The respiratory chain components that make the greatest contribution to production of free radicals are ubiquinone and cytochrome b_{566} of complex III (Cadenas et al. 1977; Nohl et al. 1978; Nohl and Hegner 1978). An increase in production of superoxide radicals by cytochrome b_{566} occurs with normal aging (Nohl 1986). In the presence of specific inhibitors of the electron transport chain, the generation of superoxide is increased (Turrens and Boveris 1980).

The vulnerability of the mitochondrial DNA to oxidative damage may be due to its limited repair mechanisms (Clayton et al. 1974), its lack of protective histones, and its close proximity to the inner mitochondrial membrane, where reactive oxygen species are generated (Linnane et al. 1989; Miguel 1991; Wallace 1992). Recent studies have demonstrated the presence of an age-dependent deletion between nucleotide positions 8470 and 13459 of the mitochondrial genome (Linnane et al. 1990; Cortopassi and Arnheim 1990; Simonetta et al.

1992). In the heart, the deletion has been detected in individuals starting at age 30 and increases exponentially with advancing age (Hattori et al. 1991; Corral-Debrinski et al. 1991). A recent quantitative study showed that the deletion was estimated at 3% and 9% in patients aged 80 and 90, respectively (Sugiyama et al. 1991). Furthermore, deletions are much more frequent in patients with ischemic heart disease (Corral-Debrinski et al. 1991). We and others have recently shown that there are marked increases in the deletion in human postmortem brain tissue with normal aging (Corral-Debrinski et al. 1992; Soong et al. 1992). The most marked increases were in the putamen, where as much as 12% of the mitochondrial DNA exhibited the mutation in a 97-year old. Intermediate levels of the deletion were found in cerebral cortex, and low levels in cerebellum, consistent with a lower rate of metabolism in the cerebellum. This finding is consistent with the suggestion that patients with defects in oxidative phosphorylation generate increased amounts of oxygen free radicals which result in mitochondrial DNA damage (Linnane et al. 1989).

Several studies show that 8-hydroxy-2-deoxyguanosine is a biomarker of oxidative DNA damage (Shigenaga et al. 1990). Of 13 base adducts formed after exposing purified mammalian chromatin to ionizing-radiation-generated free radicals, 8-hydroxy-2-deoxyguanosine is the most frequent (Dizdaroglu 1991). Several studies indicate that 8-hydroxy-2-deoxyguanosine most frequently codes correctly for cytosine, but also has the monospecific mutagenic ability to pair with adenine about 1% of the time (Kuchino et al. 1987; Cheng et al. 1992; Wood et al. 1990; Shibutani et al. 1991). It also results in misreading at adjacent residues (Kuchino et al. 1987). Inhibitors of the electron transport chain increase the amount of 8-hydroxy-2-deoxyguanosine in mitochondrial DNA (Hayakawa et al. 1991a). Concentrations of 8-hydroxy-2-deoxyguanosine increase with normal aging in several rat tissues and in mitochondrial DNA isolated from human diaphragm and heart muscle (Fraga et al. 1990; Hayakawa et al. 1991b, 1992). In heart muscle, the amount of mitochondrial deletions correlates with 8-hydroxy-2-deoxyguanosine concentrations in mitochondrial DNA (Hayakawa et al. 1992).

We have examined oxidative damage to mitochondrial DNA and nuclear DNA in human post mortem brain tissue (Mecocci et al. 1993). In this study, we determined that the amount of 8-hydroxy-2-deoxyguanosine showed an age-related increase with age in the mitochondrial DNA and nuclear DNA. Also, the levels of 8-hydroxy-2-deoxyguanosine were 10 times greater in the mitochondrial DNA than in the nuclear DNA. Age-related increases were much more marked in the mitochondrial DNA than in the nuclear DNA.

In addition to mitochondrial DNA damage, aging has also been associated with oxidative damage to proteins (Stadtman 1992). In post mortem brain tissue, protein oxidative damage increases with age (Smith et al. 1991; Stadtman 1992). The protein complexes involved in oxidative phosphorylation may be parti-cularly susceptible to oxidative damage since free radicals are generated by oxi-dative phosphorylation and free radical levels may thereby be especially elev-ated near the mitochondrial inner membrane. Studies with submitochondrial particles have demonstrated differential vulnerability to reactive oxygen species of the complexes involved in oxidative phosphorylation (Zhang et al. 1990). Complex I was particularly sensitive to hydroxyl radical and superoxide anion; only limited studies were conducted with complex IV. Studies of *in vivo* peroxidative stress induced by 2-cyclohexene-1-one indicate that complex IV is the most vulnerable but that complexes I and II are also significantly affected (Benzi et al. 1991, 1992).

Like reactive oxygen species, nitric oxide may interact with oxidative phosphorylation complexes to reduce activity. While nitric oxide regulates vasodilation and may play a role in mediating glutamate toxicity, it also inhibits complexes I and II and the mitochondrial matrix enzyme aconitase (Hibbs et al. 1988; Stadler et al. 1991). The effects of nitric oxide on these mitochondrial enzymes may be due to an interaction with iron-sulfur prosthetic groups to produce inactive iron-nitric oxide complexes. Nitric oxide may also react with superoxide to produce peroxynitrite anion, a free radical generator (Beckman et al. 1990). However, the significance of peroxynitrite is not clear at this time since the superoxide-induced formation of peroxynitrite may actually be a mechanism for inactivating nitric oxide (Oury et al. 1992).

Finally, peroxidative damage to lipids in brain also increases with age (Tappel 1973). The mitochondrial membrane lipid composition undergoes changes with aging, with cardiolipin exhibiting a decrease in content in mitochondria from aged rat heart and brain (Paradies and Ruggiero 1990; Ruggiero et al. 1992). Several of the oxidative phosphorylation complexes are sensitive to the lipids in the environment, especially cardiolipin (Fry and Green 1980, 1981). Also, since the proteins of the oxidative phosphorylation system are located in the inner mitochondrial membrane, these proteins may be more vulnerable than matrix proteins to free radicals generated by lipids.

The fact that the oxidative phosphorylation system itself generates free radicals, and that the mitochondrial DNA encodes for polypeptides involved in oxidative phosphorylation, allows for several possible cycling mechanisms that may produce slowly progressive impairment of mitochondrial function. A minor defect in oxidative phosphorylation may produce mildly increased levels of free radicals, which may then damage mitochondrial DNA, proteins, and lipids, resulting in a more impaired oxidative phosphorylation system that may generate even greater levels of free radicals. In this manner, a defect in oxidative phosphorylation that is initially minor may become amplified over time. In addition, different genetic and environmental factors that influence oxidative damage and mitochondrial function may result in variable rates of amplification in different individuals, and thereby produce variable degrees of impairment of oxidative phosphorylation with age. Finally, these cycling mechanisms suggest that defects in mitochondrial function and defects that increase oxidative damage may share a final common pathway that results in cell death.

Evidence for Impaired Energy Metabolism in AD

The largest body of evidence suggesting an impairment of energy metabolism in AD has come from studies of glucose metabolism using positron emission tomography. The major difficulty with these studies is determining whether alterations play a role in the disease process or are merely secondary to neuronal loss. Studies of cerebral blood flow, oxygen utilization and glucose metabolism show consistent decreases in AD in a temporo-parietal pattern (Haxby et al. 1986). Comparisons of patients with early and more advanced dementia showed that a substantial decrease in cerebral glucose metabolism may precede cognitive impairment. Several reports showed reduced glucose transport in microvessels of AD patients (Kalaria and Harik 1989); however, this does not appear to be sufficient to account for the decrease in glucose metabolism (Jagust et al. 1991).

Additional studies by Hoyer (1993) suggest that an impairment of energy metabolism occurs in AD. He examined the cerebral metabolic rates of oxygen, CO_2, glucose, and lactate using a modified Kety-Schmidt technique. In these studies AD patients showed decreased oxygen and glucose utilization, and decreased ATP production. Neurochemical studies have also suggested that energy metabolism may be impaired in AD. Sims and colleagues (1983) studied cerebral biopsies and found that the adenylate energy charge was unchanged, but oxygen uptake was significantly increased under conditions of submaximal metabolic activity, consistent with uncoupling of mitochondrial energy metabolism. This result, however, is not consistent with a defect in electron transport, which would result in decreased oxygen uptake.

Electron microscopic studies of cortical biopsies in AD show abnormal mitochondria with increased matrix density and paracrystalline inclusions in the intercristal space (Saraiva et al. 1985). This finding is of interest due to the observation of paracrystalline inclusions in the mitochondria of patients with known mitochondrial diseases. Mitochondrial dysfunction is also suggested by studies showing 70–100% reductions in activity of the thiamine-dependent mitochondrial enzymes pyruvate dehydrogenase and 2-ketoglutarate dehydrogenase (Gibson et al. 1988; Sorbi et al. 1983). Parker and colleagues (1990) reported a deficiency in cytochrome oxidase (complex IV) activity in mitochondria isolated from AD platelets. A recent study showed reduced cytochrome oxidase activity in several cortical regions in AD postmortem brain tissue (Kish et al. 1992). Paradoxically, however, an increase in expression of cytochrome oxidase subunit 3 mRNA was reported in AD brain (Albert et al. 1992). An increase in expression could occur as a compensatory response to an electron transport chain defect. The biochemical studies to date are inconsistent; some studies suggest uncoupling of mitochondria, whereas other studies indicate electron transport chain enzyme deficits or defects in tricarboxylic acid cycle enzymes.

The role of point mutations in mitochondrial DNA in AD has recently been examined. It was reported that point mutations in subunit 2 of NADH dehydrogenase may be associated with AD (Lin et al. 1992). This point muta-tion, however, was subsequently reported to be a normal polymorphism (Pet-ruzzella et al. 1992; Shoffner et al. 1993). Shoffner and colleagues, however, found three point mutations in mitochondrial DNA of patients with either AD, Parkinson's disease (PD) or AD with PD (Shoffner et al. 1993). The most frequent was a tRNA^{Gln} gene mutation found in 5.2% of patients, but only 0.7% of Caucasian controls. An ND1 point mutation in an evolutionarily highly conserved region was found in two unrelated patients who had AD with PD. A third mutation was an insertion in the 12s rRNA gene. The significance of these mutations remains to be clarified, but they may be analogous to the situation in Leber's disease, in which some mutations are high risk factors for the illness whereas others increase one's risk but are not sufficient by themselves to cause the illness (Brown et al. 1992).

Increases in protein oxidation products (carbonyl groups) occur in aged controls and AD brain samples as compared with young controls (Smith et al. 1991). The activity of glutamine synthetase is particularly susceptible to free radical damage. There is a loss of enzyme activity with normal aging in gerbil brain (Floyd 1991). In AD, there is a significant decrease in activity in the frontal pole but not in the occipital pole as compared with age-matched controls (Smith et al. 1991). This finding has been interpreted as supporting increased oxidative damage in AD. There is also evidence that lipid peroxidation is increased in AD cerebral cortex (Hajimohammadreza and Brammer 1990; Subbaro et al. 1990).

Regional Localization of Cytochrome Oxidase

Recent studies of Chandrasekaran and colleagues (1992a) have examined the ·localization of cytochrome oxidase activity and cytochrome oxidase mRNA in the hippocampus and entorhinal cortex of monkey brain. Within the hippocam-pal formation, the terminal field of the perforant pathway showed the highest levels of cytochrome oxidase activity while cytochrome oxidase subunit 2 (COX II) mRNA was mainly localized to neuronal cell bodies. Within the entorhinal cortex COX II mRNA was particularly high in layers II and IV, which are known to be predisposed to neurofibrillary tangle formation in AD. In the hippocampus COX II mRNA was particularly high in the CA3 and CA1 regions. The expression of mRNAs for mitochondrially encoded cytochrome oxidase subunits is higher in frontal pole, as well as association cortex, as compared to primary visual and somatosensory cortex (Chandrasekaran et al. 1992b). More recently cytochrome oxidase activity and COX II mRNA were localized in the perirhinal and superior temporal sulci of rhesus monkey brain (Chandrasekaran et al. 1993). Cytochrome oxidase activity was highest in layers I and IV, whereas COX II mRNA was localized to cell bodies. In the perirhinal region, COX II mRNA was found in cell bodies of layers III and V–VÍ. A similar distribution was found in the superior temporal cortex. Therefore, these studies show that COX II mRNA is preferentially localized to layer 2 and 4 neurons in the entorhinal cortex and in those involved in cortico-cortical connections in superior temporal cortex. These neurons are known to be particularly vulnerable to neurofibrillary tangle formation in AD.

Amyloid and Energy Metabolism

An interesting issue is whether defects in energy metabolism could play either a primary or secondary role in the pathogenesis of AD. A defect in energy metabolism may lead to the production of free radicals by mitochondria as discussed above. In this circumstance several amino acid residues of β-amyloid may be oxidized, leading to increased aggregability of amyloid (Dyrks et al. 1992). A progressive decline in energy metabolism associated with normal aging could therefore play a crucial role in amyloid deposition.

The potential neurotoxic role of amyloid is much more speculative. We and others had demonstrated that β-amyloid can exert neurotoxic effects in vivo (Kowall et al. 1992). However, whether this has any relevance to the pathogensis of AD is unclear. The distribution of neurofibrillary tangles in AD does not bear any close relationship to the distribution of amyloid deposition. Nevertheless, both in vitro and in vivo studies show that amyloid, particularly in its aggregated state, can exert neurotoxic effects. Interestingly, these neurotoxic effects are worsened by energy deprivation in vitro (Copani et al. 1991). In cell culture, amyloid also enhances glutamate neurotoxicity (Koh et al. 1990; Mattson et al. 1992).

We examined the effects of injections of β-amyloid or reverse peptide in both young adult and aged rhesus monkeys (Kowall et al. 1992). In the young adult monkeys, we found that β-amyloid injections produced some neuronal toxicity, however, no Alz-50 or thioflavin positive lesions were observed. In contrast, in aged primates the cortex surrounding the β (1–40) lesions contained argyrophilic, thioflavin S fluorescent, Alz 50, and ubiquitin immunoreactive perikaryal and neuritic alterations. The morphologies of these alterations closely resembled those associated with AD in human brains.

Therefore, these studies show that aged as opposed to young primate cerebral cortex is vulnerable to neurotoxic effects of β-amyloid, which results in lesions which show many characteristic features of AD. We hypothesize that the increased vulnerability of these aged monkeys may be a consequence of the decline in energy metabolism which accompanies normal aging.

Conclusion

The studies discussed above show that mitochondrial DNA is particularly susceptible to free radical damage. An increase in oxidative damage to mitochondrial DNA occurs with normal aging. A consequence of this may be a decrease in the activity of specific complexes of the oxidative phosphorylation system. This decline in functional activity may play a crucial role in enhancing the neurotoxicity of both glutamate and β-amyloid. As a result, the deterioration in mitochondrial energy metabolism which occurs with normal aging may play a role in the age-dependent incidence of AD.

References

Alberts MJ, Ioannu P, Deucher R, Gilbert J, Lee J, Middleton L, Roses AD (1992) Isolation of a cytochrome oxidase gene overexpressed in Alzheimer's disease brain. Mol Cell Neurosci 3:461–470

Beckman JJ, Beckman TW, Chen J, Marshall PA, Freeman BA (1990) Apparent hydroxyl radical production by peroxynitrite: implications for endothelial injury from nitric oxide and superoxide. Proc Natl Acad Sci USA 87:1620–1624

Benzi G, Curti D, Pastoris O, Marzatico F, Villa RF, Dagani F (1991) Sequential damage in mitochondrial complexes by peroxidative stress. Neurochem Res 16:1295–1302

Benzi G, Pastoris O, Marzatico F, Villa RF, Daggani F, Curti D (1992) The mitochondrial electron transfer alteration as a factor involved in the brain aging. Neurobiol Aging 13:361–368

Bowling AC, Mutisya EM, Walker LC, Price DL, Cork LC, Beal MF (1993) Age-dependent impairment of mitochondrial function in primate brain. J Neurochem 60:1964–1967

Brown MD, Voljavec AS, Lott MT, MacDonald I, Wallace DC (1992) Leber's hereditary optic neuropathy: a model for mitochondrial neurodegenerative diseases. FASEB J 6:2791–2799

Brown WM, George MJR, Wilson AC (1979) Rapid evolution of animal mitochondrial DNA. Proc Natl Acad Sci USA 76:1967–1971

Cadenas E, Boveris A, Ragan CI, Stoppani AOM (1977) Production of superoxide radicals and hydrogen peroxide by NADH-ubiquinone reductase and ubiquinol-cytochrome c reductase from beef heart mitochondria. Arch Biochem Biophys 180:248–257

Chandrasekaran K, Stoll J, Brady DR, Rappoport SI (1992a) Localization of cytochrome oxidase (COX) activity and COX mRNA in the hippocampus and entorhinal cortex of the monkey brain: correlation with specific neuronal pathways. Brain Res 579:333–356

Chandrasekaran K, Stoll J, Giordano T, Atack JR, Matocha MF, Brady DR, Rapoport SI (1992b) Differential expression of cytochrome oxidase genes in different regions of monkey brain. J Neurosci Res 32:415–523

Chandrasekaran K, Stoll J, Rapoport ST, Brady DR (1993) Localization of cytochrome oxidase (COX) activity and COX mRNA in the perirhinal and superior temporal sulci of the monkey brain. Brain Res 606:213–219

Cheng KC, Cahill DS, Kasai H, Nishimura S, Loeb LA (1992) 8-hydroxy-2-deoxyguanosine, an abundant form of oxidative DNA damage causes G—T and A—C substitutions. J Biol Chem 267:166–172

Clayton DA, Doda JN, Freiberg EC (1974) The absence of a pyrimidine dimer repair mechanism in mammalian mitochondria. Proc Natl Acad Sci USA 71:2777–2781

Cooper JM, Mann VM, Schapira AHV (1992) Analyses of mitochondrial respiratory chain function and mitochondrial DNA deletion in human skeletal muscle: effect of aging. J Neurol Sci 13:91–98

Copani A, Koh J-Y, Cotman CW (1991) β-Amyloid increases neuronal susceptibility to injury by glucose deprivation. Neuro Report 2:763–765

Corral-Debrinski M, Stepien G, Shoffner JM, Lott MT, Kanter K, Wallace DC (1991) Hypoxemia is associated with mitochondrial DNA damage and gene induction: implications for cardiac disease. JAMA 1991; 266:1812–1816

Corral-Debrinski M, Horton T, Lott MT, Shoffner JM, Beal MF, Wallace DW (1992) Mitochondrial deletions in human brain: regional variability and increase with advanced age. Nature Genetics 2:324–329

Cortopassi GA, Arnheim N (1990) Detection of a specific mitochondrial DNA deletion in tissues of older humans. Nucleic Acids Res 18:6927–6933

Curti D, Giangare MC, Redolfi ME, Fugaccia I, Benzi G (1990) Age-related modifications of cytochrome c oxidase activity in discrete brain regions. Mech Aging Dev 55:171–180

Dizdaroglu M (1991) Chemical determination of free radical-induced damage to DNA. Free Radical Biol Med 10:225–242

Dyrks T, Dyrks E, Hartmann T, Masters C, Beyreuther K (1992) Amyloidogenicity of βA4 and βA4-bearing amyloid protein precursor fragments by metal-catalyzed oxidation. J Biol Chem 267:18210–19217

Evans DA, Funkenstein HH, Albert MS, Scher PA, Cook NR, Chown MJK, Hebert LE, Henneken SCH, Taylor JO (1989) Prevalence of Alzheimer's disease in a community population of older persons. JAMA 262:2551–2556

Floyd RA (1991) Oxidative damage to behavior during aging. Science 254:1597

Fraga CG, Shigenaga MK, Park J-W, Degan P, Ames BN (1990) Oxidative damage to DNA during aging: 8-hydroxy-2-deoxyguanosine in rat organ DNA and urine. Proc Natl Acad Sci 87:4533–4537

Fry M, Green DE (1980) Cardiolipin requirement by cytochrome oxidase and the catalytic role of phospholipid. Biochem Biophys Res Commun 93:1238–1246

Fry M, Green DE (1981) Cardiolopin requirement for electron transfer in complex I and III of the mitochondrial respiratory chain. J Biol Chem 256:1874–1880

Gibson GE, Sheu K-FR, Blass JP, Baker A, Carlson KC, Harding B, Perrino P (1988) Reduced activities of thiamine-dependent enzymes in the brains and peripheral tissues of patients with Alzheimer's disease. Arch Neurol 45:836–840

Hajimohammadreza I, Brammer M (1990) Brain membrane fluidity and lipid peroxidation in Alzheimer's disease. Neurosci Lett 112:333–337

Harmon HJ, Nank S, Floyd RA (1987) Age-dependent changes in rat brain mitochondria of synaptic and non-synaptic origins. Mech Agin Dev 38:167–177

Hattori K, Tanaka M, Sugiyama S, Obayash T, Ito T, Satake T, Hanaki Y, Asai J, Nagano M, Ozawa T (1991) Age-dependent increase in deleted mitochondrial DNA in the human heart: possible contributory factor to presbycardia. Am Heart J 121:1735–1742

Haxby JV, Grady CL, Duara R, Schlageter N, Berg G, Rapoport SI (1986) Neocortical metabolic abnormalites precede non-memory cognitive deficits in early Alzheimer type dementia. Arch Neurol 43·882–885

Hayakawa M, Ogawa T, Sugiyama S, Tanaka M, Ozawa T (1991a) Massive conversion of guanosine to 8-hydroxy-2-deoxyguanosine in mouse liver mitochondrial DNA by administration of azidothymidine. Biochem Biophys Res Comm 176:87–93

Hayakawa M, Torii K, Sugiyama S, Tanaka M, Ozawa T (1991b) Age-associated accumulation of 8-hydroxy-2-deoxyguanosine in mitochondrial DNA of human diaphragm. Biochem Biophys Res Comm 179:1023–1029

Hayakawa M, Hattori K, Sugiyama S, Ozawa T (1992) Age-associated oxygen damage and mutations in mitochondrial DNA in human hearts. Biochem Biophys Res Comm 189:979–985

Hibbs JB, Taintor RR, Vavrin Z, Rachlin EM (1988) Nitric oxide: a cytotoxic activated macrophage effector molecule. Biochem Biophys Res Commun 157:87–94

Hoyer S (1993) Intermediary metabolism disturbance in AD/SDAT and its relation to molecular events. Prog Neuro-Psychopharmacol Biol Psychiat 17:199–225

Jagust WJ, Seab JP, Huesman RH, Valk PE, Mathis CA, Reed BR, Coxson PG, Budinger TF (1991) Diminished glucose transport in Alzheimer's disease: dynamic PET studies. J Cereb Blood Flow Metab 11:323–330

Kalaria RN, Harik SI (1989) Reduced glucose transporter at the blood-brain barrier and in cerebral cortex in Alzheimer disease. J Neurochem 53:1083–1088

Kish SJ, Bergeron C, Rajput A, Dozic S, Mastrogiacomo F, Chang LJ, Wilson JM, DiStefano LM, Nobrega JN (1992) Brain cytochrome oxidase in Alzheimer's disease. J Neurochem 59:776–779

Koh J-Y, Yang LL, Cotman CW (1990) β-Amyloid protein increases the vulnerability of cultured cortical neurons to excitotoxic damage. Brain Res 533:315–320

Kowall NW, McKee AC, Yankner BA, Beal MF (1992) In vivo neurotoxicity of beta-amyloid [β(1–40)] and the β(25–35) fragments. Neurobiol Aging 13:537–542

Kuchino Y, Mori F, Kasai H, Inoue H, Iwai S, Miura K, Ohtsuka E, Nishimura S (1987) Misreading of DNA templates containing 8-hydroxy-2-deoxyguanosine at the modified base and at the adjacent residues. Nature 327:77–79

Lin F-H, Lin R, Wisniewski HM, Hwang Y-W, Grundke-Iqbal I, Healy-Louie G, Iqbal K (1992) Detection of point mutations in codon 331 of mitochondrial NADH dehydrogenase subunit 2 in Alzheimer's brains. Biochem Biophys Res Comm 182:238–246

Linnane AW, Marzuki S, Ozawa T, Tanaka M (1989) Mitochondrial DNA mutations as an important contribution to aging and degenerative diseases. Lancet i: 642–645

Linnane AW, Baumer A, Maxwell RJ, Preston H, Zhang C, Marzuki S (1990) Mitochondrial gene mutation: the aging process and degenerative diseases. Biochem Int 22:1067–1076

Mattson MP, Cheng B, Davis D, Bryant K, Lieberburg I, Rydel RE (1992) β-Amyloid peptides destabilize calcium homeostasis and render human cortical neurons vulnerable to excitotoxicity. J Neurosci 12:376–389

Mecocci P, MacGarvey U, Kaufman A, Koontz D, Shoffner JM, Wallace DC, Beal MF (1993) Oxidative damage to mitochondrial DNA shows marked age-dependent increases in human brain. Ann Neurol, 34:609–616

Miquel J (1991) An integrated theory of aging as the result of mitochondrial-DNA mutation in differentiated cells. Arch Gerontol Geriatr 12:99–117

Muller-Hocker J (1989) Cytochrome-c-oxidase deficient cardiomyocytes in the human heart, an age-related phenomenon. Am J Pathol 134:1167–1173

Nohl H (1986) Oxygen radical release in mitochondria: influence of age. In: Johnson JE Jr, Walford R, Harman D, Miquel J (eds) Free radicals, aging, and degenerative diseases. Alan R. Liss, New York, pp 77–97

Nohl H, Hegner D (1978) Do mitochondria produce oxygen radicals in vivo? Eur J Biochem 82:563–567

Nohl H, Breuninger V, Hegner D (1978) Influence of mitochondrial radical formation of energy-linked respiration. Eur J Biochem 90:385–390

Oury TD, Ho Y-S, Piantadosi CA, Crapo JD (1992) Extracellular superoxide dismutase, nitric oxide, and central nervous system O2 toxicity. Proc Natl Acad Sci USA 89:9715–9719

Paradies G, Ruggiero FM (1990) Age-related changes in the activity of the pyruvate carrier and in the lipid composition in rat-heart mitochondria. Biochim Biophys Acta 1016:207–212

Parker WD, Filley CM, Parks JM (1990) Cytochrome oxidase deficiency in Alzheimer's disease. Neurology 40:1302–1303

Petruzzella V Chen X, Schon EA (1992) Is a point mutation in the mitochondrial ND2 gene associated with Alzheimer's disease? Biochem Biophys Res Comm 186:491–497

Richter C, Park J-W, Ames BN (1988) Normal oxidative damage to mitochondrial and nuclear DNA is extensive. Proc Natl Acad Sci USA 85:6465–6467

Ruggiero FM, Cafagna F, Petruzzella V, Gadaleta MN, Quagliariello E (1992) Lipid composition in synaptic and nonsynaptic mitochondria from rat brains and aging. J Neurochem 59:487–491

Saraiva AA, Borges MM, Madeira MD, Tavares MA, Paula-Barbosa MM (1985) Mitochondrial abnormalities in cortical dendrites from patients with Alzheimer's disease. J Submicrosc Cytol 17:459–464

Shibutani S, Takeshita M, Grollman AP (1991) Insertion of specific bases during DNA synthesis past the oxidation damage base 8-OXOdG. Nature 349:431–434

Shigenaga MR, Park J-W, Cundy KC, Gimeno CJ, Ames BN (1990) In vivo oxidative DNA damage: measurement of 8-hydroxy-2-deoxyguanosine in DNA and urine by high-performance liquid chromatography with electrochemical detection. Methods Enzymol 186:521–530

Shoffner JM, Brown MD, Torroni A, Lott MT, Cabell P, Mirra SS, Beal MF, Yang C-C, Gearing M, Salvo R, Watts R, Juncos JL, Hanson LA, Crain BJ, Fayad M, Wallace DW. (1993) Mitochondrial DNA mutations associated with Alzheimer's and Parkinson's disease. Genomics 17:171–184

Simonetta S, Chen X, DiMauro S, Schon EA (1992) Accumulation of deletions in human mitochondrial DNA during normal aging: analysis by quantitative PCR. Biochim Biophys Acta 1180:113–122

Sims NR, Bowen DM, Neary D, Davison AN (1983) Metabolic processes in Alzheimer's disease: adenine nucleotide content and production of $^{14}CO_2$ from [U-^{14}C] glucose in vitro in human neocortex. J Neurochem 41:1329–1334

Smith CD, Carney JM, Starke-Reed PE, Oliver CN, Stadtman ER, Floyd RA, Markesberry WR (1991) Excess brain protein oxidation and enzyme dysfunction in normal aging and in Alzheimer disease. Proc Natl Acad Sci 88:10540–10543

Soong NW, Hinton DR, Cortopassi G, Arnheim N (1992) Mosaicism for a specific somatic mitochondrial DNA mutation in adult human brain. Nature Genet 2:318–323

Sorbi S, Bird ED, Blass JP (1983) Decreased pyruvate dehydrogenase complex activity in Huntington and Alzheimer brain. Ann Neurol 13:72–78

Stadler J, Billiar TR, Curran RD, Stuehr DJ, Ochog JB, Simmons RL (1991) Effect of exogenous and endogenous nitric oxide in mitochondrial respiration in rat hepatocytes. Am J Physiol 260:C91–C916

Stadtman E (1992) Protein oxidation and aging. Science 257:1220–1224

Subbaro KV Richardson JS, Ang LC (1990) Autopsy samples of Alzheimer's cortex show increased peroxidation in vitro. J Neurochem. 55:342–345

Sugiyama S, Hattori K, Hayakawa M, Ozawa T (1991) Quantitative analysis of age-associated accumulation of mitochondrial DNA with deletion in human hearts. Biochem Biophys Res Comm 180:894–899

Tappel AL (1973) Lipid peroxidation damage to cell components. Fed Proc 32:1870–1874

Torii K, Sugiyama S, Takagi K, Satake T, Ozawa T (1992) Age-related decreases in respiratory muscle mitochondrial function in rats. Am J Resp Cell Molec Biol 6:88–92

Trounce I, Byrne E, Marzuki S (1989) Decline in skeletal muscle mitochondrial respiratory chain function: possible factor in aging. Lancet 1:637–639

Turrens JF, Boveris A (1980) Generation of superoxide anion by the NADH dehydrogenase of bovine heart mitochondria. Biochem J 191:421–427

Wallace DC (1986) Mitochondrial genes and disease. Hosp Prac 21:77–92

Wallace DW (1992) Mitochondrial genetics: a paradigm for aging and degenerative diseases? Science 256:628 632

Wood ML, Dizdaroglu M, Gajewski E, Essigmann JM (1990) Mechanistic studies of ionizing radiation and oxidative mutagenesis: genetic effects of a single 8-hydroxyguanine residue inserted at a unique site in a viral genome. Biochemistry 29:7024–7032

Yen T-C, Chen Y-S, King K-L, Yeh S-H, Wei Y-H (1989) Liver mitochondrial respiratory functions decline with age. Biochem Biophys Res Comm 165:994–1003

Zhang Y, Marcillat O, Giulivi C, Ernster L, Davies KJA (1990) The oxidative inactivation of mitochondrial electron transport chain components and ATPase. J Biol Chem 265:16330–16336

Zoccarato F, Cavallini L, Deana, R, Alexandre A (1988) Pathways of hydrogen peroxide generation in guinea pig cerebral cortex mitochondria. Biochem Biophys Res Commun 154:727–734

Molecular Biology and Genetics of Human Prion Diseases and PrP Amyloid Plaque Formation

*S. B. Prusiner**

Summary

Prion diseases include kuru, Creutzfeldt-Jakob disease (CJD) and Gerstmann-Sträussler-Scheinker disease (GSS) of humans, as well as scrapie and bovine spongiform encephalopathy (BSE) of animals. For many years, the prion diseases were thought to be caused by viruses, despite intriguing evidence to the contrary (Alper et al. 1966, 1967, 1978). The unique characteristic common to all of these disorders, whether sporadic, dominantly inherited or acquired by infection, is that they involve the aberrant metabolism of the prion protein (PrP; Prusiner 1991). In many cases, the cellular prion protein (PrP^C) is converted into the scrapie isoform (PrP^{Sc}) by a post-translational process which involves a conformational change. Often, the human prion diseases are transmissible to experimental animals (Gajdusek et al. 1966; Gibbs et al. 1968; Masters et al. 1981a; Tateishi et al. 1992) and all of the inherited prion diseases segregate with PrP gene mutations (Dlouhy et al. 1992; Gabizon et al. 1993; Hsiao et al. 1989a; Petersen et al. 1992; Poulter et al. 1992).

Introduction

Advances in understanding of neurodegeneration in humans and animals caused by prions have been unexpected and striking. For more than 25 years, two uncommon human diseases and several animal disorders were labeled transmissible encephalopathies, spongiform encephalopathies or slow virus diseases (Gajdusek 1977, 1985; Sigurdsson 1954). These illnesses were transmissible to experimental animals after a prolonged incubation period and some features of the transmissible pathogen resembled those of viruses. Yet, early attempts to characterize the infectious pathogen causing scrapie of sheep and goats argued that these transmissible agents differed from both viruses and viroids (Alper et al. 1967, 1966, 1978; Hunter 1972).

A set of remarkable discoveries in the past three decades has led to the molecular and genetic characterization of the transmissible pathogen causing

---

* Departments of Neurology and of Biochemistry and Biophysics, University of California, San Francisco, CA 94143, USA

C.L. Masters et al. (Eds.)
Amyloid Protein Precursor in Development,
Aging and Alzheimer's Disease
© Springer-Verlag Berlin Heidelberg 1994

scrapie in animals and a trio of human illnesses: kuru, Creutzfeldt-Jakob disease (CJD), Gerstmann-Sträussler-Scheinker disease (GSS; Prusiner 1991). To distinguish this pathogen from viruses and viroids, the term "prion" was introduced to emphasize its proteinaceous and infectious nature (Prusiner 1982). An abnormal isoform of the prion protein (PrP), PrP^{Sc}, is the only known component of the prion (Prusiner et al. 1981, 1984). PrP is encoded by a gene on the short arm of chromosome 20 in humans (Sparkes et al. 1986). PrP^{Sc} differs physically from the normal, cellular isoform PrP^C by its insolubility in detergents, its propensity to aggregate and its relative resistance to proteolysis (Meyer et al. 1986; Oesch et al. 1985).

Accumulation of PrP^{Sc} in the brain has been found in most of the human prion diseases. The presence of PrP^{Sc} implicates prions in the pathogenesis of these diseases. However, in rare patients and in some transgenic mice which appear to have low or undetectable amounts of PrP^{Sc} neurodegeneration appears, at least in part, to be caused by abnormal metabolism of mutant PrP (Hsiao et al. 1990). In these cases, horizontal transmission of neurodegeneration from such patients to experimental animals may not be demonstrable (Tateishi et al. 1992). Whether it will be useful to distinguish between those prion diseases in which transmission can be demonstrated and those in which it cannot with current animal models remains to be established (Hsiao and Prusiner 1990). As our knowledge of the prion diseases increases and more is learned about the molecular and genetic characteristics of prion proteins, these disorders will undoubtedly undergo modification with respect to their classification. Indeed, the discovery of the PrP and the identification of pathogenic PrP gene mutations have already forced us to view these illnesses from perspectives not previously imagined.

Clinical Manifestations of Prion Diseases

The human prion diseases are manifest as infectious, inherited, and sporadic disorders and are often referred to as kuru, CJD, GSS and fatal familial insomnia (FFI), depending upon the clinical and neuropathological findings (Table 1).

Table 1. Human prion disease

Disease	Etiology
Kuru	Infection
Creutzfeldt-Jakob disease	
Iatrogenic	Infection
Sporadic	Unknown
Familial	PrP mutation
Gerstmann-Sträussler-Scheinker disease	PrP mutation
Fatal familial insomnia	PrP mutation

Infectious forms of prion diseases result from the horizontal transmission of the infectious prions, as occurs in iatrogenic CJD and kuru. Inherited forms, notably GSS, familial CJD and FFI comprise 10–15% of all cases of prion disease. A mutation in the open reading frame (ORF) or protein coding region of the PrP gene has been found in all reported kindreds with inherited human prion disease (Bertoni et al. 1992; Dlouhy et al. 1992; Doh-ura et al. 1989; Gabizon et al. 1993; Goldfarb et al. 1990b, 1991c, 1992b; Goldgaber et al. 1989; Hsiao et al. 1989a; Kitamoto et al. 1993a,b; Medori et al. 1992b; Petersen et al. 1992; Poulter et al. 1992). Sporadic forms of prion disease comprise most cases of CJD and possibly some cases of GSS (Masters et al. 1978). How prions arise in patients with sporadic forms is unknown but has been hypothesized to involve horizontal transmission, somatic mutation of the ORF of the PrP gene as well as the spontaneous conversion of PrP^C into PrP^{Sc} (Gajdusek 1977; Hsiao et al. 1991a; Prusiner 1989). Numerous attempts to establish an infectious link between sporadic CJD and a preexisting prion disease in animals or humans have been unrewarding (Bobowick et al. 1973; Brown et al. 1987; Cousens et al. 1990; Harries-Jones et al. 1988; Malmgren et al. 1979).

Diagnosis of Human Prion Diseases

Human prion disease should be considered in any patient who develops a progressive subacute or chronic decline in cognitive or motor function. Adults between 40 and 70 years of age often exhibit clinical features helpful in providing a premorbid diagnosis of prion disease, particularly sporadic CJD (Brown et al. 1986a; Roos et al. 1973). There is as yet no specific diagnostic test for prion disease in the cerebrospinal fluid. A definitive diagnosis of human prion disease, which is invariably fatal, can usually be made from the examination of brain tissue. Over the past four years, knowledge of the molecular genetics of prion diseases has made it possible to diagnose inherited prion disease in living patients using peripheral tissues.

A broad spectrum of neuropathological features in human prion diseases precludes a precise neuropathological definition. The classic neuropathological features of human prion disease include spongiform degeneration, gliosis, and neuronal loss in the absence of an inflammatory reaction. When present, amyloid plaques which stain with α-PrP antibodies are diagnostic.

The presence of protease-resistant PrP (PrP^{Sc} or PrP^{CJD}) in the infectious and sporadic forms and most of the inherited forms of these diseases implicates prions in their pathogenesis. However, in some patients with inherited prion disease, PrP^{Sc} is barely detectable or undetectable (Brown et al. 1992c; Little et al. 1986; Manetto et al. 1992; Medori et al. 1992a), a situation mimicked in transgenic mice which express a mutant PrP gene and spontaneously develop neurologic illness indistinguishable from experimental murine scrapie (Hsiao et al. 1990).

In humans and transgenic mice which have no detectable protease-resistant PrP but express mutant PrP, neurodegeneration may, at least in part, be caused by abnormal metabolism of mutant PrP. Because molecular genetic analyses of PrP genes in patients with unusual dementing illnesses are readily performed, the diagnosis of inherited prion disease can often be established where there was either little or no neuropathology (Collinge et al. 1990), atypical neuro-degenerative disease (Medori et al. 1992a), or misdiagnosed neurodegenerative diseases (Azzarelli et al. 1985; Heston et al. 1966), including Alzheimer's disease. Although horizontal transmission of neurodegeneration to experimental hosts was for a time the "gold standard" of prion disease, it can no longer be used as such. Some investigators have reported that transmission of the inherited prion diseases from human to experimental animals is frequently negative using rodents, despite the presence of a pathogenic mutation in the PrP gene (Tateishi et al. 1992), while others state that this is not the case with apes and monkeys as hosts (Brown et al. 1993).

The hallmark common to all of the prion diseases, whether sporadic, dominantly inherited or acquired by infection, is that they involve the aberrant metabolism of the prion protein (Prusiner 1991).

Making a definitive diagnosis of human prion disease can be rapidly accomplished if PrP^{Sc} can be detected immunologically. Frequently PrP^{Sc} can be detected by either dot blot method or Western immunoblot analysis of brain homogenates, where samples were subjected to limited proteolysis to remove PrP^{C} prior to immunostaining (Bockman et al. 1985, 1987; Brown et al. 1986b; Serban et al. 1990). The dot blot method exploits enhancement of PrP^{Sc} immunoreactivity following denaturation in the chaotropic salt, guanidinium chloride. Because of regional variations in PrP^{Sc} concentration, methods using homogenates prepared from small brain regions can give false negative results. Alternatively, PrP^{Sc} may be detected in situ in cryostat sections bound to nitrocellulose membranes followed by limited proteolysis to remove PrP^{C} and guanidinium treatment to denature PrP^{Sc} and thus, enhance its avidity for α-PrP antibodies (Taraboulos et al. 1992). Denaturation of PrP^{Sc} in situ prior to immunostaining has also been accomplished by autoclaving fixed tissue sections (Kitamoto et al. 1992).

In the familial forms of the prion diseases, molecular genetic analyses of PrP can be diagnostic and performed on DNA extracted from blood leucocytes ante mortem. Unfortunately, such testing is of little value in the diagnosis of the sporadic or infectious forms of prion disease. Although the first missense PrP mutation was discovered when the two PrP alleles of a patient with GSS were cloned from a genomic library and sequenced (Hsiao et al. 1989a), all subsequent novel missense and insertional mutations have been identified in PrP open reading frames (ORF) amplified by polymerase chain reaction (PCR) and sequenced. The 759 base pairs encoding the 253 amino acids of PrP reside in a single exon of the PrP gene, providing an ideal situation for the use of PCR. Amplified PrP ORFs may be screened for known mutations using one of several methods, the most reliable of which is allele-specific oligonucleotide hybridization. If known mutations are absent, then novel mutations may be found when the PrP ORF is sequenced.

When PrP amyloid plaques in brain are present, they are diagnostic for prion disease as noted above. Unfortunately, they are thought to be present in only ~ 10% of CJD cases, and by definition all cases of GSS. The amyloid plaques in CJD are compact (kuru plaques). Those in GSS are either multi-centric (diffuse) or compact. The amyloid plaques in prion diseases contain PrP (Kitamoto et al. 1986; Roberts et al. 1986, 1988). The multicentric amyloid plaques which are pathognomonic for GSS may be difficult to distinguish from the neuritic plaques of Alzheimer's disease except by immunohistology (Ghetti et al. 1989; Ikeda et al. 1991; Nochlin et al. 1989). In these kindreds the diagnosis of Alzheimer's disease was excluded because the amyloid plaques failed to stain with β-amyloid antiserum but stained with PrP antiserum. In subsequent studies, missense mutations were found in the PrP genes of these kindreds.

In summary, the diagnosis of prion or prion protein disease may be made in patients on the basis of 1) the presence of PrP^{Sc}, 2) mutant PrP genotype or 3) appropriate immunohistology, and should not be excluded in patients with atypical neurodegenerative diseases until one or preferably two of these exam-inations have been performed (Collinge et al. 1990, 1992; Lantos et al. 1992).

Molecular Genetics of Inherited Human Prion Diseases

Genetics were first thought to have a role in CJD with the recognition that ~ 10% of cases are familial (Gajdusek 1977; Masters et al. 1981b; Rosenthal et al. 1976). Like sheep scrapie, the relative contributions of genetic and infectious etiologies in the human prion diseases remained puzzling. The discovery of the PrP gene and its linkage to scrapie incubation times in mice (Carlson et al. 1986) raised the possibility that mutation might feature in the hereditary human prion diseases. A proline (P) → leucine (L) mutation at codon 102 was shown to be linked genetically to development of GSS with a LOD score exceeding 3 (Fig. 1); Hsiao et al. 1989a). This mutation may be due to the deamination of a methyl-ated CpG in a germline PrP gene resulting in the substitution of a thymine (T) for cytosine (C). The P102L mutation has been found in ten different families in nine different countries including the original GSS family (Doh-ura et al. 1989; Goldgaber et al. 1989; Kretzschmar et al. 1991a, b).

An insert of 144 bp at codon 53 containing six octarepeats has been de-scribed in patients with CJD from four families all residing in southern England (Fig. 1); Collinge et al. 1989, 1990, 1992; Crow et al. 1990; Owen et al. 1989, 1990b, 1991; Poulter et al. 1992). This mutation must have arisen through a complex series of events since the human PrP gene contains only five oc-tarepeats, indicating that a single recombination event could not have created the insert. Genealogic investigations have shown that all four families are related, arguing for a single founder born more than two centuries ago (Crow et al. 1990). The LOD score for this extended pedigree exceeds 11. Studies from

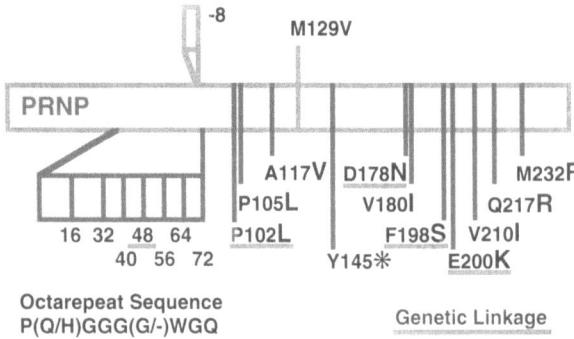

Fig. 1. Human prion protein gene (PRNP). The open reading frame (ORF) is denoted by the large gray rectangle. Human PRNP wild-type polymorphisms are shown above the rectangle, whereas mutations that segregate with the inherited prion diseases are depicted below. The wild-type human PrP gene contains five octarepeats [P(Q/H)GGG(G/-)WGQ] from codons 51 to 91 (Kretzschmar et al. 1986). Deletion of a single octarepeat at codon 81 or 82 is not associated with prion disease (Laplanche et al. 1990; Puckett et al. 1991; Vnencak-Jones and Phillips 1992); whether this deletion alters the phenotypic characteristics of a prion disease is unknown. There are common polymorphisms at codons 117 (Ala → Ala) and 129 (Met → Val); homozygosity for Met or Val at codon 129 appears to increase susceptibility to sporadic CJD (Palmer et al. 1991). Octarepeat inserts of 16, 32, 40, 48, 56, 64, and 72 amino acids at codons 67, 75 or 83 are designated by the small rectangle below the ORF. These inserts segregate with familial CJD and significant genetic linkage has been demonstrated where sufficient specimens from family members are available (Collinge et al. 1989, 1990; Crow et al. 1990; Goldfarb et al. 1990c, 1991a; Owen et al. 1989, 1990b; Palmer et al. 1993). Point mutations are designated by the wild-type amino acid preceding the codon number and the mutant residue follows, i.e., P102L. These point mutations segregate with the inherited prion diseases, and significant genetic linkage (underlined mutations) has been demonstrated where sufficient specimens from family members are available. Mutations at codons 102 (Pro → Leu), 117 (Ala → Val), 198 (Phe → Ser) and 217 (Gln → Arg) are found in patients with GSS (Doh-ura et al. 1989; Goldfarb et al. 1990a, 1990c, 1990d; Goldgaber et al. 1989; Hsiao et al. 1989a,b, 1991b; Hsiao and Prusiner 1990; Tateishi et al. 1990). Point mutations at codons 178 (Asp → Asn), 200 (Glu → Lys) and 210 (Val → Iso) are found in patients with familial CJD (Gabizon et al. 1991; Goldfarb et al. 1990b, 1991c; Hsiao et al. 1991a; Ripoll et al. 1993). Point mutations at codons 198 (Phe → Ser) and 217 (Gln → Arg) are found in patients with GSS who have PrP amyloid plaques and neurofibrillary tangles (Dlouhy et al. 1992; Hsiao et al. 1992). Additional point mutations at codons 145 (Tyr → Stop), 105 (Pro → Leu), 180 (Val → Iso) and 232 (Met → Arg) have been recently reported (Kitamoto et al. 1993a,b). Single letter code for amino acids is as follows: A, Ala; D, Asp; E, Glu; F, Phe; I, Iso; K, Lys; L, Leu; M, Met; N, Asn; P, Pro; Q, Gln; R, Arg; S, Ser; T, Thr; and V, Val

several laboratories have demonstrated that two, four, five, six, seven, eight or nine octarepeats in addition to the normal five are found in individuals with inherited CJD (Brown 1992; Collinge et al. 1989, 1990; Goldfarb et al. 1991a; Owen et al. 1989, 1990b, 1992), whereas deletion of one octarepeat has been identified without the neurologic disease (Laplanche et al. 1990; Palmer et al. 1993; Vnencak-Jones and Phillips 1992).

For many years the unusually high incidence of CJD among Israeli Jews of Libyan origin was thought to be due to the consumption of lightly cooked sheep brain or eyeballs (Alter and Kahana 1976; Herzberg et al. 1974; Kahana et al.

1974, 1991; Neugut et al. 1979; Zilber et al. 1991). Recent studies have shown that some Libyan and Tunisian Jews in families with CJD have a PrP gene point mutation at codon 200 resulting in a glutamate (E) → lysine (K) substitution (Gabizon et al. 1991; Goldfarb et al. 1990d; Hsiao et al. 1991a). One patient was homozygous for the E200K mutation but her clinical presentation was similar to that of heterozygotes (Hsiao et al. 1991a), arguing that familial prion diseases are true autosomal dominant disorders like Huntington's disease (Wexler et al. 1987). The E200K mutation has also been found in Slovaks originating from Orava in North Central Czechoslovakia (Goldfarb et al. 1990d), in a cluster of familial cases in Chile (Goldfarb et al. 1991b) and in a large German family living in the United States (Bertoni et al. 1992). Some investigators have argued that the E200K mutation originated in a Sephardic Jew whose descendants migrated from Spain and Portugal at the time of the inquisition (Goldfarb et al. 1991b). It is more likely that the E200K mutation has arisen independently multiple times by the deamidation of a methylated CpG as described above the codon 102 mutation (Hsiao et al. 1989a, 1991a). In support of this hypothesis are historical records of Libyan and Tunisian Jews indicating that they are descended from Jews living on the island of Jerba, where Jews first settled around 500 B.C., and not from Sephardim (Udovitch and Valensi 1984).

Many families with CJD have been found to have a point mutation at codon 178 resulting in an aspartic acid (D) → asparagine (N) substitution (Brown et al. 1992b; Fink et al. 1991; Goldfarb et al. 1991c, 1992c; Haltia et a. 1991). In these patients as well as those with the E200K mutation PrP amyloid plaques are rare; the neuropathologic changes generally consist of widespread spongiform degeneration. Recently a new prion disease which presents with insomnia has been described in three Italian families with the D178N mutation (Medori et al. 1992a). The neuropathology in these patients with fatal familial insomnia is restricted to selected nuclei of the thalamus. It is unclear whether all patients with the D178N mutation or only a subset present with sleep disturbances. It has been proposed that the allele with the D178N mutation encodes a methionine at position 129 in fatal familial insomnia, whereas a valine is encoded at position 129 in familial CJD (Goldfarb et al. 1992c). The discovery that fatal familial insomnia is an inherited prion disease clearly widens the clinical spectrum of these disorders and raises the possibility that many other degenerative diseases of unknown etiology may be caused by prions (Johnson 1992; Medori et al. 1992a).

Like the E200K and D178N (V129) mutations, a valine (V) → isoleucine (I) mutation at PrP codon 210 produces CJD with classic symptoms and signs (Pocchiari et al. 1993; Ripoll et al. 1993). It appears that this V210I mutation is also incompletely penetrant.

Other point mutations at codons 105, 117, 145, 198, 217 and possibly 232 also segregate with inherited prion diseases (Brown 1992; Doh-ura et al. 1989; Hsiao et al. 1991b, 1992; Kitamoto et al. 1993a,b; Tranchant et al. 1992). Patients with a dementing or telencephalic form of GSS have a mutation at codon 117. These patients as well as some in other families were once thought to have familial Alzheimer's disease, but are now known to have prion diseases on the basis of PrP immunostaining of amyloid plaques and PrP gene mutations (Farlow et al. 1989; Ghetti et al. 1989; Giaccone et al. 1990; Nochlin et al. 1989). Patients with the codon 198 mutation have numerous neurofibrillary tangles that stain with antibodies to τ and have amyloid plaques (Farlow et al. 1989; Ghetti et al. 1989; Giaccone et al. 1990; Nochlin et al. 1989) that are composed largely of a PrP fragment extending from residues 58 to 150 (Tagliavini et al. 1991). A genetic linkage study of this family produced a LOD score exceeding 6 (Dlouhy et al. 1992). The neuropathology of two patients of Swedish ancestry with the codon 217 mutation (Ikeda et al. 1991) was similar to that of patients with the codon 198 mutation.

Patients with GSS who have a substitution of leucine for proline at PrP codon 105 have been reported (Kitamoto et al. 1993b). One patient with a prolonged neurologic illness spanning almost two decades with PrP amyloid plaques was found to have an amber mutation of the PrP gene resulting in a stop codon at residue 145 (Kitamoto et al. 1993a). Staining of the plaques with α-PrP peptide antisera suggested that they might be composed exclusively of the truncated PrP molecules. That a PrP peptide ending at residue 145 polymerizes in amyloid filaments is to be expected since an earlier study noted above showed that the major PrP peptide in plaques from patients with the F198S mutation was an 11 kDa PrP peptide beginning at codon 58 and ending at ~ 150 (Tagliavini et al. 1991). Furthermore, synthetic PrP peptides adjacent to and including residues 109 to 122 readily polymerize into rod-shaped structures with the tinctorial properties of amyloid (Come et al. 1993; Forloni et al. 1993; Gasset et al. 1992; Goldfarb et al. 1993b; Verga et al. 1992).

Nomenclature for the Inherited Human Prion Diseases

Although each of the PrP mutations is associated with a typical clinical presentation as noted above, there are a sufficient number of exceptions that a particular mutation in a single pedigree can present with symptom complexes typical of CJD in some patients and GSS in others. Since we now know the molecular basis of the disorders, it seems preferable to name them according to the mutation and no longer refer to them as familial CJD, GSS or FFI. Once the PrP gene has been determined, then we suggest that Prion Disease (D102L) be used in place of ataxic GSS such as that found in the original GSS family (Gerstmann et al. 1936; Kretzschmar et al. 1991a), Prion Disease (E200K) instead of familial CJD in Libyan Jews, and Prion Disease (D178N, M129) instead of FFI (Table 2). These designations describe the precise etiologies of the disorders and remove any possible ambiguities. While some investigators argue against these changes in terminology on the grounds that they will diminish the esteem in which we hold such historical figures as Creutzfeldt, Jakob and Gerstmann (Brown et al. 1992a, 1993), using the most concise and clear descriptors of the diseases available would seem to be the only approach consistent

Table 2. Inherited prion diseases of humans

Proposed Designation	Alternative Name
Inherited prion disease (P102L)	GSS
Inherited prion disease (P105L)	GSS
Inherited prion disease (A117V)	GSS
Inherited prion disease (Y145Stop)	GSS
Inherited prion disease (D178N)	familial CJD, FFI
Inherited prion disease (V180I)	GSS
Inherited prion disease (F198S)	GSS
Inherited prion disease (E200K)	familial CJD
Inherited prion disease (V210I)	familial CJD
Inherited prion disease (Q217R)	GSS
Inherited prion disease (octarepeat insert)	familial CJD

with the goals of modern medicine, which identify the molecular basis of disease and create effective therapies.

The need to designate the inherited prion diseases by their mutations (molecular lesions) is emphasized by the vastly different clinical presentations and post mortem neuropathologies observed in four afflicted members of a family with Prion Disease (6 octarepeat insert; Collinge et al. 1992). One of the four family members with the insert presented a classical case of CJD and had pronounced spongiform change in the cerebral cortex whereas another presented with ataxia and had numerous PrP amyloid plaques at autopsy. The second case might have been called GSS with hesitation. The third and fourth members of the family died in hospitals with the diagnosis of dementia but had no spongiform change at autopsy and were not given the diagnosis of CJD.

Human PrP Gene Polymorphisms

At PrP codon 129, an amino acid polymorphism for the methionine (M) or valine (V) (Fig. 1) has been identified (Owen et al. 1990a). This polymorphism appears able to influence prion disease expression not only in inherited forms, but also in iatrogenic and sporadic forms of prion disease.

Susceptibility to infection may be partially determined by the PrP codon 129 genotype (Collinge et al. 1991), analogous in principle to the incubation-time alleles in mice (Carlson et al. 1986; Collinge et al. 1991). Population frequencies for the codon 129 polymorphism in Caucasians are 12% V/V, 37% M/M, and 51% M/V (Collinge et al. 1991). In 16 patients (15 Caucasian, one Afro-American) from the UK, USA, and France with iatrogenic CJD from contaminated growth hormone extracts, eight (50%) were V/V, five (31%) were M/M, and three (19%) were M/V (Brown et al. 1992d; Buchanan et al. 1991; Collinge et al. 1991; Fradkin et al. 1991; Goldfarb et al. 1993a). Thus, a disproportionate number of patients with iatrogenic CJD were homozygous for valine at PrP codon 129. Heterozygosity at codon 129 may provide partial protection. Whether these associations are strongly significant awaits statistical analysis of larger samples. Thousands of children who received pituitary growth hormone extracts are still at risk for the development of CJD. Fortunately, the use of genetically engineered growth hormone will eliminate this form of iatrogenic CJD.

No specific mutations have been identified in the PrP gene of patients with sporadic CJD. However, patients with sporadic CJD are largely homozygous at codon 129 (Hardy 1991; Palmer et al. 1991). This finding supports a model of prion production which favors PrP interactions between homologous proteins, as appears to occur in transgenic mice expressing Syrian hamster PrP inoculated with either hamster prions or mouse prions (Prusiner et al. 1990; Scott et al. 1989), as well as transgenic mice expressing a chimeric mouse/hamster PrP transgene inoculated with "artificial" prions (Scott et al. 1993).

Approximately 15% of patients with sporadic CJD develop ataxia as an early sign, accompanied by dementia (Brown et al. 1984). Most but not all patients with ataxia have compact (kuru) plaques in the cerebellum (Pearlman et al. 1988). Patients with ataxia and compact plaques exhibit a protracted clinical course which may last up to three years. The molecular basis for the differences between CJD of shorter and longer duration has not yet been fully elucidated. However, some preliminary analyses have suggested that patients with protracted, atypical clinical courses are more likely to be heterozygous at codon 129 (Collinge and Palmer 1991; Doh-ura et al. 1991).

Homozygosity at codon 129 has been reported to be associated with an earlier age of onset in the inherited prion disease by the six octarepeat insert but not by the E200K mutation in Libyan Jews (Baker et al. 1991; Gabizon et al. 1993). As noted above, the FFI phenotype is found in patients with the D178N mutation who encode a methionine at codon 129 on the mutant allele, whereas those with dementing illness (familial CJD) encode a valine at 129 (Goldfarb et al. 1992c). Homozygosity for either M or V at codon 129 is thought to be associated with an earlier age of onset for the D178N mutation.

De Novo Synthesis of Prions in Tg(MoPrP-P101L)H Mice

The codon 102 point mutation found in GSS patients was introduced into the mouse (Mo) PrP gene and Tg(MoPrP-P101L)H mice were created expressing high (H) levels of the mutant transgene product. The Tg(MoPrP-P101L)H mice spontaneously developed CNS degeneration, characterized by clinical signs indistinguishable from experimental murine scrapie and neuropathology consisting of widespread spongiform morphology and astrocytic gliosis (Hsiao et al. 1990) and PrP amyloid plaques. Brain extracts prepared from Tg(MoPrP-P101L)H mice transmitted CNS degeneration to inoculated recipients. Although inoculated CD-1 Swiss mice failed to develop illness, some Syrian hamsters and many Tg196 mice expressing low levels of the P101L mutant trangene product did become ill. By inference, these results contend that PrP mutations cause GSS and familial CJD. It is unclear whether the low levels of protease-resistant PrP in the brains of Tg mice with the GSS mutation is PrP^{Sc} or residual PrP^C. Undetectable or low levels of PrP^{Sc} in the brains of these Tg mice are consistent with the results of transmission experiments that suggest low titers of infectious prions (K.K. Hsiao et al., in preparation). These findings argue that prions are devoid of foreign nucleic acid, in accord with many studies that use other experimental approaches (Bellinger-Kawahara et al. 1987a, 1987b; Diedrich et al. 1987; Diener et al. 1982; Duguid et al. 1988; Gabizon et al. 1988a; Kellings et al. 1992; McKinley et al. 1983; Meyer et al. 1991; Neary et al. 1991; Oesch et al. 1988; Weitgrefe et al. 1985).

One view of the PrP gene mutations has been that they render individuals susceptible to a common "virus" (Aiken and Marsh 1990; Chesebro 1992; Kimberlin 1990). In this scenario, the putative scrapie virus is thought to persist within a worldwide reservoir of humans, animals or insects without causing detectable illness. Yet $1/10^6$ individuals develop sporadic CJD and die from a lethal "infection", whereas $\sim$ 100% of people with PrP point mutations or inserts appear eventually to develop neurologic dysfunction. That germline mutations found in the PrP genes of patients and at-risk individuals are the cause of familial prion diseases is supported by experiments with the Tg(MoPrP-P101L) mice described above (Hsiao and Prusiner 1990; Hsiao et al. 1991c; Weissmann 1991). The Tg mouse studies also argue that sporadic CJD might arise from the spontaneous conversion of PrP^C to PrP^{CJD} due to either a somatic mutation of the PrP gene or rare event involving modification of wild-type PrP^C (Prusiner 1991).

Species Barriers for Transmission of Prion Diseases

The passage of prions between species is a stochastic process characterized by prolonged incubation times (Pattison 1965, 1966; Pattison and Jones 1967). Prions synthesized *de novo* reflect the sequence of the host PrP gene and not that of the PrP^{Sc} molecules in the inoculum (Bockman et al. 1987). On subsequent passage in a homologous host, the incubation time shortens to that recorded for all subsequent passages and it becomes a nonstochastic process. The species barrier concept is of practical importance in assessing the risk for humans of developing CJD after consumption of scrapie-infected lamb or BSE beef (Dealler and Lacey 1990; Goldmann et al. 1991; Hope et al. 1988; Prusiner et al. 1993; Wilesmith et al. 1992a,b).

To test the hypothesis that differences in PrP gene sequences might be responsible for the species barrier, Tg mice expressing Syrian hamster (SHa) PrP were constructed (Prusiner et al. 1990; Scott et al. 1989). The PrP genes of Syrian hamsters and mice encode proteins differing at 16 positions. Incubation times in four lines of Tg(SHaPrP) mice inoculated that Mo prions were prolonged compared to those observed for non-Tg, control mice (Fig. 2A). Inoculation of Tg(SHaPrP) mice with SHa prions demonstrated abrogation of the species barrier resulting in abbreviated incubation times due to a nonstochastic process (Fig. 2B; Prusiner et al. 1990; Scott et al. 1989). The length of the incubation time after inoculation with SHa prions was inversely proportional to the level of SHaPrP^C in the brains of Tg(SHaPrP) mice (Fig. 2B and 2C; Prusiner et al. 1990). SHaPrP^{Sc} levels in the brains of clinically ill mice were similar in all four Tg(SHaPrP) lines inoculated with SHa prions (Fig. 2D). Bioassays of brain extracts from clinically ill Tg(SHaPrP) mice inoculated with Mo prions revealed that only Mo prions and no SHa prions were produced (Fig. 2E). Conversely, inoculation of Tg(SHaPrP) mice with SHa prions led to the synthesis of only SHa prions (Fig. 2F). Thus, the *de novo* synthesis of prions is species-specific and reflects the genetic origin of the inoculated prions. Similarly, the neuropathology of Tg(SHaPrP) mice is determined by the genetic origin of prion inoculum. Mo prions injected into Tg(SHaPrP) mice produced a neuropathology character-istic of mice with scrapie. A moderate degree of vacuolation in both the gray and white matter was found, whereas amyloid plaques were rarely detected (Fig. 2G; Table 3). Inoculation of Tg(SHaPrP) mice with SHa prions produced intense vacuolation of the gray matter, sparing of the white matter and numerous SHaPrP amyloid plaques characteristic of Syrian hamsters with scrapie (Fig. 2H).

The foregoing investigations indicate that PrP transgenes modulate virtually all phases of scrapie including; 1) replication of prions, 2) incubation times, 3) synthesis of PrP^{Sc}, 4) species barrier, and 5) neuropathologic changes.

PrP Amyloid

The discovery of PrP 27–30 in fractions enriched for scrapie infectivity was accompanied by the identification of rod-shaped particles (Prusiner et al. 1982, 1983). The rods are ultrastructurally indistinguishable from many purified amyloids and display the tinctorial properties of amyloids (Prusiner et al. 1983). These findings were followed by the demonstration that amyloid plaques in prion diseases contain PrP, as determined by immunoreactivity and amino acid sequencing (Bendheim et al. 1984; DeArmond et al. 1985; Kitamoto et al. 1986; Roberts et al. 1988). Some investigators believe that scrapie-associated fibrils are synonymous with the prion rods and are composed of PrP even though these fibrils can be distinguished ultrastructurally and tinctorially from amyloid polymers (Diener 1987; Diringer et al. 1983; Kimberlin 1990; Merz et al. 1981, 1983, 1984, 1987; Somerville et al. 1989).

The formation of prion rods require limited proteolysis in the presence of detergent (McKinley et al. 1991). Thus, the prion rods in fractions enriched for scrapie infectivity are largely, if not entirely, artifacts of the purification proto-col. Solubilization of PrP 27–30 into liposomes with retention of infectivity (Gabizon et al. 1987) demonstrated that large PrP polymers are not required for

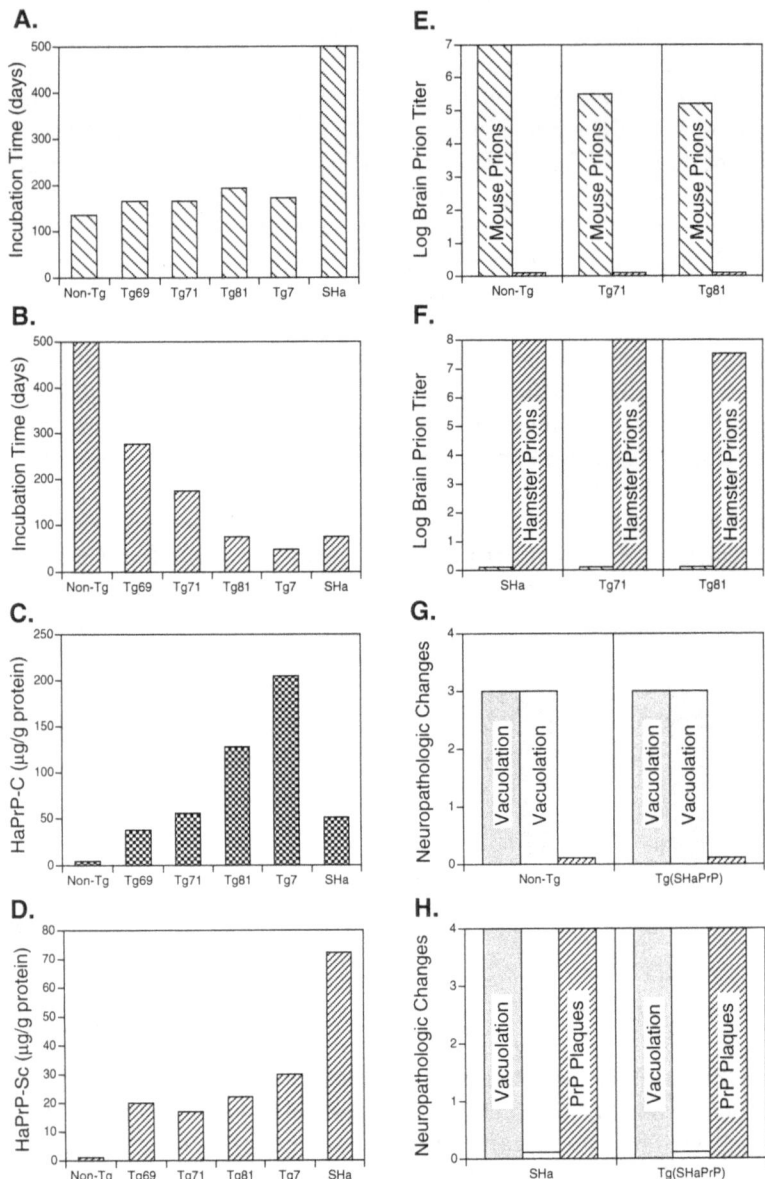

Fig. 2. Transgenic (Tg) mice expressing Syrian hamster (SHa) prion protein exhibit species-specific scrapie incubation times, infectious prion synthesis and neuropathology (Prusiner et al. 1990). **A** Scrapie incubation times in non-transgenic mice (Non-Tg) and four lines of Tg mice expressing SHaPrP and Syrian hamsters inoculated intracerebrally with $\sim 10^6$ ID_{50} units of Chandler Mo prions serially passaged in Swiss mice. The four lines of Tg mice have different numbers of transgene copies: Tg69 and 71 mice have two to four copies of the SHaPrP transgene, whereas Tg81 have 30 to 50 and Tg7 mice have > 60. Incubation times are number of days from inoculation to onset of neurologic dysfunction. **B** Scrapie incubation times in mice and hamsters inoculated with $\sim 10^7$

Table 3. Species-specific prion inocula determine the distribution of spongiform change and deposition of PrP amyloid plaques in transgenic mice

Animal	SHa prions					Mo prions			
	Spongiform change[a]			PrP plaques[b]		Spongiform change[a]			PrP plaques[b]
	n^c	Gray	White	Frequency	Diameters[d]	n^c	Gray	White	Frequency
Non-Tg	N.D.¶			N.D.		10	+	+	−
Tg 69	6	+	−	Numerous	6.5 ± 3.1 (389)	2	+	+	−
Tg 71	5	+	−	Numerous	8.1 ± 3.6 (345)	2	+	+	−
Tg 81	7	+	−	Numerous	8.3 ± 3.0 (439)	3	+	+	Few
Tg 7	3	+	−	Numerous	14.0 ± 8.3 (19)	4	+	+	−
SHa	3	+	−	Numerous	5.7 ± 2.7 (247)	N.D.			N.D.

[a] Spongiform change evaluated in hippocampus, thalamus, cerebral cortex and brainstem for gray matter and the deep cerebellum for white matter.
[b] Plaques in the subcallosal region were stained with SHaPrP mAb 13A5, anti-PrP rabbit antisera R073 and trichrome stain.
[c] n, number of brains examined.
[d] Mean diameter of PrP plaques given in microns ± standard error with the number of observations in parentheses.
N.D., not determined. +, present; −, not found.

infectivity and permitted the immunoaffinity copurification of PrP^{Sc} and infectivity (Gabizon et al. 1988b; Gabizon and Prusiner 1990).

By comparing the amino acid sequences of 11 mammalian and one avian prion protein, structural analyses predicted four α-helical regions (Huang et al. 1994; Cohen et al. 1986). Peptides corresponding to these regions of the SHaPrP were synthesized and, contrary to predictions, three of the four spontaneously formed amyloids, as shown by electron microscopy and Congo red staining (Gasset et al. 1992). By infrared spectroscopy, these amyloid peptides were found to exhibit a secondary structure comprised largely of β-sheets. The first of the predicted

---

ID$_{50}$ units of Sc237 prions serially passaged in Syrian hamsters and as described in (A). **C** Brain SHaPrP^c in Tg mice and hamsters. SHaPrP^c levels were quantified by an enzyme-linked immunoassay. **D** Brain SHaPrP^{Sc} in Tg mice and hamsters. Animals were killed after exhibiting clinical signs of scrapie. SHaPrP^{Sc} levels were determined by immunoassay. **E** Prion titers in brains of clinically ill animals after inoculation with Mo prions. Brain extracts from Non-Tg, Tg71, and Tg81 mice were bioassayed for prions in mice (left) and hamsters (right). **F** Prion titers in brains of clinically ill animals after inoculation with SHa prions. Brain extracts from Syrian hamsters as well as Tg71 and Tg81 mice were bioassayed for prions in mice (left) and hamsters (right). **G** Neuropathology in Non-Tg mice and Tg(SHaPrP) mice with clinical signs of scrapie after inoculation with Mo prions. Vacuolation in gray (left) and white matter (center); PrP amyloid plaques (right). Vacuolation score: 0 = none, 1 = rare, 2 = modest, 3 = moderate, 4 = intense. **H** Neuropathology in Syrian hamsters and transgenic mice inoculated with SHa prions. Degree of vacuolation and frequency of PrP amyloid plaques as described in (G). Adapted from Prusiner, 1991

helices is the 14-residue peptide correspond ing to SHaPrP codons 109–122; this peptide and the overlapping 15-residue sequence 113–127 both form amyloid. The most highly amyloidogenic peptide is the sequence AGAAAAGA corresponding to PrP codons 113–120. This peptide is in a region of PrP that is conserved across all known species. Two other predicted α-helices correspond-ing to SHaPrP codons 178–191 and 202–218 form amyloids and exhibit considerable β-sheet structure when synthesized as peptides. These findings suggest the possibility that the conversion of PrP^C to PrP^{Sc} involves the transition of one or more putative PrP α-helices into β-sheets. Infrared spectro-scopy of PrP 27–30 has shown a high β-sheet content (Caughey et al. 1991) which decreased when PrP 27–30 was denatured and scrapie infectivity dimin-ished concomitantly (Gasset et al. 1993).

Some investigators have suggested that scrapie agent multiplication pro-ceeds through a crystallization process involving PrP amyloid formation (Gaj-dusek 1988, 1990; Gajdusek and Gibbs 1990). Arguing against this hypothesis is the absence or rarity of amyloid plaques in many prion diseases, as well as the inability to identify any amyloid-like polymers in cultured cells chronically synthesizing prions (McKinley et al. 1991; Prusiner et al. 1990). Purified infec-tious preparations isolated from scrapie-infected hamster brains exist as amor-phous aggregates; only if PrP^{Sc} is exposed to detergents and limited proteolysis does it then polymerize into prion rods exhibiting the ultrastructural and tinctorial features of amyloid (McKinley et al. 1991). Furthermore, dispersion of prion rods into detergent-lipid-protein complexes results in a 10- to 100-fold increase in scrapie titer, and no rods could be identified in these fractions by electron microscopy (Gabizon et al. 1987).

Perspectives and Conclusions

The knowledge accrued from the study of prion diseases may provide an effective strategy for defining the etiologies and dissecting the molecular pathogenesis of the more common neurodegenerative disorders such as Al-zheimer's disease, Parkinson's disease and amyotrophic lateral sclerosis (ALS). Advances in the molecular genetics of Alzheimer's disease and ALS suggest that, like the prion diseases, an important subset are caused by mutations that result in nonconservative amino acid substitutions in proteins expressed in the CNS (Goate et al. 1991; Levy et al. 1990; Mullan et al. 1992; Rosen et al. 1993; Schellenberg et al. 1992; St George-Hyslop et al. 1992; Van Broeckhoven et al. 1990, 1992).

Currently, there are no effective therapies for treatment of prion diseases. These diseases are invariably fatal. The inherited prion diseases can be pre-vented by genetic counseling coupled with prenatal DNA screening, but such testing presents ethical problems. For example, during the child-bearing years, the parents are generally symptom free and may not want to know their own genotype. The apparent incomplete penetrance of some of the inherited prion diseases makes predicting the future for an asymptomatic individual uncertain (Gabizon et al. 1993; Hsiao et al. 1991a).

Unexpectedly, ablation of the PrP gene in Tg(Prn-p$^{0/0}$) mice has not affected the development of these animals, and they remain healthy at almost two years of age (Büeler et al. 1992). Since Prn-p$^{0/0}$ mice are resistant to prions and do not propagate scrapie infectivity (Büeler et al. 1993; Prusiner et al. 1993), gene therapy or antisense oligonucleotides might ultimately provide an effective therapeutic approach. Mice that were heterozygous (Prn-p$^{0/+}$) for ablation of the PrP gene had prolonged incubation times when inoculated with mouse prions. This finding is in accord with studies on Tg(SHaPrP) mice, where increased SHaPrP expression was accompanied by diminished incubation times (Prusiner et al. 1990).

Because the absence of PrP^C expression does not provoke disease, it seems reasonable to conclude that scrapie and other prion diseases are a consequence of PrP^{Sc} accumulation rather than an inhibition of PrP^C function. The function of PrP^C remains unknown, to date. These findings suggest that perhaps the most effective therapy may evolve from the development of drugs which block the conversion of PrP^C into PrP^{Sc}.

Acknowledgments. This work was supported by grants from the National Institutes of Health (NS 14069, AG08967, AG02132 and NS22786) and the American Health Assistance Foundation, as well as by gifts from Sherman Fairchild Foundation, Bernard Osher Foundation and National Medical Enterprises.

References

Aiken JM, Marsh RF (1990) The search for scrapie agent nucleic acid. Microbiol Rev 54:242–246

Alper T, Cramp WA, Haig DA, Clarke MC (1967) Does the agent of scrapie replicate without nucleic acid? Nature 214:764–766

Alper T, Haig DA, Clarke MC (1966) The exceptionally small size of the scrapie agent. Biochem Biophys Res Commun 22:278–284

Alper T, Haig DA, Clarke MC (1978) The scrapie agent: evidence against its dependence for replication on intrinsic nucleic acid. J Gen Virol 41:503–516

Alter M, Kahana E (1976) Creutzfeldt-Jakob disease among Libyan Jews in Israel. Science 192:428

Azzarelli B, Muller J, Ghetti B, Dyken M, Conneally PM (1985) Cerebellar plaques in familial Alzheimer's disease (Gerstmann-Sträussler-Scheinker variant?). Acta Neuropathol (Berl) 65:235–246

Baker HF, Poulter M, Crow TJ, Frith CD, Lofthouse R, Ridley RM (1991) Amino acid polymorphism in human prion protein and age at death in inherited prion disease. Lancet 337:1286

Bellinger-Kawahara C, Cleaver JE, Diener TO, Prusiner SB (1987a) Purified scrapie prions resist inactivation by UV irradiation. J Virol 61:159–166

Bellinger-Kawahara C, Diener TO, McKinley MP, Groth DF, Smith DR, Prusiner SB (1987b) Purified scrapie prions resist inactivation by procedures that hydrolyze, modify, or shear nucleic acids. Virology 160:271–274

Bendheim PE, Barry RA, DeArmond SJ, Stites DP, Prusiner SB (1984) Antibodies to a scrapie prion protein. Nature 310:418–421

Bertoni JM, Brown P, Goldfarb L, Gajdusek D, Omaha NE (1992) Familial Creutzfeldt-Jakob disease with the PRNP codon 200^{lys} mutation and supranuclear palsy but without myoclonus or periodic EEG complexes. Neurology 42 [No 4, Suppl 3]: 350 (Abstr)

Bobowick AR, Brody JA, Matthews MR, Roos R, Gajdusek DC (1973) Creutzfeldt-Jakob disease: a case-control study. Am J Epidemiol 98: 381–394

Bockman JM, Kingsbury DT, McKinley MP, Bendheim PE, Prusiner SB (1985) Creutzfeldt-Jakob disease prion proteins in human brains. N Engl J Med 312: 73–78

Bockman JM, Prusiner SB, Tateishi J, Kingsbury DT (1987) Immunoblotting of Creutzfeldt-Jakob disease prion proteins: host species-specific epitopes. Ann Neurol 21: 589–595

Brown P (1992) The clinico-pathological features of transmissible human spongiform encephalopathy, with a discussion of recognized risk factors and preventive strategies. International Meeting on Transmissible Spongiform Encephalopathies, Impact on Animal and Human Health, June 23–24, 1992. International Association of Biological Standardization, Heidelberg, Germany (Abstr)

Brown P, Cathala F, Castaigne P, Gajdusek DC (1986a) Creutzfeldt-Jakob disease: clinical analysis of a consecutive series of 230 neuropathologically verified cases. Ann Neurol 20: 597–602

Brown P, Cathala F, Raubertas RF, Gajdusek DC, Castaigne P (1987) The epidemiology of Creutzfeldt-Jakob disease: conclusion of 15-year investigation in France and review of the world literature. Neurology 37: 895–904

Brown P, Coker-Vann M, Pomeroy K, Franko M, Asher DM, Gibbs CJ Jr, Gajdusek DC (1986b) Diagnosis of Creutzfeldt-Jakob disease by Western blot identification of marker protein in human brain tissue. N Engl J Med 314: 547–551

Brown P, Gálvez S, Goldfarb LG, Nieto A, Cartier L, Gibbs CJ Jr, Gajdusek DC (1992a) Familial Creutzfeldt-Jakob disease in Chile is associated with the codon 200 mutation of the PRNP amyloid precursor gene on chromosome 20. J Neurol Sci 112: 65–67

Brown P, Goldfarb LG, Kovanen J, Haltia M, Cathala F, Sulima M, Gibbs CJ Jr, Gajdusek DC (1992b) Phenotypic characteristics of familial Creutzfeldt-Jakob disease associated with the codon 178^{Asn} PRNP mutation. Ann Neurol 31: 282–285

Brown P, Goldfarb LG, McCombie WR, Nieto A, Squillacote D, Sheremata W, Little BW, Godec MS, Gibbs CJ Jr, Gajdusek DC (1992c) A typical Creutzfeldt-Jakob disease in an American family with an insert mutation in the PRNP amyloid precursor gene. Neurology 42: 422–427

Brown P, Preece MA, Will RG (1992d) "Friendly fire" in medicine: hormones, homografts, and Creutzfeldt-Jakob disease. Lancet 340: 24–27

Brown P, Kaur P, Sulima MP, Goldfarb LG, Gibbs CJ Jr, Gajdusek DC (1993) Real and imagined clinicopathological limits of "prion dementia". Lancet 341: 127–129

Brown P, Rodgers-Johnson P, Cathala F, Gibbs CJ Jr, Gajdusek DC (1984) Creutzfeldt-Jakob disease of long duration: clinicopathological characteristics, transmissibility, and differential diagnosis. Ann Neurol 16: 295–304

Buchanan CR, Preece MA, Milner RDG (1991) Mortality, neoplasia and Creutzfeldt-Jakob disease in patients treated with pituitary growth hormone in the United Kingdom. Br Med J 302: 824–828

Büeler H, Fischer M, Lang Y, Blüthmann H, Lipp H-L, DeArmond SJ, Prusiner SB, Aguet M, Weissmann C (1992) The neuronal cell surface protein PrP is not essential for normal development and behavior of the mouse. Nature 356: 577–582

Büeler H, Aguzzi A, Sailer A, Greiner R, Autenried P, Aguet M, Weissmann C (1993) Mice devoid of PrP are resistant to scrapie. Cell 73: 1339–1347

Carlson GA, Kingsbury DT, Goodman PA, Coleman S, Marshall ST, DeArmond SJ, Westaway D, Prusiner SB (1986) Linkage of prion protein and scrapie incubation time genes. Cell 46: 503–511

Caughey BW, Dong A, Bhat KS, Ernst D, Hayes SF, Caughey WS (1991) Secondary structure analysis of the scrapie-associated protein PrP 27–30 in water by infrared spectroscopy. Biochemistry 30: 7672–7680

Chesebro B (1992) PrP and the scrapie agent. Nature 356: 560

Cohen FE, Abarbanel RM, Kuntz ID, Fletterick RJ (1986) Turn prediction in proteins using a pattern-matching approach. Biochemistry 25: 266–275

Collinge J, Palmer M (1991) CJD discrepancy. Nature 352: 802

Collinge J, Brown J, Hardy J, Mullan M, Rossor MN, Baker H, Crow TJ, Lofthouse R, Poulter M, Ridley R, Owen F, Bennett C, Dunn G, Harding AE, Quinn N, Doshi B, Roberts GW, Honavar N, Janota I, Lantos PL (1992) Inherited prion disease with 144 base pair gene insertion. 2. Clinical and pathological features. Brain 115: 687–710

Collinge J, Harding AE, Owen F, Poulter M, Lofthouse R, Boughey AM, Shah T, Crow TJ (1989) Diagnosis of Gerstmann-Sträussler syndrome in familial dementia with prion protein gene analysis. Lancet 2: 15–17

Collinge J, Owen F, Poulter H, Leach M, Crow T, Rosser M, Hardy J, Mullan H, Janota I, Lantos P (1990) Prion dementia without characteristic pathology. Lancet 336: 7–9

Collinge J, Palmer MS, Dryden AJ (1991) Genetic predisposition to iatrogenic Creutzfeldt-Jakob disease. Lancet 337: 1441–1442

Come JH, Fraser PE, Lansbury PT Jr (1993) A Kinetic model for amyloid formation in the prion diseases: importance of seeding. Proc Natl Acad Sci USA, 90: 5959–5963

Cousens SN, Harries-Jones R, Knight R, Will RG, Smith PG, Matthews WB (1990) Geographical distribution of cases of Creutzfeldt-Jakob disease in England and Wales 1970–84. J Neurol Neurosurg Psychiat 53: 459–465

Crow TJ, Collinge J, Ridley RM, Baker HF, Lofthouse R, Owen F, Harding AE (1990) Mutations in the prion gene in human transmissible dementia. Seminar on Molecular Approaches to Research in Spongiform Encephalopathies in Man. Medical Research Council, London (Abstr)

Dealler SF, Lacey RW (1990) Transmissible spongiform encephalopathies: the threat of BSE to man. Food Microbiol 7: 253–279

DeArmond SJ, McKinley MP, Barry RA, Braunfeld MB, McColloch JR, Prusiner SB (1985) Identification of prion amyloid filaments in scrapie-infected brain. Cell 41: 221–235

Diedrich J, Weitgrefe S, Zupancic M, Staskus K, Retzel E, Haase AT, Race R (1987) The molecular pathogenesis of astrogliosis in scrapie and Alzheimer's disease. Microb Pathog 2: 435–442

Diener TO (1987) PrP and the nature of the scrapie agent. Cell 49: 719–721

Diener TO, McKinley MP, Prusiner SB (1982) Viroids and prions. Proc Natl Acad Sci USA 79: 5220–5224

Diringer H, Gelderblom II, Hilmert II, Ozel M, Edelbluth C, Kimberlin RII (1983) Scrapie infectivity, fibrils and low molecular weight protein. Nature 306: 476–478

Dlouhy SR, Hsiao K, Farlow MR, Foroud T, Conneally PM, Johnson P, Prusiner SB, Hodes ME, Ghetti B (1992) Linkage of the Indiana kindred of Gerstmann-Straussler-Scheinker disease to the prion protein gene. Nature Genet 1: 64–67

Doh-ura K, Kitamoto T, Sakaki Y, Tateishi J (1991) CJD discrepancy. Nature 353: 801–802

Doh-ura K, Tateishi J, Sasaki H, Kitamoto T, Sakaki Y (1989) Pro → Leu change at position 102 of prion protein is the most common but not the sole mutation related to Gerstmann-Sträussler syndrome. Biochem Biophys Res Commun 163: 974–979

Duguid JR, Rohwer RG, Seed B (1988) Isolation of cDNAs of scrapie-modulated RNAs by subtractive hybridization of a cDNA library. Proc Natl Acad Sci USA 85: 5738–5742

Farlow MR, Yee RD, Dlouhy SR, Conneally PM, Azzarelli B, Ghetti B (1989) Gerstmann-Sträussler-Scheinker disease. I. Extending the clinical spectrum. Neurology 39: 1446–1452

Fink JK, Warren JT Jr, Drury I, Murman D, Peacock BA (1991) Allele-specific sequencing confirms novel prion gene polymorphism in Creutzfeldt-Jakob disease. Neurology 41: 1647–1650

Forloni G, Angeretti N, Chiesa R, Monzani E, Salmona M, Bugiani O, Tagliavini F (1993) Neurotoxicity of a prion protein fragment. Nature 362: 543–546

Fradkin JE, Schonberger LB, Mills JL, Gunn WJ, Piper JM, Wysowski DK, Thomson R, Durako S, Brown P (1991) Creutzfeldt-Jakob disease in pituitary growth hormone recipients in the United States. JAMA 265: 880–884

Gabizon R, Prusiner SB (1990) Prion liposomes. Biochem J 266: 1–14

Gabizon R, McKinley MP, Groth DF, Kenaga L, Prusiner SB (1988a) Properties of scrapie prion liposomes. J Biol Chem 263:4950–4955

Gabizon R, McKinley MP, Groth DF, Prusiner SB (1988b) Immunoaffinity purification and neutralization of scrapie prion infectivity. Proc Natl Acad Sci USA 85:6617–6621

Gabizon R, McKinley MP, Prusiner SB (1987) Purified prion proteins and scrapie infectivity copartition into liposomes. Proc Natl Acad Sci USA 84:4017–4021

Gabizon R, Meiner Z, Cass C, Kahana E, Kahana I, Avrahami D, Abramsky O, Scarlato G, Prusiner SB, Hsiao KK (1991) Prion protein gene mutation in Libyan Jews with Creutzfeldt-Jakob disease. Neurology 41:160 (Abstr)

Gabizon R, Rosenman H, Meiner Z, Kahana I, Kahana E, Shugart Y, Ott J, Prusiner SB (1993) Mutation and polymorphism of the prion protein gene in Libyan Jews with Creutzfeldt-Jakob disease. Am J Hum Genet 33:828–835

Gajdusek DC (1977) Unconventional viruses and the origin and disappearance of kuru. Science 197:943–960

Gajdusek DC (1985) Subacute spongiform virus excephalopathies caused by unconventional viruses. In: Maramorosch K, McKelvey JJ Jr (eds) Subviral pathogens of plants and animals: viroids and prions. Academic Press, Orlando, pp 483–544

Gajdusek DC (1988) Transmissible and non-transmissible amyloidoses: autocatalytic post-translational conversion of host precursor protein to β-pleated sheet configurations. J Neuroimmunol 20:95–110

Gajdusek DC (1990) Subacute spongiform encephalopathies: transmissible cerebral amyloidoses caused by unconventional viruses. In: Fields BN, Knipe DM, Chanock RM, Hirsch MS, Melnick JL, Monath TP, Roizman B (eds) Virology, 2nd Ed. Raven Press, New York, pp 2289–2324

Gajdusek DC, Gibbs CJ Jr (1990) Brain amyloidoses-precursor proteins and the amyloids of transmissible and nontransmissible dementias: scrapie-kuru-CJD viruses as infectious polypeptides or amyloid enhancing vector. In: Goldstein A (ed) Biomedical advances in aging. Plenum Press, New York, pp 3–24

Gajdusek DC, Gibbs CJ Jr, Alpers M (1966) Experimental transmission of a kuru-like syndrome to chimpanzees. Nature 209:794–796

Gasset M, Baldwin MA, Fletterick RJ, Prusiner SB (1993) Perturbation of the secondary structure of the scrapie prion protein under conditions associated with changes in infectivity. Proc Natl Acad Sci USA 90:1–5

Gasset M, Baldwin MA, Lloyd D, Gabriel J-M, Holtzman DM, Cohen F, Fletterick R, Prusiner SB (1992) Predicted α-helical regions of the prion protein when synthesized as peptides form amyloid. Proc Natl Acad Sci USA 89:10940–10944

Gerstmann J, Sträussler E, Scheinker I (1936) Über eine eigenartige hereditär-familiäre Erkrankung des Zentralnervensystems zugleich ein Beitrag zur Frage des vorzeitigen lokalen Alterns. Z Neurol 154:736–762

Ghetti B, Tagliavini F, Masters CL, Beyreuther K, Giaccone G, Verga L, Farlo MR, Conneally PM, Dlouhy SR, Azzarelli B, Bugiani O (1989) Gerstmann-Sträussler-Scheinker disease. II. Neurofibrillary tangles and plaques with PrP-amyloid coexist in an affected family. Neurology 39:1453–1461

Giaccone G, Tagliavini F, Verga L, Frangione B, Farlow MR, Bugiani O, Ghetti B (1990) Neurofibrillary tangles of the Indiana kindred of Gerstmann-Sträussler-Scheinker disease share antigenic determinants with those of Alzheimer disease. Brain Res 530:325–329

Gibbs CJ Jr, Gajdusek DC, Asher DM, Alpers MP, Beck E, Daniel PM, Matthews WB (1968) Creutzfeldt-Jakob disease (spongiform encephalopathy): transmission to the chimpanzee. Science 161:388–389

Goate A, Chartier-Harlin M-C, Mullan M, Brown J, Crawford F, Fidani L, Giuffra L, Haynes A, Irving N, James L, Mant R, Newton P, Rooke K, Roques P, Talbot C, Pericak-Vance M, Roses A, Williamson R, Rossor M, Owen M, Hardy J (1991) Segregation of a missense mutation in the amyloid precursor protein gene with familial Alzheimer's disease. Nature 349:704–706

Goldfarb L, Brown P, Goldgaber D, Garruto R, Yanaghiara R, Asher D. Gajdusek DC (1990a) Identical mutation in unrelated patients with Creutzfeldt-Jakob disease. Lancet 336:174–175

Goldfarb L, Korczyn A, Brown P, Chapman J, Gajdusek DC (1990b) Mutation in codon 200 of scrapie amyloid precursor gene linked to Creutzfeldt-Jakob disease in Sephardic Jews of Libyan and non-Libyan origin. Lancet 336:637–638

Goldfarb LG, Brown P, Goldgaber D, Asher DM, Rubenstein R. Brown WT, Piccardo P, Kascsak RJ, Boellaard JW, Gajdusek DC (1990c) Creutzfeldt-Jakob disease and kuru patients lack a mutation consistently found in the Gerstmann-Sträussler-Scheinker syndrome. Exp Neurol 108:247–250

Goldfarb LG, Brown P, Gajdusek DC (1993a) The molecular genetics of human transmissible spongiform encephalopathy. In: Prusiner SB, Collinge J, Powell J, Anderton B (eds) Prion diseases of humans and animals. Ellis Horwood, London, pp 139–153

Goldfarb LG, Brown P, Haltia M, Cathala F, McCombie WR, Kovanen J, Cervenakova L, Goldin L, Nieto A, Godec MS, Asher DM, Gajdusek DC (1992a) Creutzfeldt-Jakob disease cosegregates with the codon 178^{Asn} PRNP mutation in families of European origin. Ann Neurol 31:274–281

Goldfarb LG, Brown P, Haltia M, Ghiso J, Frangione B, Gajdusek DC (1993b) Synthetic peptides corresponding to different mutated regions of the amyloid gene in familial Creutzfeldt-Jakob disease show enhanced in vitro formation of morphologically different amyloid fibrils. Proc Natl Acad Sci USA 90:4451–4454

Goldfarb LG, Brown P, McCombie WR, Goldgaber D, Swergold GD, Wills PR, Cervenakova L, Baron H, Gibbs CJJ, Gajdusek DC (1991a) Transmissible familial Creutzfeldt-Jakob disease associated with five, seven, and eight extra octapeptide coding repeats in the PRNP gene. Proc Natl Acad Sci USA 88:10926–10930

Goldfarb LG, Brown P, Mitrova E. Cervenakova L, Goldin L, Korczyn AD, Chapman J, Galvez S, Cartier L, Rubenstein R, Gajdusek DC (1991b) Creutzfeldt-Jakob disease associated with the PRNP codon 200^{Lys} mutation: an analysis of 45 families. Eur J Epidemiol 7:477–486

Goldfarb LG, Brown P, Vrbovská A, Baron H, McCombie WR, Cathala F, Gibbs CJ Jr, Gajdusek DC (1992b) An insert mutation in the chromosome 20 amyloid precursor gene in a Gerstmann-Sträussler-Scheinker family. J Neurol Sci 111:189–194

Goldfarb LG, Haltia M, Brown P, Nieto A, Kovanen J, McCombie WR, Trapp S, Gajdusek DC (1991c) New mutation in scrapie amyloid precursor gene (at codon 178) in Finnish Creutzfeldt-Jakob kindred. Lancet 337:425

Goldfarb LG, Mitrova E, Brown P, Toh BH, Gajdusek DC (1990d) Mutation in codon 200 of scrapie amyloid protein gene in two clusters of Creutzfeldt-Jakob disease in Slovakia. Lancet 336:514–515

Goldfarb LG, Petersen RB, Tabaton M, Brown P, LeBlanc AC, Montagna P, Cortelli P, Julien J, Vital C, Pendelbury WW, Haltia M, Wills PR, Hauw JJ, McKeever PE, Monari L, Schrank B, Swergold GD, Autilio-Gambetti L, Gajdusek DC, Lugaresi E, Gambetti P (1992c) Fatal familial insomnia and familial Creutzfeldt-Jakob disease: disease phenotype determined by a DNA polymorphism. Science 258:806–808

Goldgaber D, Goldfarb LG, Brown P, Asher DM, Brown WT, Lin S, Teener JW, Feinstone SM, Rubenstein R, Kascsak RJ, Boellaard JW, Gajdusek DC (1989) Mutations in familial Creutzfeldt-Jakob disease and Gerstmann-Sträussler-Scheinker's syndrome. Exp Neurol 106:204–206

Goldmann W, Hunter N, Martin T, Dawson M, Hope J (1991) Different forms of the bovine PrP gene have five or six copies of a short, G-C-rich element within the protein-coding exon. J Gen Virol 72:201–204

Haltia M, Kovanen J, Goldfarb LG, Brown P, Gajdusek DC (1991) Familial Creutzfeldt-Jakob disease in Finland: Epidemiological, clinical, pathological and molecular genetic studies. Eur J Epidemiol 7:494–500

Hardy J (1991) Prion dimers—a deadly duo. Trends Neurosci 14:423–424

Harries-Jones R, Knight R, Will RG, Cousens S, Smith PG, Matthews WB (1988) Creutzfeldt-Jakob disease in England and Wales, 1980–1984: a case-control study of potential risk factors. J Neurol Neurosurg Psychiat 51:1113–1119

Herzberg L, Herzberg BN, Gibbs CJ Jr, Sullivan W, Amyx H, Gajdusek DC (1974) Creutzfeldt-Jakob disease: hypothesis for high incidence in Libyan Jews in Israel. Science 186:848

Heston LL, Lowther DLW, Leventhal CM (1966) Alzheimer's disease: a family study. Arch Neurol 15:225–233

Hope J, Reekie LJD, Hunter N, Multhaup G, Beyreuther K, White H, Scott AC, Stack MJ, Dawson M, Wells GAH (1988) Fibrils from brains of cows with new cattle disease contain scrapie-associated protein. Nature 336:390–392

Hsiao K, Prusiner SB (1990) Inherited human prion diseases. Neurology 40:1820–1827

Hsiao K, Baker HF, Crow TJ, Poulter M, Owen F, Terwilliger JD, Westaway D, Ott J, Prusiner SB (1989a) Linkage of a prion protein missense variant to Gerstmann-Sträussler syndrome. Nature 338:342–345

Hsiao KK, Doh-ura K, Kitamoto T, Tateishi J, Prusiner SB (1989b) A prion protein amino acid substitution in ataxic Gerstmann-Sträussler syndrome. Ann Neurol 26:137

Hsiao K, Meiner Z, Kahana E, Cass C, Kahana I, Avrahami D, Scarlato G, Abramsky O, Prusiner SB, Gabizon R (1991a) Mutation of the prion protein in Libyan Jews with Creutzfeldt-Jakob disease. N Engl J Med 324:1091–1097

Hsiao KK, Cass C. Schellenberg GD, Bird T, Devine-Gage E, Wisniewski H, Prusiner SB (1991b) A prion protein variant in a family with the telecephalic form of Gerstmann-Sträussler-Scheinker syndrome. Neurology 41:681–684

Hsiao KK, Groth D, Scott M, Yang S-L, Serban A, Rapp D. Foster D. Torchia M, De Armond SJ, Prusiner SB (1991c) Neurologic disease of transgenic mice which express GSS mutant prion protein is transmissible to inoculated recipient animals. Prion Diseases of Humans and Animals Symposium, London, Sept. 2–4 (Abstr)

Hsiao KK, Scott M, Foster D, Groth DF, DeArmond SJ, Prusiner SB (1990) Spontaneous neurodegeneration in transgenic mice with mutant prion protein of Gerstmann-Sträussler syndrome. Science 250:1587–1590

Hsiao K, Dloughy S, Ghetti B, Farlow M, Cass C, Da Costa M, Conneally M, Hodes ME, Prusiner SB (1992) Mutant prion proteins in Gerstmann-Sträussler-Scheinker disease with neurofibrillary tangles. Nature Genet 1:68–71

Huang Z, Gabriel J-M, Baldwin MA, Fletterick RJ, Prusiner SB, Cohen FE (1994) Proposed three-dimensional structure for the cellular prion protein. Proc Natl Acad Sci USA, in press

Hunter GD (1972) Scrapie: a prototype slow infection. J Infect Dis 125:427–440

Ikeda S, Yanagisawa N, Allsop D, Glenner GG (1991) A variant of Gerstmann-Sträussler-Scheinker disease with β-protein epitopes and dystrophic neurites in the peripheral regions of PrP-immunoreactive amyloid plaques. In: Natvig JB, Forre O, Husby G, Husebekk A, Skogen B, Sletten K, Westermark P (eds) Amyloid and amyloidosis 1990. Kluwer Academic Publishers, Dordrecht, pp 737–740

Johnson RT (1992) Prion disease. N Engl J Med 326:486–487

Kahana E, Milton A, Braham J, Sofer D (1974) Creutzfeldt-Jakob disease: focus among Libyan Jews in Israel. Science 183:90–91

Kahana E, Zilber N, Abraham M (1991) Do Creutzfeldt-Jakob disease patients of Jewish Libyan origin have unique clinical features? Neurology 41:1390–1392

Kellings K, Meyer N, Mirenda C, Prusiner SB, Riesner D (1992) Further analysis of nucleic acids in purified scrapie prion preparations by improved return refocussing gel electrophoresis (RRGE). J Gen Virol 73:1025–1029

Kimberlin RH (1990) Scrapie and possible relationships with viroids. Semin Virol 1:153–162

Kitamoto T, Iizuka R, Tateishi J (1993a) An amber mutation of prion protein in Gerstmann-Sträussler syndrome with mutant PrP plaques. Biochem Biophys Res Commun 192:525–531

Kitamoto T, Ohta M, Doh-ura K, Hitoshi S, Terao Y, Tateishi J (1993b) Novel missense variants of prion protein in Creutzfeldt-Jakob disease or Gerstmann-Sträussler syndrome. Biochem Biophys Res Commun 191:709–714

Kitamoto T, Shin R-W, Doh-ura K, Tomokane N, Miyazono M, Muramoto T. Tateishi J (1992) Abnormal isoform of prion proteins accumulates in the synaptic structures of the central nervous system in patients with Creutzfeldt-Jakob disease. Am J Pathol 140:1285–1294

Kitamoto T, Tateishi J, Tashima I, Takeshita I, Barry RA, DeArmond SJ, Prusiner SB (1986) Amyloid plaques in Creutzfeldt-Jakob disease stain with prion protein antibodies. Ann Neurol 20:204–208

Kretzschmar HA, Stowring LE, Westaway D, Stubblebine WH, Prusiner SB, DeArmond SJ (1986) Molecular cloning of a human prion protein cDNA. DNA 5:315–324

Kretzschmar HA, Honold G, Seitelberger F, Feucht M, Wessely P, Mehraein P, Budka H (1991a) Prion Protein mutation in family first reported by Gerstmann, Straussler, and Scheinker. Lancet 337:1160

Kretzschmar HA, Kufer P, Riethmuller G, DeArmond SJ, Prusiner SB, Schiffer D (1991b) Prion protein mutation at codon 102 in an Italian family Gerstmann-Sträussler-Scheinker syndrome. Neurology 42:809–810

Lantos PL, McGill IS, Janota I, Doey LJ, Collinge J, Bruce MT, Whatley SA, Anderton BH, Clinton J, Roberts GW, Rossor MN (1992) Prion protein immunocytochemistry helps to establish the true incidence of prion diseases. Neurosci Lett 147:67–71

Laplanche J-L, Chatelain J, Launay J-M, Gazengel C, Vidaud M (1990) Deletion in prion protein gene in a Moroccan family. Nucleic Acids Res 18:6745

Levy E, Carman MD, Fernandez-Madrid IJ, Power MD, Lieberburg I, van Duinen SG, Bots GTAM, Luyendijk W, Frangione B (1990) Mutation of the Alzheimer's disease amyloid gene in hereditary cerebral hemorrhage, Dutch type. Science 248:1124–1126

Little BW, Brown PW, Rodgers-Johnson P, Perl DP, Gajdusek DC (1986) Familial myoclonic dementia masquerading as Creutzfeldt-Jakob disease. Ann Neurol 20:231–239

Malmgren R, Kurland L, Mokri B, Kurtzke J (1979) The epidemiology of Creutzfeldt-Jakob disease. In: Prusiner SB, Hadlow WJ (eds) Slow transmissible diseases of the nervous system, Vol 1. Academic Press, New York, pp 93–112

Manetto V, Medori R, Cortelli P, Montagna P, Tinuper P, Baruzzi A, Rancurel G, Hauw J-J, Vanderhaeghen J-J, Mailleux P, Bugiani O, Tagliavini F, Bouras C, Rizzuto N, Lugaresi E, Gambetti P (1992) Fatal familial insomnia: clinical and pathological study of five new cases. Neurology 42:312–319

Masters CL, Gajdusek DC, Gibbs CJ Jr (1981a) Creutzfeldt-Jakob disease virus isolations from the Gerstmann-Sträussler syndrome. Brain 104:559 588

Masters CL, Gajdusek DC, Gibbs CJ Jr (1981b) The familial occurrence of Creutzfeldt-Jakob disease and Alzheimer's disease. Brain 104:535–558

Masters CL, Harris JO, Gajdusek DC, Gibbs CJ, Jr, Bernouilli C, Asher DM (1978) Creutzfeldt-Jakob disease: patterns of worldwide occurrence and the significance of familial and sporadic clustering. Ann Neurol 5:177–188

McKinley MP, Masiarz FR, Isaacs ST, Hearst JE, Prusiner SB (1983) Resistance of the scrapie agent to inactivation by psoralens. Photochem Photobiol 37:539–545

McKinley MP, Meyer R, Kenaga L, Rahbar F, Cotter R, Serban A, Prusiner SB (1991) Scrapie prion rod formation *in vitro* requires both detergent extraction and limited proteolysis. J Virol 65:1440–1449

Medori R, Montagna P, Tritschler HJ, LeBlanc A, Cortelli P, Tinuper P, Lugaresi E, Gambetti P (1992a) Fatal familial insomnia: a second kindred with mutation of prion protein gene at codon 178. Neurology 42:669–670

Medori R, Tritschler H-J, LeBlanc A, Villare F, Manetto V, Chen HY, Xue R, Leal S, Montagna P, Cortelli P, Tinuper P, Avoni P, Mochi M, Baruzzi A, Hauw JJ, Ott J, Lugaresi E, Autilio-Gambetti L, Gambetti P (1992b) Fatal familial insomnia, a prion disease with a mutation at codon 178 of the prion protein gene. N Engl J Med 326:444–449

Merz PA, Kascsak RJ, Rubenstein R, Carp RI, Wisniewski HM (1987) Antisera to scrapie-associated fibril protein and prion protein decorate scrapie-associated fibrils. J Virol 61:42–49

Merz PA, Rohwer RG, Kascsak R, Wisniewski HM, Somerville RA, Gibbs CJ Jr, Gajdusek DC (1984) Infection-specific particle from the unconventional slow virus disease. Science 225:437–440

Merz PA, Somerville RA, Wisniewski HM, Iqbal K (1981) Abnormal fibrils from scrapie-infected brain. Acta Neuropathol (Berl) 54:63–74

Merz PA, Wisniewski HM, Somerville RA, Bobin SA, Masters CL, Iqbal K (1983) Ultrastructural morphology of amyloid fibrils from neuritic and amyloid plaques. Acta Neuropathol (Berl) 60:113–124

Meyer N, Rosenbaum V, Schmidt B, Gilles K, Mirenda C, Groth D, Prusiner SB, Riesner D (1991) Search for a putative scrapie genome in purified prion fractions reveals a paucity of nucleic acids. J Gen Virol 72:37–49

Meyer RK, McKinley MP, Bowman KA, Braunfeld MB, Barry RA, Prusiner SB (1986) Separation and properties of cellular and scrapie prion proteins. Proc Natl Acad Sci USA 83:2310–2314

Mullan M, Houlden H, Windelspecht M, Fidani L, Lombardi C, Diaz P, Rossor M, Crook R, Hardy J, Duff K, Crawford F (1992) A locus for familial early-onset Alzheimer's disease on the long arm of chromosome 14, proximal to the α1-antichymotrypsin gene. Nature Genet 2:340–342

Neary K, Caughey B, Ernst D, Race RE, Chesebro B (1991) Protease sensitivity and nuclease resistance of the scrapie agent propagated in vitro in neuroblastoma-cells. J Virol 65:1031–1034

Neugut RH, Neugut AI, Kahana E, Stein Z, Alter M (1979) Creutzfeldt-Jakob disease: familial clustering among Libyan-born Israelis. Neurology 29:225–231

Nochlin D, Sumi SM, Bird TD, Snow AD, Leventhal CM, Beyreuther K, Masters CL (1989) Familial dementia with PrP-positive amyloid plaques: a variant of Gerstmann-Sträussler syndrome. Neurology 39:910–918

Oesch B, Groth DF, Prusiner SB, Weissmann C (1988) Search for a scrapie-specific nucleic acid: a progress report. In: Book G, Marsh J (eds) Novel infectious agents and the central nervous system, Ciba Foundation Symposium 135. John Wiley and Sons, Chichester, UK, pp 209–223

Oesch B, Westaway D, Wälchli M, McKinley MP, Kent SBH, Aebersold R, Barry RA, Tempst P, Teplow DB, Hood LE, Prusiner SB, Weissmann C (1985) A cellular gene encodes scrapie PrP 27–30 protein. Cell 40:735–746

Owen F, Poulter M, Collinge J, Crow TJ (1990a) Codon 129 changes in the prion protein gene in Caucasians. Am J Hum Genet 46:1215–1216

Owen F, Poulter M, Collinge J, Leach M, Lofthouse R, Crow TJ, Harding AE (1992) A dementing illness associated with a novel insertion in the prion protein gene. Mol Brain Res 13:155–157

Owen F, Poulter M, Collinge J, Leach M, Shah T, Lofthouse R, Chen YF, Crow TJ, Harding AE, Hardy J (1991) Insertions in the prion protein gene in atypical dementias. Exp Neurol 112:240–242

Owen F, Poulter M, Lofthouse R, Collinge J, Crow TJ, Risby D, Baker HF, Ridley RM, Hsiao K, Prusiner SB (1989) Insertion in prion protein gene in familial Creutzfeldt-Jakob disease. Lancet 1:51–52

Owen F, Poulter M, Shah T, Collinge J, Lofthouse R, Baker H, Ridley R, McVey J, Crow T (1990b) An in-frame insertion in the prion protein gene in familial Creutzfeldt-Jakob disease. Mol Brain Res 7:273–276

Palmer MS, Dryden AJ, Hughes JT, Collinge J (1991) Homozygous prion protein genotype predisposes to sporadic Creutzfeldt-Jakob disease. Nature 352:340–342

Palmer MS, Mahal SP, Campbell TA, Hill AF, Sidle KCL, Laplanche J-L, Collinge J (1993) Deletions in the prion protein gene are not associated with CJD. Hum Mol Genet 2:541–544

Pattison IH (1965) Experiments with scrapie with special reference to the nature of the agent and the pathology of the disease. In: Gajdusek DC, Gibbs CJ Jr, Alpers MP (eds) Slow, latent and temperate virus infections, NINDB Monograph 2. US Government Printing, Washington DC, pp 249–257

Pattison IH (1966) The relative susceptibility of sheep, goats and mice to two types of the goat scrapie agent. Res Vet Sci 7:207–212

Pattison IH, Jones KM (1967) The possible nature of the transmissible agent of scrapie. Vet Rec 80:1–8

Pearlman RL, Towfighi J, Pezeshkpour GH, Tenser RB, Turel AP (1988) Clinical significance of types of cerebellar amyloid plaques in human spongiform encephalopathies. Neurology 38:1249–1254

Petersen RB, Tabaton M, Berg L, Schrank B, Torack RM, Leal S, Julien J, Vital C, Deleplanque B, Pendlebury WW, Drachman D, Smith TW, Martin JJ, Oda M, Montagna P, Ott J, Autilio-Gambetti L, Lugaresi E, Gambetti P (1992) Analysis of the prion protein gene in thalamic dementia. Neurology 42:1859–1863

Pocchiari M, Salvatore M, Cutruzzola F, Genuardi M, Travaglini Allocatelli C, Masullo C, Macchi G, Alema G, Galgani S, Xi YG, Petraroli P, Silvestrini MC, Brunori M (1993) A new point mutation of the prion protein gene in Creutzfeldt-Jakob disease. Ann Neurol 34:802–807

Poulter M, Baker HF, Frith CD, Leach M, Lofthouse R, Ridley RM, Shah T, Owen F, Collinge J, Brown G, Hardy J, Mullan MJ, Harding AE, Bennett C, Doshi R, Crow TJ (1992) Inherited prion disease with 144 base pair gene insertion. 1. Genealogical and molecular studies. Brain 115:675–685

Prusiner SB (1982) Novel proteinaceous infectious particles cause scrapie. Science 216:136–144

Prusiner SB (1989) Scrapie prions. Annu Rev Microbiol 43:345–374

Prusiner SB (1991) Molecular biology of prion diseases. Science 252:1515–1522

Prusiner SB, Bolton DC, Groth DF, Bowman KA, Cochran SP, McKinley MP (1982) Further purification and characterization of scrapie prions. Biochemistry 21:6942–6950

Prusiner SB, Fuzi M, Scott M, Serban D, Serban H, Taraboulos A, Gabriel J-M, Wells G, Wilesmith J, Bradley R, DeArmond SJ, Kristensson K (1993) Immunologic and molecular biological studies of prion proteins in bovine spongiform encephalopathy. J Infect Dis 167:602–613

Prusiner SB, Groth DF, Bolton DC, Kent SB, Hood LE (1984) Purification and structural studies of a major scrapie prion protein. Cell 38:127–134

Prusiner SB, Groth D, Serban A, Koehler R, Foster D, Torchia M, Burton D, Yang S-L, DeArmond SJ (1993) Ablation of the prion protein (PrP) gene in mice prevents scrapie and facilitates production of anti-PrP antibodies. Proc Natl Acad Sci USA 90:10608–10612

Prusiner SB, McKinley MP, Bowman KA, Bolton DC, Bendheim PE, Groth DF, Glenner GG (1983) Scrapie prions aggregate to form amyloid-like birefringent rods. Cell 35:349–358

Prusiner SB, McKinley MP, Groth DF, Bowman KA, Mock NI, Cochran SP, Masiarz FR (1981) Scrapie agent contains a hydrophobic protein. Proc Natl Acad Sci USA 78:6675–6679

Prusiner SB, Scott M, Foster D, Pan K-M, Groth D, Mirenda C, Torchia M, Yang S-L, Serban D, Carlson GA, Hoppe PC, Westaway D, DeArmond SJ (1990) Transgenetic studies implicate interactions between homologous PrP isoforms in scrapie prion replication. Cell 63:673–686

Puckett C, Concannon P, Casey C, Hood L (1991) Genomic structure of the human prion protein gene. Am J Hum Genet 49:320–329

Ripoll L, Laplanche J-L, Salzmann M, Jouvet A, Planques B, Dussaucy M, Chatelain J, Beaudry P, Launay J-M (1993) A new point mutation in the prion protein gene at codon 210 in Creutzfeldt-Jakob disease. Neurology, 43:1934–1938

Roberts GW, Lofthouse R, Brown R, Crow TJ, Barry RA, Prusiner SB (1986) Prion-protein immunoreactivity in human transmissible dementias. N Engl J Med 315:1231–1233

Roberts GW, Lofthouse R, Allsop D, Landon M, Kidd M, Prusiner SB, Crow TJ (1988) CNS amyloid proteins in neurodegenerative diseases. Neurology 38:1534–1540

Roos R, Gajdusek DC, Gibbs CJ Jr (1973) The clinical characteristics of transmissible Creutzfeldt-Jakob disease. Brain 96:1–20

Rosen DR, Siddique T, Patterson D, Figiewicz DA, Sapp P, Hentati A, Donaldson D, Goto J, O'Regan JP, Deng H, Rahmani Z, Krizus A, McKenna-Yasek D, Cayabyab A, Gaston SM, Berger R, Tanzi RE, Halperin JJ, Herzfeldt B, Van den Bergh R, Hung W-Y, Bird T, Deng G, Mulder DW, Smyth C, Laing NG, Soriano E, Pericak-Vance MA, Haines J, Rouleau GA, Gusella JS, Horvitz HR, Brown RH Jr (1993) Mutations in Cu/Zn superoxide dismutase gene are associated with familial amyotrophic lateral sclerosis. Nature 362:59–62

Rosenthal NP, Keesey J, Crandall B, Brown WJ (1976) Familial neurological disease associated with spongiform encephalopathy. Arch Neurol 33:252–259

Schellenberg GD, Bird TD, Wijsman EM, Orr HT, Anderson L, Nemens E, White JA, Bonnycastle L, Weber JL, Alonso ME, Potter H, Heston LL, Martin GM (1992) Genetic linkage evidence for a familial Alzheimer's disease locus on chromosome 14. Science 258:668–671

Scott M, Foster D, Mirenda C, Serban D, Coufal F, Wälchli M, Torchia M, Groth D, Carlson G, DeArmond SJ, Westaway D, Prusiner SB (1989) Transgenic mice expressing hamster prion protein produce species-specific scrapie infectivity and amyloid plaques. Cell 59:847–857

Scott M, Groth D, Foster D, Torchia M, Yang S-L, DeArmond SJ, Prusiner SB (1993) Propagation of prions with artificial properties in transgenic mice expressing chimeric PrP genes. Cell 73:979–988

Serban D, Taraboulos A, DeArmond SJ, Prusiner SB (1990) Rapid detection of Creutzfeldt-Jakob disease and scrapie prion proteins. Neurology 40:110–117

Sigurdsson B (1954) Rida, a chronic encephalitis of sheep with general remarks on infections which develop slowly and some of their special characteristics. Br Vet J 110:341–354

Somerville RA, Ritchie LA, Gibson PH (1989) Structural and biochemical evidence that scrapie-associated fibrils assemble *in vivo*. J Gen Virol 70:25–35

Sparkes RS, Simon M, Cohn VH, Fournier REK, Lem J. Klisak I, Heinzmann C, Blatt C, Lucero M, Mohandas T, DeArmond SJ, Westaway D. Prusiner SB, Weiner LP (1986) Assignment of the human and mouse prion protein genes to homologous chromosomes. Proc Natl Acad Sci USA 83:7358–7362

St. George-Hyslop P, Haines J, Rogaev E, Mortilla M, Vaula G, Pericak-Vance M, Foncin J-F, Montesi M, Bruni A, Sorbi S, Rainero I, Pinessi L, Pollen D, Polinsky R, Nee L, Kennedy J, Macciardi F, Rogaeva E, Liang Y, Alexandrova N, Lukiw W, Schlumpf K, Tanzi R, Tsuda T, Farrer L, Cantu J-M, Duara R, Amaducci L, Bergamini L, Gusella J, Roses A, McLachlan DC (1992) Genetic evidence for a novel familial Alzheimer's disease locus on chromosome 14. Nature Genet 2:330–334

Tagliavini F, Prelli F, Ghisto J, Bugiani O, Serban D, Prusiner SB, Farlow MR, Ghetti B, Frangione B (1991) Amyloid protein of Gerstmann-Sträussler-Scheinker disease (Indiana kindred) is an 11-kd fragment of prion protein with an N-terminal glycine at codon 58, EMBO J 10:513–519

Taraboulos A, Jendroska K, Serban D, Yang S-L, DeArmond SJ, Prusiner SB (1992) Regional mapping of prion proteins in brains. Proc Natl Acad Sci USA 89:7620–7624

Tateishi J, Doh-ura K, Kitamoto T, Tranchant C, Steinmetz G, Warter JM, Boellaard JW (1992) Prion protein gene analysis and transmission studies of Creutzfeldt-Jakob disease. *In*: Prusiner SB, Collinge J, Powell J, Anderton B (eds) Prion disease of humans and animals. Ellis Horwood, London, pp 129–134

Tateishi J, Kitamoto T, Doh-ura K, Sakaki Y, Steinmetz G, Tranchant C, Warter JM, Heldt N (1990) Immunochemical, molecular genetic, and transmission studies on a case of Gerstmann-Sträussler-Scheinker syndrome. Neurology 40:1578–1581

Tranchant C, Doh-ura K, Warter JM, Steinmetz G, Chevalier Y, Hanauer A, Kitamoto T, Tateishi J (1992) Gerstmann-Sträussler-Scheinker disease in an Alsatian family: clinical and genetic studies. J Neurol Neurosurg Psychiat 55:185–187

Udovitch AL, Valensi L (1984) The last Arab Jews: the communities of Jerba, Tunisia. Harwood Academic Publishers, London

Van Broeckhoven C, Backhovens H, Cruts M, De Winter G, Bruyland M, Cras P, Martin J-J (1992) Mapping of a gene predisposing to early-onset Alzheimer's disease to chromosome 14q24.3. Nature Genet 2:335–339

Van Broeckhoven C, Haan J, Bakker E, Hardy JA, Van Hul W, Wehnert A, Vegter-Van der Vlis M, Roos RA (1990) Amyloid β protein precursor gene and hereditary cerebral hemorrhage with amyloidosis (Dutch). Science 248:1120–1122

Verga L, Giaccone G, Salmona M, Prelli F, Frangione B, Bugiani O, Tagliavini F (1992) Synthetic peptides homologous to prion protein fragments form amyloid-like fibrils *in vitro*. Neurobiol Aging 13 (Suppl I): 103

Vnencak-Jones CL, Phillips JA (1992) Identification of heterogeneous PrP gene deletions in controls by detection of allele-specific heteroduplexes (DASH). Am J Human Genet 50:871–872

Weissmann C (1991) Spongiform encephalopathies — the prion's progress. Nature 349:569–571

Weitgrefe S, Zupancic M, Haase A, Chesebro B, Race R, Frey W II, Rustan T, Friedman RL (1985) Cloning of a gene whose expression is increased in scrapie and in senile plaques. Science 230:1177–1181

Wexler NS, Young AB, Tanzi RE, Travers H, Starosta-Rubinstein S, Penney JB, Snodgrass SR, Shoulson I, Gomez F, Ramos Arroyo MA, Penchaszadeh GK, Moreno H, Gibbons K, Faryniarz A, Hobbs W, Anderson MA, Bonilla E, Conneally PM, Gusella JF (1987) Homozygotes for Huntington's disease. Nature 326:194–197

Wilesmith JW, Hoinville LJ, Ryan JBM, Sayers AR (1992a) Bovine spongiform encephalopathy: aspects of the clinical picture and analyses of possible changes 1986–1990. Vet Rec 130:197–201

Wilesmith JW, Ryan JBM, Hueston WD, Hoinville LJ (1992b) Bovine spongiform encephalopathy: epidemiological features 1985 to 1990. Vet Rec 130:90–94

Zilber N, Kahana E, Abraham MPH (1991) The Libyan Creutzfeldt-Jakob disease focus in Israel: An epidemiologic evaluation. Neurology 41:1385–1389

Subject Index

Springer-Verlag
and the Environment

We at Springer-Verlag firmly believe that an international science publisher has a special obligation to the environment, and our corporate policies consistently reflect this conviction.

We also expect our business partners – paper mills, printers, packaging manufacturers, etc. – to commit themselves to using environmentally friendly materials and production processes.

The paper in this book is made from low- or no-chlorine pulp and is acid free, in conformance with international standards for paper permanency.